FREUD, THE CONTEMPORARY SUPER-EGO, AND WESTERN MORALITY

Freud, the Contemporary Super-ego, and Western Morality traces the origins of the relationship between the morality of the super-ego and the destructive impulse of the death drive in the liberal democracies of the 21st century.

Giosuè Ghisalberti begins by refuting the analysis by contemporary social theorists of the phenomenon described as "the return of the religious," presenting instead a comprehensive set of ideas as outlined by Freud in the writings of the 1920s and the analysis of a contemporary theological-political unconscious. Ghisalberti argues that the psyche of the liberal West has regressed to an infantile and primitive present, driven by an unconscious hostility towards the Oedipus complex and, more comprehensively, to Western civilization as a whole. The book re-examines Freud's psychoanalytic ideas on the nature of obsessions, interpreted first from the murder of the primal father in *Totem and Taboo*, and turns to his grounding ideals of intelligence, creativity, and freedom as the affirmation of the coming-to-be-human in modernity.

Freud, the Contemporary Super-ego, and Western Morality will be of great interest to psychoanalysts in practice and in training. It will also be key reading for academics and scholars of psychoanalytic studies, philosophy, political theory, and the humanities.

Giosuè Ghisalberti is a professor of philosophy at Humber College, Toronto, Canada.

FREUD, THE CONTEMPORARY SUPER-EGO, AND WESTERN MORALITY

An Essay on Psychopolitics

Giosuè Ghisalberti

Routledge
Taylor & Francis Group
LONDON AND NEW YORK

Designed cover image: Cover image by Giosuè Ghisalberti

First published 2024
by Routledge
4 Park Square, Milton Park, Abingdon, Oxon OX14 4RN

and by Routledge
605 Third Avenue, New York, NY 10158

Routledge is an imprint of the Taylor & Francis Group, an informa business

British Library Cataloguing-in-Publication Data
A catalogue record for this book is available from the British Library

Library of Congress Cataloguing-in-Publication Data
Names: Ghisalberti, Giosuè, 1958- author.
Title: Freud, the contemporary super-ego, and Western morality : an essay on psychopolitics / Giosuè Ghisalberti.
Description: Abingdon, Oxon ; New York, NY : Routledge, 2024. | Includes bibliographical references. |
Identifiers: LCCN 2023018756 | ISBN 9781032532134 (hardback) | ISBN 9781032532127 (paperback) | ISBN 9781003410911 (ebook)
Subjects: LCSH: Political psychology--Western countries. | Liberalism--Psychological aspects. | Social ethics--Western countries. | Psychoanalysis--Political aspects. | Freud, Sigmund, 1856-1939.
Classification: LCC JA74.5 .G526 2024 | DDC 320.01/9--dc23/eng/20230718
LC record available at https://lccn.loc.gov/2023018756

ISBN: 978-1-032-53213-4 (hbk)
ISBN: 978-1-032-53212-7 (pbk)
ISBN: 978-1-003-41091-1 (ebk)

DOI: 10.4324/9781003410911

Typeset in Times New Roman
by MPS Limited, Dehradun

To my father, for his 90th birthday

CONTENTS

WORKS CITED

Sigmund Freud

All References are from the *Standard Edition of the Complete Psychological Works of Sigmund Freud.* Ed. James Strachey. London: Vintage Books.

"The Aetiology of Hysteria." SE 3:187–221.
"Analysis Terminable and Interminable." SE 23:209–253.
An Autobiographical Study. SE 20:77–175.
Beyond the Pleasure Principle. SE 18:3–64.
Civilization and its Discontents. SE 21:57–145
"Charcot," SE 3:7–23.
"'Civilized' Sexual Morality and Modern Nervous Illness." SE 9:177–204.
"The Claims of Psycho-Analysis to Scientific Interest." SE 13: 163–190.
Delusions and Dreams in Jensen's 'Gradiva.' SE 9.
"The Dissolution of the Oedipus Complex." SE 19:171–179.
"The Disposition to Obsessional Neurosis: A Contribution to the Problem of Choice of Neurosis." SE 12:
"The Economic Problem of Masochism." SE 19:157–170.
The Ego and the Id. SE 19:1–66.
The Interpretation of Dreams. SE 4-5:1–626.
Introductory Lectures on Psycho-analysis. SE 16.
"Family Romances." SE 9.
Five Lectures on Psychoanalysis. SE 11:3–55.
"Further Remarks on the Neuro-Psychoses of Defense." SE 3:157–185.
Fragment of an Analysis of a Case of Hysteria. SE 7:1–122.
The Future of an Illusion. SE 21:1–56.
"The Future Prospects of Psychoanalytic Therapy." SE 11:139–151.
"The Goethe Prize." SE 21:205–212.

Group Psychology and the Analysis of the Ego. SE 18:65–143.

Inhibitions, Symptoms and Anxiety. SE 20:87–172.

"Instincts and their Vicissitudes." SE 14:111–140.

Introductory Lectures on Psycho-analysis. SE 15.

Leonardo da Vinci and a Memory of his Childhood. SE 11:59–137.

"The Loss of Reality in Neurosis and Psychosis." SE 19:181–187.

Mourning and Melancholia. SE 14:237–258l.

Moses and Monotheism. SE 23:1–137.

"The Moses of Michelangelo." SE 13: 209–222.

"Negation." SE 19:235–242.

"The Neuro-Psychoses of Defense." SE 3:43–61.

"Observations on Transference Love. (Further Recommendations on the Technique of Psychoanalysis III)" SE 12:157–171.

"Obsessions and Phobias: Their Mechanisms and their Aetiology." SE 3:71–84.

"Obsessive Actions and Religious Practices." SE 9.

"On the History of the Psycho-Analytic Movement." SE 14:7–66.

On Narcissism: An Introduction. SE 14:67–102.

"On the Psychical Mechanism of Hysterical Phenomena: A Lecture." SE 3:287–297.

"On Psychoanalysis." SE 12.

"On Psychotherapy." SE 7:257–268."Preface to Reik's Ritual: Psycho-Analytic Studies." SE 17.

"The Question of Lay Analysis." SE 20:183–258.

"The Uncanny." SE 17:219–252.

"Remembering, Repeating, and Working-Through (Further Recommendations on the Technique of Psychoanalysis II)." SE 12.

"The Resistances to Psychoanalysis." SE 19:213–222.

"Screen Memories." SE 3:301–322.

"Some Psychical Consequences of the Anatomical Distinction between the Sexes. SE 19:243–258.

"Splitting of the Ego in the Process of Defense." SE 23:271–278.

Three Essays on the Theory of Sexuality. SE 7:125–243.

"To Romain Rolland." SE 20.

Totem and Taboo. SE 13:1–162.

"Two Encyclopedia Articles." SE 18:233–259.

The Complete Letters of Sigmund Freud to Wilhelm Fliess, 1887-1904. Tr. And Ed. Jeffrey Moussaieff Masson. Cambridge: The Belknap Press of Harvard University Press, 1985.

Breuer, Josef and Freud, Sigmund. *Studies on Hysteria*. SE 2:3–311.

INTRODUCTION

The Illusion of Secularism and the Theological-Political Unconscious of Liberalism

> An obsessional neurosis is a caricature of religion.
>
> *Totem and Taboo*

The emergence of a widely used phrase among philosophers and social theorists before and after the turn of the 21st century has been expressed with a certain alarm and aversion. Contempt has not been lacking; indignation and other, more aggressive sentiments are now the norm. The warnings, of a political danger, have been urgent. From all appearances, a phenomenon has returned to threaten the secularism of our times and its freedom from the well-known traditions of dogmatic thinking and life. "*The return of the religious*" can be read as an ominous sign for our times and with the most serious implications for social and political life: the achievements of liberal societies, above all being independent from traditional prejudices and orthodoxies, metaphysical and otherwise, are once again susceptible to somehow being undermined by a threatening revival. The well-established confidence of reason, scientific and technological, and without forgetting the considerable promotion it receives from the state and capital and their various dependents (along with all the techno-narcissistic gadgets so widely available to make life more convenient and perhaps slightly too fast, too busy, too self-involved for our own good), has become vulnerable from the possible effects of a religious return that looks and feels, precisely, *haunting*. The transferences of more than a few spirited metaphors invoking the dead – ghosts, phantasms, and specters – has become almost commonplace in various academic discourses, for a number of reasons, not all of them obvious in meaning or fully explained beyond their rhetoric. Their appearances, nevertheless, will be telling.

DOI: 10.4324/9781003410911-1

Whether one philosopher alone re-initiated a discussion on the theme of "specters" after the demise of the Soviet Union as a state and communism as an idea, and with many acknowledging the "death," mourning, or commemoration of Karl Marx as well as the ethos of revolution, are not at all central to the discussion at hand. One direction among others has to be, necessarily, set aside: the critique of political economy is a materialist axiom and secondary to psychoanalytic discoveries about the infantile and primitive psyche and what it has projected into the world. The economies and the dynamics of the psyche will be primary. Richard Rorty has made a claim about "Marxism" being "more of a religion than a secularist program for social change."[1] The connection has been well known at least since Marx's Paris Manuscripts of 1844; but the religion/secular bind remains extant, with outstanding qualities in very changed circumstances in our time. My psychopolitical essay does not examine if (or how) the return of the religious is, also, a consequence of the re-organization of political states after 1991 or, more enigmatically, to what Jacques Derrida calls, philosophically and with a double-improbability, the "messianic without messianism." The former is geopolitical and involves a number of critical factors – the re-drawing of borders, ethnic self-assertion (and, in some cases, as in the former Yugoslavia, pathological fantasies of "cleansing") – the latter is much too metaphysical and/or rhetorical and caught up in the complexities of deconstruction; in any case, the desire for autonomy and sovereignty is only partial when, merely, political. In *Specters of Marx*, Derrida asks: "could we *address ourselves in general* if already some ghost did not come back?"[2] The question, instead of being answered, in a simple yes or no, can bring us towards another sense of his subtitled theme of "debt" (what psychoanalysis believes is inseparable from moral guilt as a product of the super-ego) and its tie to both mourning and melancholia. Remembering the dead will be, in our day and age and according to certain unconscious drives, much worse than a depressive and paralyzing emotional state; the diagnosis, of specific social and political ailments, can be sufficiently recovered only through an in-depth psychoanalytic investigation. Carl Raschke adds: "the question of the return of the "religious" today continues concomitantly to haunt, fascinate, and discomfit us."[3] My interest, at first, focuses on this religious haunting and whether the phenomenon has, in fact, been correctly identified; or if other, more concealed, more unconscious energies are at work from our infantile and primitive psyche. *How* the return has manifested itself, well-disguised and screened-off and so much different than its promoted visibility, will in large part be the focus of my psychopolitical essay.[4]

Only Sigmund Freud, and the contributions made by the most astute of psychoanalysts after him, has given us the resources to begin to interpret how the return of the religious and our present-day obsession with morality in liberal democracies, as a "mechanism of psychical *displacement*" which "dominates the mental processes of obsessional neurosis,"[5] has an origin in the most complex dynamics of the super-ego and in the power of the death drive working, antithetically, on two fronts: the cultural and the biological in its nihilistic confrontation with the history of (Western) civilization and the human body. Can we identify the process of displacement and its result in one singular symptom to begin with – of obsessional neurosis, which Freud analyzed, in one way, as a caricature of religion? The manner in which certain "ghosts" – revived from history, and with the reminiscences of hysterical fantasies – have been idealized, introjected, and then projected into the world to re-make it in a new image will be essential in providing a psychoanalysis of the *morbidity* of the times and an erotic intimacy between death and political idealism. How has the displacement occurred? What were the conditions necessary for its development? No theory, of the political kind, has in my estimate been able to adequately interpret the inter-related factors of the illusion of secularism and the *theological-political unconscious* of contemporary liberalism; remote and archaic depths have been inaccessible unless examined, for example, in the splitting of the super-ego and by taking note of super-moral demands at the same time as the manifestation of the contemporary death drive. The proximity of morality and destruction are motivated by entirely different impulses, with symptoms that Freud traced to their origins and effects. The compulsions of moral absolutes and the re-shaping of both the individual and society remains to be diagnosed by Freud, as dangerous delusions and in a number of works during the 1920s that would start with an unsparing analysis in *Group Psychology and the Analysis of the Ego* (including the assessment of the ideals of justice, equality, and rights in the "Postscript") and culminate with the discontents of civilization. Conventional ideals are not spared, especially in our times when they have become imperious. His comprehensive working-out of the many symptoms evident to him are more true today than a century ago; other psychoanalysts have pointed out just how severe the ailments have become. A few philosophers have done likewise. The ailments have resulted in collective identities that, in some instances, are showing signs of the "morbid process" evident in schizoid, paranoid, and megalomaniacal conditions. The psychoanalytic remedies, however, are no less evident, as long as they can be re-affirmed at a time when so much negation opposes them.

Peter Sloterdijk opens one of his tomes with: "A *spectre* is haunting the Western world – the spectre of religion. All over the country we hear that after an extended absence, it has now returned and is among people of the modern world, and that one would do well to reckon seriously with its renewed presence."[6] In one of his own beginnings, Slavoj Žižek adds: "one of the most deplorable aspects of the postmodern era and its so-called 'thought' is the return of the religious dimension in all its different guises."[7] Identifying the "guises" will be the perpetual work of interpretation; the masquerades are many and are not disguised well enough for them to be hidden from psychoanalytic perception. The masks worn by characters on the stage of Greek tragedies revealed who they were, as people. Our present is no different; identities crave attention, acknowledgement for being, and so make spectacles of themselves, reminiscent of the classical era when an actor was called a *hypokrites*. Quentin Meillassoux uses two terms (reason and religion) and gives one more explanation for the origin of a return along with another commonplace assumption, now revisable, about the end of metaphysics: "*by forbidding reason any claims to the absolute, the end of metaphysics has taken the form of an exacerbated return of the religious*."[8] Whether *post*-modernity and the presumed *end* of metaphysics have been collaborative illusions from the philosophy of the last century and into our own cannot be easily discounted. One first question, and from the perspective of the psychoanalytic thesis of regression, the theme of our first chapter: how can we even presume to be modern when, psychically, the regression to infantile and primitive fantasies of the super-ego has barely been perceived and the projections, which are split between taboo restrictions and the other extreme of an almost all-out permissiveness, have become binding realities in the world of a new liberal order? By starting with Freud's analysis of group regression we can begin to wonder if modernity has been realized at all, or if its possibilities have been reversed by powerful unconscious drives and fixated on an irreconcilable conflict on the post-natal subject.

One of Charles Taylor's doubts comes near the end of his monumental study in *A Secular Age*. "We are not necessarily as 'modern' as we think we are."[9] He has not been alone. When Bruno Latour presents a compelling argument that *we have never been modern*[10] (which, in part, accurately reflects the nature of our psyche and its regressions) only Freud and the outstanding individual figures of psychoanalysis and philosophy provide us with the resources of interpretation, conceptually and affectively, to understand the entire range of a transformation in the individual and in society. One summing-up has been more decisive, dispirited, and perhaps too final. Rémi Brague believes modernity has failed and, therefore, there needs to be an "enterprise of rescuing premodern ideas."[11] Has modernity failed, definitively, or has it been unconsciously paralyzed by a number of fixations? How the present has been characterized by an unconscious repetition of an archaic event, as Freud conceived it, will be a starting-point towards understanding our predicament. Only the mythic – as narrated, and in the remnants of our selves – can offer an interpretation capable of identifying the force and compulsion of an epoch. To Jean-François Lyotard's *question,* (*Can we?*) the answer requires not the slightest pause. "Is it in our power, our strength, and our competence to perpetuate the project of modernity? The question suggests that to be sustained, such a project would call for strength and competence, and that these things have failed us."[12] Two philosophers, of quite different persuasions, believe the failure has already occurred; but what if psychoanalysis, at least giving itself the time for reflection and by turning back to the always necessary reading of Freud and his interpretations of us as individuals and a civilization, could (today) reveal something new to us and perhaps even re-invigorate ourselves towards another commitment? Strength and competence have not been obliterated; and neither have two of Freud's enduring virtues: courage and originality, which can be expressed by a conscious ego aware of its itself and the external conditions of life.

Alain Badiou introduces his own summing up of the last century and its persistence into our own; the continuity, once gradual, has increased in rhythm and intensity. The drive today is relentless. While he does not mention the difference between rights and duties, the analytically minded will not forget one or the other and how, today, they function – or don't, and can't, because the first has become inviolable and the second practically non-existent. In *The Century*, he writes: "These days – that is, in the fourth year of the twenty-first century – we hear nothing save for human rights and the return of the religious."[13] While contemporary thinkers provide us with explanations for one or more possible meanings for the return of the religious, there is one alternative that will give us much more to think about than the either/or distinction between the religious and the secular, faith and reason, the material and the metaphysical. Badiou has returned to one theme with consistency. He has been, to my mind, one unique contemporary philosopher who demonstrates the capacity to so clearly place two phenomena side by side. A reference has to be necessarily made to Nietzsche and his announcement that "God is dead" and, equally as important as one of his enduring testimonies, the consequences since the reality has been more or less accepted as a verifiable fact. Proof has not been necessary. If a death has occurred and society, in the liberal West, has promoted itself with this self-congratulatory perception, the outcomes have not been as readily noticed. In *Philosophy and the Event*, Badiou remarked: "For my part, I am a strict Nietzschean on this question. I really think that God is dead. If he is dead, he's dead. You have to take it seriously. The 'return of religion' masks, then, something else, I'm absolutely convinced of this. Religion is, in fact, the mask of political decomposition."[14] The relation of religion and "political decomposition" is the phenomenon in need of a more complete analysis, which Freud will provide, with exacting details and beginning, in *Group Psychology*, with the temporal/psychical symptom of regression. One statement may have to be modified: is politics the mask of religious decomposition once it has been internalized into liberal consciousness and its polity? Badiou gives us an incomparable start to our investigation by showing us the reality of the death of God: the human subject (the individual) has suffered "disastrous effects" that can only now be fully understood once we consider Freud's work of the 1920s. His anticipations were predicated on his consciousness of the temporality of the psyche and its intrusion into history. Badiou adds:

> Regarding the God of religions, its death must simply be declared. The problem, which is *a political one in the final analysis*, is to ward off *the disastrous effects wrought by any obscure subjectivation of this death…* From then on, the dead God's spectral authority, which can always criminally bind itself to the megalomaniacal scraps of the State remains without influence and without effect on minds.[15]

Recalling the earlier reference to ghosts, specters, and hauntings, we can now add Badiou's description of the demise of a "spectral authority." A more than ephemeral presence remains. Without turning to any of the other announcements of the death of God in Nietzsche's writings and simply accepting the epochal idea as a presumably conscious fact, one of the interests guiding the four-part essay to come will be to show how secularism has been an illusion; its psychical characteristic have not been fully examined because disavowed. The once moderating limits of the church-state relation are no longer in effect. Hyperbole is not intended. But if one of the motivations of the work to come is made explicit, then it is hard to avoid recognizing how Freud was prophetic by allowing us to see, with a detailed prognosis, the future of our illusions – which were caught in a religious/secular bind and ordered according to the vagaries of a 21st century psyche. The theme of the religious has been primary. The supplement comes from others who have not been convinced by either appearances – whether it was the return of the religious or, more explicitly, how the secular world and its reality in liberal democracies has not recognized a hidden and active dynamic. In *Psychopolitics*, Byung-Chul Han writes: "Emancipation from a transcendent order – that is, an order grounded in religious premises – is the hallmark of modern politics."[16] How the ideals of modern *politics* towards emancipation have led to far from beneficial effects will be the purpose of the four-part essay to come. Indeed, in his sub-titled "A Psychopolitical Investigation,"[17] Sloterdijk isolates the phenomenology of rage (along with resentment) rather than transcendence as the defining feature of our politicized time.

The American philosopher Adrian Johnston warns us about the all-too-easy assumptions about the death of God as an event, again with a reference to ghosts. Such a belief, in secularity as an achievement, "risks blinding one to the multifarious manner in which *ghostly unconscious religious beliefs* continue to enjoy a psychical afterlife in the aftermath of the supposed accession to atheism at the level of self-consciousness."[18] The philosophical perception is pivotal once psychoanalysis is taken into consideration. What does the phrase "the return of the religious" actually mean for us today when we set out from Freud's arguments in the 1920s? Exemplary thinkers have not been lacking to show us the nature of the psychopathology of everyday life. Rereading Freud at this particular historical time sems to be indispensable because especially revealing since the problems he was analyzing can only be fully appreciated today. There is, no doubt, the return of the religious in an unconscious form within politics; from all appearances, it has been duly noted, by a few individuals, and yet almost completely ignored as a social reality and as a selective memory becomes more regulated by moral objections to Western history and its *accomplishments*. Hysterical reminiscences have been validated to become an exclusive, and highly deceptive because one-dimensional, truth.

"It is because the various forms of rationalism," Jean-Pierre Dupuy writes, "deny having any relationship at all to the sacred that they cannot help but reflect it; only they do so in a distorted fashion that is often illogical and self-contradictory."[19] One of the intents of a psychopolitical investigation will be to outline how the *distortions* of religion have been adopted, unconsciously, as irrepressible drives of the super-ego and the destructive forms of the death drive, into the bureaucratic policies of *institutions* in liberal democracies and with effects on freedom that have become increasingly dominating. The self-contradictions are specific; they can be analyzed. Everyone who has made the same observation, in passing or with some attention to detail, deserves to be commended; their metaphors, when compared to each other, are hardly incidental. There have, by this point, been enough to make some remarks on a general trend. The examples of *spirited* metaphors – of haunting, of specters, of ghosts – gives us one indication of the persistence and also the remains of a phenomenon. The event of death appears to be less than final. Our *metaphysics*, that is, our conception of reality, remains as compelling as when the idea first appeared, in thought or in Aristotle's categorical writing. We are nowhere near "the end of metaphysics" because we continue to be permeated, through and through, with a historical and phantasmatic reality that will not (never) be overcome unless the still-not-modern individual of today learns, *against himself*, to make the super-ego more present to consciousness – and to come to the aid the resiliency of our *ego*, its strength and courage and independence, which is today being undermined by a number of protesters.

Briefly mentioning Hobbes' *Leviathan* can be one reference point; he is, after all, a representative of modernity at one of its inceptions. His short Introduction gave us two precepts, with translations from the Latin, that are suggestive for us once we turn to the question of how to best read Freud. *Salus populis* is not, for me, the *safety* of the people, but rather their psychological *health*. The second, "*Nosce teipsum*, Read *thy self*,"[20] repeating a classical dictum and Platonic truism, alerts us to the obligation to interpret, both ourselves and, concurrently, how we read others, from the past and today. Reading *like an analysand* will have hermeneutic benefits; interpretation will have to a double-task – for the sake of any writing, and the self as it develops its perception, internal and externally. How, then, will health and interpretation be re-affirmed again as a criteria? Freud's language is, as always, intriguing. His presence in any further discussion on the matter can be moved to its deserved place of prominence. "It is surely possible to throw oneself into a line of thought and to follow it wherever it leads out of simple scientific curiosity, or, if the reader prefers, as an *advocatus diaboli*."[21] "Throwing oneself," however, is not as reckless as it sounds; on the contrary, to be an advocate – for the layers of Freud's writing, addressed to analysands and readers – will be a constant responsibility. The theological *diaboli* has an additional meaning; the emphasis placed on *ad-vocatus*, *speaking for*, which is a reminder of the irrepressible duty of *free* association, involves being a witness – in our case, from the present towards the mythic and as presented in *Totem and Taboo*. After our initial awareness of ghosts and their haunting, Freud takes us to another primal scene when a murder was committed. A cadaver can be easily disposed of; one ghostly presence, among others, continues to have considerable effects.

Living in an age of a viral and moral pandemic calls for a renewed attention to psychoanalysis and, so too, its own kind of return – to Freud's mythic origin of civilization and, much more important than a hypothesis about archaic events in history, its meaning for us today once we begin to consider how a primal murder has been repeated, that is, unconsciously thought-out. One repetition compulsion has been devastating. *Totem and Taboo* has been justifiably regarded as one of the essential writings of Freud's turn toward a broader set of interests. Its importance for our coming argument cannot be stressed enough since his reconstruction of the origins of civilization allows us to connect his speculations to our present day and to recognize our history as a fateful repetition, unconscious and therefore more insidious, more exploitable, and much more dangerous in its effects. Once the 1913 work serves as an introduction to an analysis of the psychopolitics of our age, the moralizing drive of our super-ego and the death drive can be anticipated. In the context of an introduction, only the most outstanding points will be mentioned, the ones acting as a foundation to so much of the character of our contemporary situation, as individuals and as a collective in liberal democracies.[22] In *Totem and Taboo*, Freud gives us one sense of how a conception of reality can be made and *enforced*. "The projection outwards of internal perception is a *primitive* mechanism, to which, for instance, our sense perceptions are subject, and which therefore plays a very large part in determining the form taken by our external world."[23] One particular mechanism can be traced, both to its disparate origins and its effects. Our life-experience, viscerally, tells us that a *theory* of evolution along imprecise aeons and epochal periods no longer give us any assurance at all about ourselves as a species, as a society, or as individuals. A scientific *truth* is proving to be almost irrelevant for us; evolution has become, merely, veridical and by no means secure if one pays the slightest attention to revisionists. The power of the psyche has dislodged, unconsciously, even Charles Darwin from his pre-eminent place in our civilization. The primitive mechanisms of the psyche are more immediately instrumental in defining the level of reality and of manipulating others to serve specific ends. Defining the meaning of "illiberal" (as a merely political phenomenon) will not be enough. Any attempt to think about freedom, which was of paramount importance for Freud and for psychoanalysis as a therapy, has to go far beyond any political conception: our illiberalism has become pathological because the initiatives – ideally, to supposedly make a better, more just, more equitable society – are proving to be different, and often much worse, than any conscious intentions.

Psychoanalysis as a discipline remains independent because of its rightful separation from the institution of the university. Laying out the different sections of a psychopolitical essay with the commitment of an *analysand* (rather than a "theorist" in an academic department of the humanities) will have several benefits. Being able to *speak one's mind, freely*, and not to dismiss the controversial or the politically troubling will be one; there will be no reluctance when it becomes necessary to undermine the most deeply held values of the times and to be sceptical about our social categorical orthodoxies, the ones enjoying consensus privileges. *Theoretical* realities have become exclusive; and binding because they are serving a function beyond their persuasions. D. W. Winnicott made a comment for academics: "This matter of *illusion* is one that belongs inherently to human beings and no individual finally solves for himself or herself, although a *theoretical* understanding of it may provide a *theoretical* solution."[24] Winnicott's awareness, of the relation of illusion to theory, can be extended: has the theoretical today exacerbated the illusion and made it possible to make the "solution" deceptive? In *Group Psychology*, Freud gave us one illustration. The neurotic "creates his own world of the imagination for himself, his own religion, his own system of delusions, and thus recapitulates the institutions of humanity in a distorted way" (18:142). One institution has made itself conspicuous – for reasons that are more related to its social place in the present than its moral high-mindedness.

Our associations will be free; they will neither be censored nor editorialized, and they will be written, equally as important, with the consciousness of an intentional transference, for an individual reader and for the purpose of a transmission. An analysand and a reader will be collaborative in the turn to Freud, again, and from the primal story – of a murder – he set out from until it reached the present day. Hanna Segal gives us one psychoanalytic foundation: "Even though psychoanalytic ideas gained some general acceptance, the battle for freedom of thought has to be fought individually with every analysand on the couch, as well as within one's self."[25] The struggle, *in ourselves*, can begin with once again acknowledging the primacy of a *creative* myth as opposed to the limits of reason as presently defined; the historical creation of a sensibility remains as important as ever. Freud's discoveries would not have been possible if uncertainly had led to indecisiveness. The return to the still unfulfilled resources of myth gave him the independence of mind (and from his times) to more effectively inquire into long-lost possibilities of civilization, for consciousness, for thought, for life. The return to the creativity of myth was a counter-force to the regression of the psychically infantile and primitive. A moment on the metaphysics of myth (which is to say, its enduring *truth and reality*, as an *inspiration* for a reader) gives Freud a place in a different kind of pantheon once we recall how it was Plato who invented the idea of *muthos* – that is, a creative, artistic story whose revelation of truth is, on our case, psychoanalytic. Julia Kristeva reminds us that "more than a hundred years ago, a rabbi's grandson, a humanist like Diderot and Goethe, and by profession a neurologist, discovered that there was truth in ancient myths."[26] The bridge between a primal myth and the work of the 1920s are going to be cross-referenced. The loss of freedom has been noted. "Illiberalism" has many causes and more symptoms than can be rightly assessed by political thought alone.

"A specter is haunting world politics: the specter of 'illiberal democracy.'"[27] How this "illiberalism" has resulted as a symptom of specific shifts in our current reality will be essential to the psychopolitical essay: how has the moral *malice* of our contemporary super-ego and its complicity with a peculiar death drive against *Western civilization* created conditions that Freud *expected* and diagnosed in a number of seminal works? Moreover, illiberal democracy will not be, solely and conveniently, attributed to one side of the political spectrum either across parliamentary aisles, democratic assemblies, or the redundant ideology in the public sphere whereby one perspective enjoys legitimacy; there are simply too many factors inter-mixed today to identify one monolithic entity. States, capital, and class divisions are no longer adequate as focus-points. Our political perceptions require a different acuity. The particular world of states and political parties, structurally organized to serve the ends and means of a certain kind of democracy, upheld by the fact of a vote and moving from one side to the other and therefore structurally protected, is again not part of my examination.[28] More significant than the right/left slide of *states*, or the disposition of groups, there is today a more pervasive phenomenon: how has the morality of our contemporary super-ego and its complicity with a peculiar death drive created conditions that Freud anticipated and diagnosed and that should be striking for us today in liberal democracies?

We can, with Freud, call them "morbid phenomena," and for more than one reason. Morbidity refers to a disease; and to an outcome when the condition becomes grave. Psychoanalysis, however, believes itself capable of making a successful intervention; for Freud, it is "the only one" capable of doing so effectively. He writes: "Putting aside for a moment the therapeutic point of view, I may also say of it that it [psychoanalysis] is the most interesting method, *the only one* which informs us at all about the origin and interrelation of morbid phenomena."[29] The thesis, as a matter of necessity, will be sustained; political solutions will be excluded. There is no question of *a* return of religious sentiments and dogmas; but in a way that can be fully understood if only the intimations of a past correlation, the theological-political, is interpreted from the findings of psychoanalysis and so to understand the reality of our present situation. The morbidity goes well beyond metaphors. The wide-ranging conceptual edifice of psychoanalysis does give us a method much more productive than mere "critique," that academic exercise that has long sustained itself by a circular confirmation, departments creating and living in their own private realities. The symptoms of a malaise have, in the 21st century, intensified. The complicity of the university is an ancillary problem; academics are not exempt from the increase in the expression of malice and in the one-sided critique of Western civilization. The university has given itself the prerogative of moral leadership, with far from conducive effects for either intelligence or the freedom of personal conscience. Dogmas and orthodoxies are campus realities. They are as fierce as they are uncompromising, and they are receiving the full co-operation of the hierarchy of the institution, which believes it can conceal its complicities with the economic and managerial by taking on the veil of the moral. The symptoms can also be outlined, as the predilections of individuals and their associated groups. Various forms of advertisements and promotions have exposed them to the point of over-saturation; social reality has taken on the characteristics of an endless moral campaign, as can be witnessed, for one, in the preposterous advertisements on television. Today, we are increasingly made to submit to a "super-morality" (*Übermoralität*, Freud's term) that has become the most noticeable feature of the authoritative drive of liberal democracies.

A conjunction can be recognized between, on the one hand, Freud's myth of the murder of the primal father from *Totem and Taboo*, and on the other, the death of God as announced by Nietzsche and the self-reckoning necessary for us as *his killers*. Described as "the greatest recent event," Nietzsche goes on. "The event itself is far too great, too distant, too remote… … Much less may one suppose that many people know as yet *what* this event really means."[30] My psychopolitical essay will show not only how Freud understood the meaning of this one death; he also recognized it to be a repetition of another original murder and so prepared us for the many consequences to follow. His analysis of the origin of morality (in hate and killing) gives us a most uncomfortable reflection of ourselves and our illusions of goodness. The diagnoses of obsessional neuroses would be more direct and prepare for a more comprehensive analysis of the nature of society. One modern danger of liberal democracies can be presented. That the statement comes from *Totem and Taboo* should make us realize how the mythic was (and is) informing the present. "The asocial nature of neuroses has its genetic origin in their fundamental purpose, which is to take flight from an unsatisfying reality into a more pleasurable world of phantasy. The real world, which is avoided in this way by neurotics, is under the sway of human society and of the institutions collectively created by it" (SE 13:74). But what happens, as is the case today, when the institutions of human society are themselves neurotic?

Two epochs, a mythical and a relatively recent one, have become mutually conferring; the unity of two disparate events are provocative to the extreme in their meaning and implications for us. The murder of the primal father, displaced from the archaic to the almost-modern, has been nothing more than a passage from the savage and primitive to the failed substitution of the divine. Replacing a god is not simply done by *fiat*. Our present exemplifies just how severe repetition compulsions can become in their affects and implications when they are *thought-out* and then unconsciously projected into reality. The displacements may be somewhat concealed; they are not, by any means, invisible. Obsessions were first observed in the daily life of patients. Freud complemented his initial discoveries, in origin and manifestation, by noting how they were active in the day to day function of social life. While many have defined "Freud as cultural critic,"[31] the term (*critic*) has become so over-saturated that it can no longer be meaningful. To critique and to diagnose are not at all the same; the latter offers remedies based on therapeutic realities, not ideals or delusions of the political sort. More importantly for us, Freud makes it possible to understand the consequences of psychological mechanisms. Obsessions have causes and consequences.

Freud reminds us, time and again, how we have arrived at this point in history by a thinking-out and repetition. "We have learnt that the patient repeats instead of remembering, and repeats it under the conditions of resistance. We may now ask what it is that he in fact repeats or acts out."[32] For us, the question can be posed, and answered, this way: the murder of the primal father by a band of brothers has been *repeated* in the almost-modern world by the murder of God – and with precisely the same consequences as Freud outlined for the archaic world but with *the horde* made up of brothers and sisters who have hardly been amicable once one authority has been dispensed with. "The dead father became stronger than the living one had been – for events took the course we so often see them follow in human affairs today" (SE 13:143) *Human affairs today*. Freud's myth is, ultimately, a veiled allegory of our present-day situation and the one he believed would become more prevalent. How we understand the periods of history and the movement from the archaic to the *attempt to become modern*, Freud's warning to us sounds more formidable today than when it was first written. One gets the sense that many of these observations have been ignored. "We shall not be surprised to find that element of filial rebelliousness also emerges, in the *later* products of religion, often in the strangest disguises and transformations" (SE 13:145). This "rebelliousness," exemplified by the political groups of our times, can serve as the transition towards Freud's first work of the 1920s once we return to the totem and taboo thesis. The sense of guilt, so intense today as an imperative, "we find it operating in an asocial manner in neurotics, and producing new moral precepts and persistent restrictions, as an atonement from crimes that have been committed and as a precautions against the committing of new ones" (SE 13:159). The archaic guilt of the murder of the primal father – and its repetition in the killing of the God of Judeo-Christian religion – is no longer the guilt that motivates the "conscience" of our political activists and their various group identities. One conclusion to *Totem and Taboo* can serve as the transition and keeping in mind both the creation of "new moral precepts" (which Freud anticipated) and an equally devastating hostility to civilization.

In "Obsessions and Phobias," Freud sets out a principle for us; the analysis of neurotic experience reaches back to an origin and an explanation. "The associated idea is *no longer the appropriate original one, related to the aetiology of the obsession, but is one which replaces it, a substitute for it.*"[33] Another observation, focusing on obsessions, deals with an inherent conflict of our time – between stages of development, for the individual and society, and the regressive character of our psychopolitics and its fixation. The infantile and the primitive will be closely related as regressive processes; at the same time, a confrontation between love and hate, as well as its intimacy, has intensified – as has one neurotic symptom in particular (super-morality), though there are others. Freud writes:

> If we consider that obsessional neurotics have to develop a *super-morality* in order to protect their object-love from the hostility lurking behind it, we shall be inclined to regard some degree of this precocity of ego development as typical of human nature and to derive the capacity for the origin of morality from the fact that in the order of development hate is the precursor of love.[34]

The analysis will have to be seen more closely along Freud's complex axis; several intersections will be analyzed, none more important than *the suppression of love* (much more significant than *the repression of sexuality* could be – which has taken up an inordinate amount of cultural attention and with far from healthy results, especially for the impressionable young) due to the instrumental obsession with certain ideals. Present-day moralism is inimical to love since it has to sustain its aggressive critique at all costs, at the expense of everything except its own justifications. The metaphors of debt are more consequential than in guilt alone. The negation inherent in critique has produced conditions of aggression and hate; they are irrepressible because justified on moral grounds and rationalized to serve the supposed ends of justice, equality, and rights. In the psychopolitical essay to come, the morality of the times will receive as much attention as possible, and with a certain intolerance in order to reject its aims without hesitation and without timidity. Freud will spare no effort in, first, presenting the consequences of a hate-love conflict; second, analyzing the many characteristics of a "super-morality" driven by the super-ego; and, third, offering the possibility of remedies for the individual if not yet, for obvious reasons, to society as a whole in order to reaffirm the values of life: love, intelligence, freedom, and creativity. Freud's early observations would lead to far-reaching developments. In 1896, he wrote: "*Obsessional* ideas are invariably transformed *self-reproaches*."[35] How, then, did the experience of a mandatory guilt lead to obsessions, a problem that will continue to preoccupy him until, for example, examining the masochistic-sadistic relation and the focus on the discontents of civilization?

If the "religious roots of secular culture"[36] can be examined, they will, as the metaphor suggests, be found below the surface and in a place Freud himself discovered; the "roots" are not, strictly speaking, religious since the social reality is already a second-order phenomenon produced from hysterical and obsessive experiences. "The characteristics peculiar to both of them – megalomania, turning away from the world of objects, increased difficulty in transference – have obliged us to conclude that their dispositional fixation is to be looked for in a stage of libidinal development *before* object-choice has been established" (12:318). Before we can inquire into religion, as a system of beliefs or an institution, Freud's direction goes to the source and the creation of the super-ego. The grounds are to be found in infantile and primitive aspects of the self in its post-natal life and as it begins the arduous task of becoming human. The conflict can be extreme and lead to severe impairment later in life. Melanie Klein prepares us for understanding one way how the super-ego and the death drive are activated: "The nucleus of the super-ego is to be found in the partial incorporation that takes place during the cannibalistic phase of development."[37] Freud's definition of hysterical identification, introjection, and projection will clarify how primitive beginnings, in the psyche, subsist into the reality of the political neurotic.

Before offering an essay on Freud's analytic understanding of a theological-political phenomenon in our time, a brief overview will contextualize the discussion to come. The analysis of all the different pathologies now evident in the 21st century will be unwavering: regressions, sadomasochistic convolutions, perversions, omnipotence, hypochondria, paranoia, and functional psychosis will all be given explanations at the right time as social and, above all, the manifest appearance of political phenomena. One instance, among many others, is important for my argument, in part to make an early distinction between the sexual and the more comprehensively amorous. Freud writes: "human beings fall ill when, as a result of external obstacles or of an internal lack of adaptation, the satisfaction of erotic needs *in reality* is frustrated. We see that they then take flight into *illness* in order that by its help they may find a satisfaction to take the place of what has been frustrated."[38] Has critical theory and negation, unaware of its built-up consequences over more than a half-century, led to the prohibition of "erotic needs" (in short, to the reality of love) and ultimately to the illness we can now witness with more severe symptoms, including peculiar psycho-somatic ones, a new kind of neurasthenia Freud diagnosed as "disturbed attention"?[39]

The loss of the ability to love will not be one among other ailments. Can a more severe symptom be imagined? Should we be surprised that the nature of compulsive critique has estranged us from our capacity to *feel* something positive instead of the incessant rationalization of rage and from a discontent that has become programmatic? Such intense pleasure can be experienced from self-righteousness; the ego fills itself up in proportion to its revolt against reality. Psychoanalytic remedies will, one hopes, be possible once the pathologies are systematically recognized. The attainable *ideals* of psychoanalysis will each be presented in due time, as antidotes. Love is one, and surely the most important; our feelings of the *comprehensively* erotic can be given priority. Freud's belief in a real instead of a projective love has been a concern since *On Narcissism*. The *healthy* narcissism of what Freud simply calls "self-regard" may have to become necessary to off-set the crushing opposition of the super-ego and the re-making of the liberal subject who has been managed to submit to strict imperatives. The ego (of the individual, as opposed to his ideal) can be re-affirmed and in opposition to the forces that have, systematically, led to its denigration.

The individual in today's liberal society is constantly experiencing the *systematic* "impoverishment of the ego," an expression repeated by Freud on a number of occasions. The propaganda of our times demands that guilt become so ingrained and overpowering as to reduce love to a mere image of itself and distorted by both libido and extra-biological fantasies. Love has been reduced to the narrowly erotic and the sexualized, with the perverse desires of the psyche making extravagant claims about altering the nature of earthly, biological reality. Freud writes: "the realization of impotence, of one's inability to love, in consequence of mental and physical disorder, has an exceedingly lowering effect upon self-regard."[40] The *diagnosis*, so crucial, is no longer limited to an individual affliction; taken as a whole, we will have to outline how the inability to love, the withering of self-regard, as well as the loss of freedom and intelligence, are some of the discontents now being experienced and due to the hyper-moralism of the 21st century. The traditional perpetrators can no longer be easily isolated. One tradition, the political and the critical, does not have a monopoly on the perception of reality. Is a monolithic capitalism, with its innumerable attacks on life, alone capable of representing our innermost malaise? The change of an external system, however egregious its global reach, will not be the last word on our interiority. Byung-Chul Han writes: "Capitalism is aggravating the pornographication of society by making everything a commodity and putting it on display. Knowing no other use for sexuality, it profanes eros – into porn."[41] However true Han's analysis may be, the factors are multiple; and some of them are not so easily attributable to the same old problems that have served as the ground of the critique of capitalism since the 19th century. There are more immediate, more internal, problems than those of a world political economy and its machinations. The globalization of capital may be a structural reality; its material exchange can also be perceived within the recesses of the psyche as it effectively mis-manages its economy, of a different sort, with objects. Daring to suspend our taken-for-granted villains may perhaps give us a chance to see *ourselves* more clearly and pause the incessant one-way drift of our attention. Freud may very well be an unparalleled thinker for today since the reliance on comfortable truths may be over-dependent and so relieve us of the responsibility to see and think and be differently than conformism demands.

It may not be immediately apparent how we can draw Freud and psychoanalysis into an involvement with the theological-political makeup of contemporary liberal societies. But all the reasons for such a *confrontation* will be, eventually made, point by point and beginning with the all-important thesis that our democracies (of disparate groups in a susceptible collective, each of them vying for recognition) are now driven by a moral drive that is unconsciously, and in a distorted form, religiously ultra-moral, in terms of its bind, in its psychical origins and guilt, in its judgment and retribution. Freud has no parallel in the analysis he presents. The psychical cross-reference of the super-ego and the death drive has formed a reality of incompatible aims. One date is fortuitous, coming, as it does, when Freud made the decision to present the tripartite psyche. In 1922, Carl Schmitt published his *Political Theology*. The most often-quoted passage opens chapter 3: "All significant concepts of the modern theory of the state are secularized theological concepts."[42] How do we respond, today, to that thesis? We can only do so by introducing Freud as a thinker who can supplement the observation and, instead of pursuing the narrowly political consequences – for *the state*, which is not as predominant as an independent society and its various groups, of ideology and propaganda and above all strict identities – first of all interpret the depth-psychological ones. The theological-political drive of the times will be explained by reading Freud's systematic analysis of *Kultur* or civilization and its expression by present-day individuals in politically motivated groups. My interests are not with the liberal state, as such, or ultimately not even with the assumptions of the political on its own, either as a fact or according to its modern theory. The function of the state has been reduced, in many ways, to a managerial one while independent groups have made incursions into policies as well as, more seriously, judicial influence outside, and independently, of the institution of the law. The relationship between morality and bureaucracy has been only one of the repercussions of a secular imperative. The avaricious policies of neo-liberal marketability have led to the abnegation of its other responsibilities. The state facilitates; it enables with such concepts as "free trade," only that the exchange of material objects is more than capable to ignoring other, more telling transferences. The urgency of the moment requires us to think about the polity and *who*, precisely, has inaugurated the return of a religious unconscious and in the guise of a punitive super-ego and, increasingly, a destructive and nihilistic death drive. Various accomplices, and methods, will be exposed. Psychoanalysis can interpret the relation (the unconscious transference of the theological *into* the political) in order to give us a better understanding of the dynamic realities involved.

Returning to Schmitt, and without forgetting Hobbes, it is not at all an individual "sovereign," (to use Schmitt's language – or Freud's, the authoritative leader, as *the exception*) who is to be the focus today, but the development of independent groups who have, by virtue of their identities, managed to insinuate themselves into position of influence and, more intrusively, extra-judicial coercion. We can no longer rely on the analysis of, first, a jurist or, second, a political philosopher, to present an adequate portrait of our situation; conditions have changed to a significant degree, to the point that Freud's understanding of the temporal variations of the psyche can give us a more in-depth sense of our reality. Leo Strauss writes: "by *political theology* we understand political teachings which are based on divine revelations."[43] Far from any awareness of a *divine revelation*, our theological politics today is, first of all, cut off from its foundations and therefore has no inkling of what a revelation could mean, either as a phenomenological experience or as one interpreted from a God/human relation. When the theological politics of our times is perverse and sadistic (and in the specific ways Janine Chasseguet-Smirgel will uniquely tell us about at the appropriate time), the consequences are proving to be more than disquieting. Her attention to the corruptions of the ego-ideal and her contributions to the "study of the malady of the ideal"[44] will lead us, more seriously, to both its illness and its malice. Her writings, on certain questions, which are highly visible today, are incomparable; making herself independent from the fervour of a historical period (Paris '68) allowed her to see disguised characteristics of a mass movement. The analyses she gives us are psychologically precise as they are uncompromising because she was aware of the inherent dangers of certain social initiatives, politically manifest and unconsciously driven. History has proven her insights to be far-reaching. A mood is prevailing; as both anxious and depressive, the political feelings have all the characteristics of both mourning and melancholia – a certain kind of "love" that has been transformed by a rigid and long-lasting (indeed, perpetual) relation to death.

Paul Kahn adds a point, for us, of contention: "The very possibility of a political theology has been displaced from *the academy* by the rise of positive political science."[45] I disagree: the displacement has occurred, slowly, incrementally, but not because of any one intellectual discipline or *away from* the university. The displacement has been (*within* the university) psychological and academic. Kahn is right to have isolated the "academy" – that is, those institutions in the past associated with "higher learning" – as the place where the theological-political would receive its sustained support and, though unconsciously, following the supposed new-found freedom of secularism. The mendacity of this "freedom" will be one more strain of the work to come; the totality of our moral convictions has hardly been conducive to *being liberal* within college and university institutions. Quite the contrary; intellectual restrictions, in the name of slogans (equality, diversity, inclusivity) have become mandatory.

Finally, in the question of "Permanence of the Theologico-Political?," Claude Lefort gives us one sense for the remnant of the theological. "Beneath the appearance of the divine," there is an "excess of Being over appearance."[46] A Freudian analysis would, and does, significantly alter the statement. My argument will be, in part, that the *beneath the appearance of the secular* there has been an impoverishment of Being due to a psychological regression to an infantile and primitive fixation that, obsessively, has compromised love, freedom and intelligence. The crucial problem, as Freud anticipated, required an analytic interpretation because of how the very process of secularism internalized (and then projected) a moral view into the world. Although *historical* research is not without its scholarly importance,[47] the conditions of the present demand a different kind of scrutiny; a prominence has to be re-studied. Once we move the exclusively political discussion to a psychoanalytic one, then we can trace the collaboration between the superego and the death drive insofar as they are determining the theological-political character of the liberal present. Jürgen Habermas makes a significant statement: "the secularization of the state is not the same as the secularization of society."[48] That distinction will be noted more than once. The secularization of society has become as potentially dangerous as the excesses of the state; the liberal state appears to be increasingly manipulated by the social forces of an all-purpose morality, by distinct groups, some more powerful than others, all of them vying for recognition and social influence. The groups who promote the often-used slogan of "empowerment" (as a virtue) are oblivious to its effects when it is *wielded*. The power of the theological-political reality today and its institutional moral drive has made serious incursions into the administration of the law and in the conception of justice. How we "take exception" to one social development in particular will require some time to contemplate. Once we come to the realization of the meaning of one example – "*political theology* is concerned not only with the appeal to a source of legitimation figured as "beyond" the law, but with the completion or closure of the law in its annihilation or displacement"[49] – Freud's interpretation of the super-ego and death drive bound together will make it possible to understand the dynamic of the 21st century and its totalizing direction.

That we can set aside any misgivings, for example, on "the presumed political irrelevance of Freudian theory"[50] will make the following essay free of any such doubt. The first topsy-turvy rectification has been made. Theological morality is the unconscious of liberal politics. Going forward, my responsibility will be to, more distinctly, and by relying on psychoanalysis as Freud developed it, define the psychical maladies of liberal societies once he alerted us to its unconscious mechanisms. To provisionally conclude our few paragraphs on the dead, specters, ghosts, and other haunting presences, we can express our "gratitude" to Howard Kaye who, in his attempt to help raise "Freud from the dead,"[51] allowed us to realize that he was, as they say, alive and well and did not need to be resurrected either by an academic or miracle-worker. Kaye's belief that a Freud relieved of his therapeutic purpose would restore him to the rightful place of being a social critic makes the fateful error of disregarding the *foundations* of his social and political thought. Freud is not a *critic* like everyone else. The definition is, in any case, under-determined when it comes to the work of psychoanalysis. As for anticipations of death, Freud was no stranger to presumptuous obituaries. "After each of these obituaries psycho-analysis regularly gained new adherents and co-workers or acquired new channels of publicity. After all, being declared dead was an advance on being buried in silence."[52]

We have still not fully distinguished, as is necessary, the clinical from the critical, a point academics lose to *their* detriment. Hubert Damisch gives us a distinction we have previously alluded to and can rely on to further the consciousness of an analysand. "My own experience, as a critic, as an art historian, and philosopher (not to mention reader of Freud!), persuaded me that "critique" is never more interesting, never more convincing, never more farsighted, than when it tends and even drifts toward "clinique."[53] The all-important distinction between *critique* and *clinique* will be maintained along with the equally important difference between the clinic and the university, the analysand and the theorist. The antinomy between clinical therapeutics and academic theorizing has reached a time of a necessary divergence; between one and the other, compatibility, and affinity, have been lost. Freud's analysis of group psychology exposes more than a few selected groups; virtually all of them have found self-confirmation in academic departments and most especially where the words political or, especially, "cultural," appear in their self-definition.

Freud has been resented because he has exposed the self-righteousness of anyone who gave themselves the illusions of being a thinker of the free while exhibiting the very worst tendencies of the authoritarian mind. Freud was fully conscious of the negative reactions of his ideas. "I have long recognized that to stir up contradiction and arouse bitterness is the inevitable fate of psycho-analysis."[54] Paying attention to the many autobiographical notes he gives the reader is instructive for us getting both a sense of Freud the individual and the history of psychoanalysis. Some have read him carefully enough to shake up any complacency on our one theme in particular. "Psychoanalysis is a peculiar protest against the casual dismissal of religion as an archaic anomaly that shall soon pass. It concordantly rejects the liberal dream of politics without theology and claims instead the political is necessarily theological."[55] Once we pursue this one contemporary reality, Freud will be understood to be much more significant than any run-of-the-mill critic and who will force us to look at our internal illusions *before* turning our attention to the external world. The question leads us to make a proposal for a re-evaluation of the concepts, to clarify its inversion: the terms, as in the following – "is theology necessarily political?"[56] – are to be set within a particular equation. How the political has become unconsciously religious – by adopting its worst characteristics, orthodoxy and absolutism – is our question at the outset and directed exclusively at our liberal inquisitorial temptations.

Has the "return of the religious" been misdiagnosed and interpreted far too one-dimensionally, in part because it was much easier to be witnesses to spectacles of destruction and to immediately identify one vulgar and pathological instance of fanatical religiosity rather than taking one or more events as signs for us to think about our own psychical characteristics? Jean-Joseph Goux gives us one of the many arguments to be considered: "There is no doubt that the Freudian discovery fits into the vast movement of decline, or of the withdrawal of religious faith… … If God is dead, a new man must be born, more responsible, more conscious of himself and of his strengths. The Freudian discovery is precisely located in *this* juncture."[57] It would be straightforward, but partial, to simply agree and not also see Goux's argument – on the vulnerability of this "new man"; but as soon as we look further into the nature of Freud's *discovery*, the obvious nature of a historical transformation, from religion to secularism, was *not* what he began to more deeply investigate. That was only the beginning. The optimism in the possibility of a "new man" has been, in many ways and to use a concept repeated and emphasized by Freud, a *regression*. Not a new human being at all; rather, one who has reduced himself to an infantile and primitive form of being, with all the defenses available to him in his helpless, his weakness, his fragility, and then the intense identification (far more powerful than a political or religious leader) he has exploited for his own benefit. The results have been devastating. The super-ego and the death drive have been in evidence before in history, one might say perpetually. The desire and the fantasy has led us to the very worst situations for human beings when the morality of two impulses become complicitous and urged on by antithetical motivations – to at once create the conditions of the good and doing so by destroying the past, indeed, with a power to nullify both the nature of civilization and, more recently, the human body insofar as sexualized and as the condition for reproduction and *life*. In our case, liberal democracies are intent on creating a new moral order but with two formidable ideologies of destruction, towards civilization and the reality of terrestrial existence. One consequence of the rise of 20th century secularism has been a slide into a noticeably *felt* regression, with psychological symptoms for social life that has been experienced, and yet without understanding either its origin or felt implications, intuitively or clearly. The many readers who have been consoled by Freud's analysis of religion, which *appears*, at the manifest level, in the form of a "critique," in *The Future of an Illusion* and elsewhere, are more than content to stop at his atheism and do not continue to investigate what he has in store for us and to make us aware of our desires. Goux adds: "on the surface, these atheisms are the complete renunciation of ancient beliefs, but in reality and in depth, they continue to operate following patterns of interpretations" (219). The "patterns," however, have been unnoticed and the interpretations have been, at best, superficial; distortion and misapprehensions have been common. Freud's manifest/latest distinction will be permanent in the analysis to come as one prerequisite. It will be the objective of the psychopolitical essay to trace how liberal democracies have developed from a social phenomenon that was intended to lead to freedom from religious binds, and instead has re-deployed the unconscious drives of dogmatism and orthodoxy and activated them through today's unforgiving super-ego and, more *dangerously* (a word Freud uses on several occasions) the impulses of the death drive. We are, remarkably, at a displaced and repetitive moment of the murder of the primal father. Our recent act, of killing God, as been our latest attempt to be both free and modern. Neither goal has been achieved. We have regressed to patterns of primitive and infantile destitution and are nowhere near being able to recognize the fact and so prepare for its overcoming. Nietzsche was the first to see what the consequences would be – for us: "those who have abandoned God cling that much more firmly to morality… the more emancipated one is from theology, the more imperativistic morality becomes."[58]

Although different kinds of neurotic suffering will be mentioned at the appropriate moments to present the severity of our cultural predicament, Freud's analysis of obsessional neurosis can, once more, be isolated due to the fact that it "displays extreme characteristics of the nature of neurosis far more glaringly."[59] These "extreme characteristics" can be outlined, first, structurally, before making the necessary turn towards their specific historical consequences today. The symptoms of obsessions have become much more numerous and severe; when added to the hysterical ones, a more complete analysis can be presented. To give but one broad example, from the *Introductory Lectures on Psycho-analysis* and "Fixation to Traumas – the Unconscious," Freud gives us a sense of the process in which an individual, and a group, can become fixated on a past occurrence and how "they could not manage to free themselves from it and were for that reason alienated from the present and the future" (SE 16:273). Fixations, as defenses, are not without psychical benefits for the infant – though they are inevitably injurious and especially limiting, and draining, for the adult with an immature ego. The ideology of traumatism and the gain from illness (in an era of easily dispensed rights) has been virtually promoted, as has the legitimacy of multi-level hypochondria. The estrangement from a full historical consciousness is one of the primary consequences of the process of regression, which is one reason for Freud highlighting that one particular process in *Group Psychology*. The moral activist of our present time is fixated on (and becomes obsessed with) a trauma that he has recollected, in fantasy *and* history, from the experience of others who have become ego-ideals. Their introjection will be consequential and one more of the many connected issues. The fixation and obsession is not – except through the process of displacement that will be later explained more fully – a *personal* experience; rather, it is recovered from one historical moment (1492, in North America the ur-example of the times) that now serves as the over-arching explanation for our *Western* history, which has never been so vilified. Civilization is one object of the death drive. The historical "trauma," fabricated from the fantasy and reality of the past, serves to justify the focus on our obsessions. As we will first notice with Freud's analysis of group psychology, the regression leads to an infantile and primitive stasis, which then justifies all the subsequent "developments" of specifically political initiatives. If Freud had only gotten as far as the psychical temporality of regression, we would have sufficient knowledge to carry out a full-fledged analysis of our contemporary situation. But he gives us much more. Because once he had established the fundamental discoveries of psychoanalysis in relation to obsessional neurosis, he made even more important advancements. The philosophical expression of metaphors of haunting can be revealed when Freud provides us with a diagnosis of a pathological form of mourning.

> A perfect model of an affective fixation to something that is past is provided by mourning, which actually involves the most complete alienation from the present and the future. But even the judgement of a layman will distinguish sharply between mourning and neurosis. There are, on the other hand, neuroses which may be described as a pathological form of mourning. It may happen, too, that a person is brought so completely to a stop by a traumatic event which shatters the foundation of his life that he abandons all interest in the present and future.
>
> (SE 16:276)

One kind of infatuation with death, and the pleasure of traumatism, as a political characteristic of the gain from illness, will be more closely examined. The *introjection of the dead* will have extreme consequences. The nature of a hysterical identification and introjection will be at the origin of a contemporary phenomenon. Mourning and melancholia (a perverse kind of love for the dead and the ensuing depression along with other chronic symptoms) is only one of the many characteristics of the liberal politics of the day. A few additions will have to be made; among the most necessary is the masochistic-sadistic bind of the political activist and how the power of the super-ego can be effectively used to rid oneself of internal pain by projecting it, with cruelty and retribution (but certainly no forgiveness) to the external world. The ensuing suffering has been visceral; by the end of the essay, in the sections on *Civilization and its Discontents*, this suffering will be traced back to a disheartening circumstance and one of our main preoccupations: *the suppression of* love as a by-product of the relentless power of critique and negation. Certain principles of being are easily forgotten if they prove to be inconvenient. How the extreme forms of aggression and psychical violence are being directed by the power of the death drive in its collaboration with the super-ego is among the most important of the tasks of the psychopolitical essay ahead to detail. The essay will point towards the possibility of a future without either the imposition of a severely punitive super-ego within liberal democracies and, equally seriously, if the character of the nihilism of our times and the increasing force of the death-drive can be minimized and, perhaps, made less dangerous because of the counter-force of life and subjectivity, that is, the ego. Despite Freud's interpretation in *Group Psychology* and the acceptance that "only a few points chosen from the whole material are to be dealt with here. And they will in fact only be a few questions with which the depth-psychology of psycho-analysis is specially concerned" (18:71), their inter-connectedness will be sufficient to provide an account of our contemporary super-ego and, perhaps, offer a compelling enough analysis to be able to, at some future date, turn away from the theological-politics of liberal democracies and remodel our sensibilities. Freud obliges us to present an *essay*, a first attempt at re-thinking psychoanalysis specifically for our modern predicament. Taking one more occasion to witness his commitment despite all the controversies and in many cases, social disapproval of psychoanalysis, he concludes one essay with: "the rest of us, I hope, will be permitted without hindrance to carry through to the conclusion our labour in the depths."[60] The following essay is an emulation of the work we have inherited from Freud and from thinkers who anticipated how wide-ranging his reflections would be for his own time and beyond. That Nietzsche writes the following in a work whose subtitle is "Thoughts on the Prejudices of Morality" allows us one more measure of awareness of how our current nihilism, as enacted so forcefully by the super-ego, is indeed *sacrificing* the individual.

There is today perhaps no more firmly credited prejudice than this:

> that one *knows* what really constitutes the moral. Today it seems to *do everyone good* when they hear that society is on the way to *adapting* the individual to general requirements, and that *the happiness and at the same time the sacrifice of the individual* lies in feeling himself to be a useful member and instrument of the whole... ... What is wanted – whether this is admitted or not – is nothing less than a fundamental remoulding, indeed weakening and abolition of the *individual*.[61]

If true, then any present work will have to devote itself to the *individual's ego* insofar as he is still capable of its essential human characteristics – freedom and intelligence, creativity and love, as the achievable goals within our reach. Freud's confrontation has been set. Psychoanalysis, as a discipline, has not avoided difficult challenges. "When a civilization, like our own, devotes itself to the task of undermining its confidence in itself, this is an act of self-destruction."[62] Paying attention to the way various groups are actively undermining civilization will be isolated as the two fundamental characteristics of the complicity of a morbid morality and nihilism. The counterforce of psychoanalysis will be presented in order to renew the vigour of the individual. Christopher Bollas has described the historical creation of psychoanalysis as *the Freudian moment*. A complement is, today, warranted; rather than noting its epochal coming-to-be, Freud gives us the promise of a reinvigorated present. In an interview, Bollas made a remark for us: "if psychoanalysis is to serve the crisis of our times, if we are to be politically effective, then we have to prove the efficacy of insight into our own political realm."[63] It is my belief that Freud's thinking and writing can "serve the crisis of our times" and offer us, over a lifetime of work and with special attention to his concentrated reflections of the 1920s, the possibility of making remedies real – cures of affective awareness that will unify the fundamental human need for freedom, intelligence, creativity, and love and as alternative ways of being to the effects of super-ego morality and death-drive destruction against Western civilization.

Notes

1 Rorty, Richard. *Achieving Our Country: Leftist Thought in Twentieth-Century America*. Cambridge, Massachusetts: Harvard University Press, 1998, 45.

2 Derrida, Jacques. *Specters of Marx: The State of Debt, the Work of Mourning and the New International*. Tr. Peggy Kamuf. New York: Routledge, 1994, 221.

3 Raschke, Carl. *Postmodernism and the Revolution in Religious Theory: Toward a Semiotics of the Event*. Charlottesville: University of Virginia Press, 2012, 1. In a chapter entitled "Postmodernism and the return of the "religious" (with an additional title of "Specters of Religion") he also asks a question directly related to

one of Derrida's concepts: "Religion today returns, but can such a *revenant* be thought?" (53) One should point out that a *revenant* is usually used for someone who has died and, in some sense, come back to life. *How* is the question.

4 One set of circumstances will most certainly not be examined. None of the proposals for understanding the return of the religious related to that one date (September 11, 2001) are neither relevant nor of any interest for me. It seems much more important to analyze *ourselves* than to focus, with some distraction, on another civilization and their internal conflicts and external aggression. The outstanding word, "clash," is not external, for *us* or *them*, as in part conceived by Samuel P. Huntington in *The Clash of Civilizations and the Remaking of World Order*. New York: Simon & Schuster, 1996. Islam may have a visceral Shia/Sunni divide (leading, each, to detonate bombs in their mosques) but we should not be self-congratulatory about our own more refined methods, which are many and exposed for a psychoanalysis of our contemporary liberal reality. For a work dedicated to this theme, see Gabrielle Rifkind's *The Psychology of Political Extremism: What Would Sigmund Freud have Thought about Islamic State*. London: Routledge, 2018. For another concentration, and on what Manlio Graziano calls the "geopolitics of religion," see *Holy Wars and Holy Alliance: The Return of Religion to the Global Political Stage*. Tr. Brian Knowlton. New York: Columbia University Press, 2017. Lastly, for a philosophical inquiry into the theme, one is Gregg Lambert's *Return Statements: The Return of Religion in Contemporary Philosophy*. Edinburgh: Edinburgh University Press, 2016. Looking at ourselves to see how we are also intent on remaking liberal democracies should, today, preoccupy us much more than any one particular opposition. The internal self-loathing of Western civilization is proving to be much more lethal than any external antipathy, however pathological their acting-out appears in terms of extreme violence.

5 Freud, Sigmund. "Obsessive Actions and Religious Practices." SE 9:126.

6 Sloterdijk, Peter. *You Must Change Your Life: On Anthropotechnics*. Tr. Wieland Hoban. Cambridge, UK: Polity, 2013, 1. Spectre is my emphasis. He adds the first of other important statements. "The return of religion after the 'failure' of the Enlightenment must be confronted with a clearer view of the spiritual facts… … the tiresome distinction between 'true religion' and superstition loses its meaning. There are only regimes that are more or less capable and worthy of propagation. The false dichotomy of believers and unbelievers becomes obsolete and is replaced by the distinction between the practising and the untrained, or those who train differently. Something is indeed returning today – but the conventional wisdom that this is religion making its reappearance is insufficient to satisfy critical inquiries," 3. What is required, after a protracted period of "critical inquiries," is something that Freud can offer us both intellectually and therapeutically.

7 Žižek, Slavoj. *The Fragile Absolute, or, Why is the Christian Legacy Worth Fighting For*. London: Verso, 2000, 1.

8 Meillassoux, Quentin. *After Finitude: An Essay on the Necessity of Contingency*. Tr. Ray Brassier. London: Bloomsbury, 2008, 45.

9 Taylor, Charles. *A Secular Age*. Cambridge: Massachusetts: Harvard University Press, 2007, 546.

10 While Bruno Latour has argued that *We Have Never Been Modern* (Tr. Catherine Porter. Cambridge: Harvard University Press, 1993) the psychoanalytic thesis of the convergence between the infantile and the primitive will be one more reasons why we have become (because of the super-ego and the death drive) *anti-modern* and, to use Nietzsche's phrase for the first time, nihilistic most especially – that is, exclusively – towards Western civilization. Modernity, for Latour, has *not begun*. This one principle can very well serve us in the study moving forward and with one

further argument: the morality of our theological-political present does not want us to begin to be modern since the secondary gain from being infantile and primitive (and neurotic) has been a most intense desire and that simply keeps in place of all the most entrenched mechanisms of defense. They, as always, cause the most harm; all the defenses of the infant, the youth, and the teenager, becomes the prolonged misery of adult life, for the individual and everyone else.

11 Brague, Rémi. *Curing Mad Truths: Medieval Wisdom for the Modern Age*. Notre Dame: Notre Dame University Press, 2019, 6. Chapter One is entitled "The Failure of the Modern Project." In principle, we should indeed "rescue" pre-modern ideas. Future work will have to be dedicated to the task of identifying, precisely, *which ones*.

12 Lyotard, Jean-François. *The Postmodern Explained: Correspondence, 1982–1985*. Tr. and Ed. by Julian Pefanis and Morgan Thomas. Minneapolis: University of Minnesota Press, 1993, 28.

13 Badiou, Alain. *The Century*. Tr. Alberto Toscano. Cambridge, UK: Polity, 2007, 165.

14 Badiou, Alain. *Philosophy and the Event*, with Fabien Tarby. Tr. Louise Burchill. Cambridge, UK: Polity, 2013, 30.

15 Badiou, Alain. *Briefings on Existence: A Short Treatise on Transitory Ontology*. Translated, edited, and with an introduction by Norman Madarasz. Albany: SUNY, 2006. 30–31, my emphasis.

16 Han, Byung-Chul. *Psychopolitics*. Tr. Erik Butler. London: Verso, 2017, 7.

17 Sloterdijk, Peter. *Rage and Time: A Psychopolitical Investigation*. Tr. Mario Wenning. New York: Columbia University Press, 2010.

18 Johnston, Adrian. *Adventures in Transcendental Materialism: Dialogues With Continental Thinkers*. Edinburgh: Edinburgh University Press, 2014, 219–220.

19 Dupuy, Jean-Pierre. *The Mark of the Sacred*. Tr. M.B. DeBevoise. Stanford: Stanford University Press, 2013, 16.

20 Hobbes, Thomas. *Leviathan*. New York: E.P. Dutton and Company, Inc., 1950, 4.

21 Freud, Sigmund. *Beyond the Pleasure Principle*. SE 18:59.

22 As for the status of *Totem and Taboo* being historically true or verifiable, the question is for me as irrelevant as asking if the first book of the Torah or Hesiod's *Theogony* are based on actual events. Critiques from the discipline of anthropology, or any other, have no bearing on the matter. My immediate response is: its *mythic truth*, allegorically speaking and for us specifically, is more important than history. Any of the numerous commentaries on the status of the 1913 work are not an issue – whether we can say with Torberg Foss that "Freud's tale" "rings somewhat true" (in "Freud 100 Years Ago: Totem and Taboo (1912–1913) 1–4 *The Scandinavian Psychoanalytic Review*, 36:12, 2013, or Robert A. Paul's even more emphatic "Yes, The Primal Crime Did Take Place: A Further Defense of Freud's Totem and Taboo," 230–249 *Ethos*, Vol. 38, Issue 2, 2010.

23 Freud, Sigmund. *Totem and Taboo*. SE 13:64.

24 Winnicott, D.W. *Playing and Reality*. London: Routledge, 1971, 13.

25 Segal, Hanna. "Psychoanalysis and Freedom of Thought," 51–63 *Dimensions of Psychoanalysis: Selected Papers Presented at the Freud Memorial Lectures*. Ed. Joseph Sandler. London: Karnac, 1989, 52–53.

26 Kristeva, Julia. *Passions of Our Time*. Tr. Constance Borde and Sheila Malovany-Chevallier. New York: Columbia University Press, 2013, 61.

27 Isaac, Jeffrey. "Liberal Democracy in Question?" 1–5 *Perspectives on Politics*, Vol. 15, No. 1 (Mar. 2017), 1. Isaac remains committed to the problems he outlined in his 2003 *The poverty of progressivism: the future of American democracy in a time of liberal decline*. His American context can be expanded considerably. The "world politics" can be narrowed.

28 As Marc F. Plattner presents in "Illiberal Democracy as the Struggle on the Right," 5–19 *Journal of Democracy*, Vol. 30, No. 1, 2019. The political analysis is as follows: "I am concerned with the threat that mainstream center-right parties will be captured by tendencies that are indifferent or even hostile to liberal democracy," 6.

29 Freud, Sigmund. "On Psychotherapy." SE 7:260, my emphasis. If Freud is right that psychoanalysis is *the only* form of thinking to be able to understand and interpret the extent of the internal (in the individual) and external *morbid* phenomena (in society), we can also be aware of the relation between what is morbid and therefore diseased and how psychoanalysis has also been unique in showing us the many ways one can be close to *mori* in life. Morbidity gives us one immediate sense of the analysis to come: the super-ego, the death drive, and its illnesses.

30 Nietzsche, Friedrich. *The Gay Science*. Tr. Walter Kaufmann. New York: Vintage Books, 1974, 279.

31 Turner, Stephen. "Freud in Many Contexts," 269–275 *Society*, Vol. 57, Issue 3 (Jun 2020).

32 Freud, Sigmund. "Remembering, Repeating, and Working-Through (Further Recommendations on the Technique of Psychoanalysis II). SE 12:151.

33 Freud, Sigmund. "Obsessions and Phobias. Their Psychological Mechanism and Their Aetiology." SE 3:74.

34 Freud, Sigmund. "The Disposition to Obsessional Neurosis: A Contribution to the Problem of Choice of Neurosis." (SE 12:325) The emphasis on super-morality is mine. Although there will be more than one occasion to introduce the specific characteristics of other neurotic afflictions (including hysteria) it is obsessional neurosis that will recur throughout the essay, in large part because its *symptoms* are so easily identifiable from the ideas and the acts of the social and political initiates of our current super-morality. That the paper was delivered in the fall of 1913 – that is, in the same year as the publication of *Totem and Taboo* – will make this one observation (on love and hate, empathy and aggression, Eros and Thanatos) foundational for many of the ideas to be analyzed in what follows.

35 Freud, Sigmund. "Further Remarks on the Neuro-Psychoses of Defense." SE 3:168. The remark comes in the section "The Nature and Mechanism of Obsessional Neurosis." This one writing can be accessed for being at the root of many of the ideas he would come to express almost three decades later. He adds: "obsessional ideas have, as it were, a compulsive [obsessional] psychical currency, not on account of their intrinsic value, but on account of the source from which they derive or which has added a contribution to their value." SE 3:171.

36 Latrie, Stijn, Van Herck, Walter, Vanheerwijck. (Eds.) *Radical Secularization? An Inquiry Into the Religious Roots of Secular Culture*. London: Bloomsbury, 2015.

37 Klein, Melanie. *The Psycho-Analysis of Children*. Tr. Alix Strachey. London: Virago Press, 1989, 136–137.

38 Freud, Sigmund. "Five Lectures on Psycho-analysis." SE 11:49.

39 Freud, Sigmund. *Introductory Lectures on Psycho-analysis*. SE 15:45.

40 Freud, Sigmund. *On Narcissism: An Introduction*. SE 14:98.

41 Han, Byung-Chul. *The Agony of Eros*. Tr. Erik Butler. Cambridge, Massachusetts: The MIT Press, 2017, 32.

42 Schmitt, Carl. *Political Theology: Four Chapters on the Concept of Sovereignty*. Tr. George Schwab. Chicago: The University of Chicago Press, 1985, 36.

43 Strauss, Leo. *What is Political Philosophy?* Chicago: The University of Chicago Press, 1959, 13. My emphasis. That the relation itself requires an important distinction is a crucial point. The emphasis has to be placed on the first term of the pair: the transference of the theological *into* the political is the process now underway. What the process, together, has produced is my main interest.

44 Chasseguet-Smirgel, Janine. *The Ego-Ideal: A Psychoanalytic Study on the Malady of the Ideal*. Tr. Paul Burrows. New York: W.W. Norton, 1985. It seems to me that her extraordinary work as a psychoanalyst and writer has become even more relevant than during her life. In her paper "The Body and the World" (13–27, *International Congress Series*, 2006) and in the memorable phrase of "the dismantling of one's own body" (which was used to define the individuals responsible for the 9/11 event), she has also made it possible for us to consider other ways in which the body can be "dismantled" and according to the perversions of our contemporary theological-political situation in liberal democracies. Has the nihilism of Western civilization gone as far as to emulate and *mimic* (allegorically and unconsciously) other forms of extreme pathological violence?
45 Kahn, Paul W. *PoliticaL Theology: Four New Chapters on the Concept of Sovereignty*. New York: Columbia University Press, 2012, 4, my emphasis.
46 Lefort, Claude. "Permanence of the Theologico-Political?" in *Democracy and Political Theory*. Tr. David Macey. Cambridge: Polity Press, 2000, 223.
47 As, for example, in the collection of essays in *Political Theology and Early Modernity*. Ed. Graham Hammill and Julia Reinhard Lupton. Chicago: The University of Chicago Press, 2012.
48 Habermas, Jürgen. "The Rational Meaning of a Questionable Inheritance of Political Theology," in *The Power of Religion in the Public Sphere*. Ed. and Introduced by Eduardo Mendieta and Jonathan Vanantwerpen. New York: Columbia University Press, 2011, 23.
49 Frank, Jason and McNulty, Tracy. "Taking Exception to the Exception," 4–11 *Diacritics*, Vol. 37, No. 2/3, Summer 2007, 4.
50 Elliott, Anthony. *Social Theory Since Freud: Traversing Social Imaginaries*. London: Routledge, 2004, 53.
51 Kaye, Howard. "Raising Freud from the Dead," 294–298 *Society*, Vol. 57, No. 3 (Jun. 2020).
52 Freud, Sigmund. "On the History of the Psycho-Analytic Movement." SE 14:35.
53 Damisch, Hubert. "Bridging the Gap Between Two Scenes," 93–95 *Whose Freud? The Place of Psychoanalysis in Contemporary Culture*. Ed. Peter Brooks and Alex Woloch. Ithaca: Cornell University Press, 2000, 95.
54 Freud, Sigmund. "On the History of the Psycho-Analytic Movement." SE 14:8.
55 Delay, Tad. *God is Unconscious: Psychoanalysis and Theology*. Eugene, Oregon: Wipf & Stock, 2015, xv.
56 Gourgoris, Stathis. *The Perils of the One*. New York: Columbia University Press, 2019, 140.
57 Goux, Jean-Joseph. "Freudian Unconscious and Secularization of Judaism," in *Disciplining Freud on Religion: Perspectives from the Humanities*. Ed. Greg Kaplan and William Parsons. Lanham: Lexington Books, 2010, 218.
58 Nietzsche, Friedrich. *The Will to Power*. Tr. Walter Kaufmann and R.J. Hollingdale. New York: Vintage Books, 1967, 16.
59 Freud, Sigmund. *Introductory Lectures on Psycho-Analysis*. SE 16:258.
60 Freud, Sigmund. "On the History of the Psycho-Analytic Movement." SE 14:66.
61 Nietzsche, Friedrich. *Daybreak: Thoughts on the Prejudices of Morality*. Tr. R.J. Hollingdale. Cambridge: Cambridge University Press, 1982, 83.
62 Schwartz, Howard S. *Society Against Itself: Political Correctness and Organizational Self-Destruction*. London: Karnac, 2010, xi.
63 Bollas, Christopher. *The Freudian Moment*. London: Karnac, 2013. The quote comes from the interview with Vincenzo Bonaminio.

1

THE REGRESSIVE PSYCHOLOGY OF GROUPS

> It might be said that the intense emotional ties which we observe in groups are quite sufficient to explain one of their characteristics – the lack of independence and initiative in their members... ... a picture of a regression of mental activity to an earlier stage such as we are not surprised to find among savages and children.
>
> *Group Psychology and the Analysis of the Ego*

(a) Love-Hate, Diminished Intelligence, Loss of Freedom

The primary three-part relation in the 1921 *Group Psychology and the Analysis of the Ego* can be introduced as a foundation to the study of the contemporary nature of the superego and the increasing force of a specifically social and political death drive as it effects the individual and liberal democratic societies as a whole. One, love-hate; two, the lessening of intelligence; and three, the loss of freedom, will be considered as inter-related processes. The characteristics of each, and their specific alteration in the 21st century, have been part of a combination of factors in creating a deeply *impoverished* individual who continues to be exposed to considerable pressure. Freud's language is cumulative and emphatic: the self who has been overwhelmed by the coercions of the group has suffered from impoverishment, loss, reduction, inhibition, and depletion. Recalling Freud's *On Narcissism* allows us to trace how the psychical energy expended to deal with neurotic conflict results in a "depleted"[1] self. More importantly for us in the present and the changed dynamics of self-absorption: how has the contemporary individual been systematically undermined by a political culture intent on promoting different

DOI: 10.4324/9781003410911-2

forms of psychical destitution (which are rationalized by an imperious morality) while unconscious of a regression to the infantile and the primitive conflicts of the psyche? The insights of "Mourning and Melancholia," once they were brought forward to group psychology and society, led Freud to recognize how the enthusiasm of a mass movement led to the "loss of capacity to love" as well as a "lowering of self-regard."[2] *Love and ego* have been eroded by a wide range of obsessive fixations. Conditions can be identified at the outset. Harry Guntrip presents us with one of the more serious diagnoses. The term "schizoid" represents a certain class of pathological individuals (for us, they will be exclusively *political*) who are afflicted by a "*profound complex inhibition of the capacity to love*."[3] This inhibition is a *direct result* of political sensibilities; none of the symptoms are new, but they are recognizable by the displacements we will trace back, as Freud did, consistently until *Civilization and its Discontents*.

Freud's findings, and his interpretation of their consequences, are essential in grounding our inquiry into the nature of the group today: no real love for others, no regard for the self, no tolerance for independence of mind. In his 1921 review of *Group Psychology*, Sandor Ferenczi noted its importance: "the investigation of the process of group psychology was capable of solving important problems of individual psychology."[4] The emotions, freedom, and intelligence of *the individual* is my main concern insofar as he can be adversely influenced (made sick, psychologically, and with other psycho-somatic effects) by the drives of powerful groups in society that are absolute in their demands. Freud's preoccupation with the psychical effects of neuroses on emotions, freedom, and intelligence will be constant right until our concluding chapter and the culmination of a decade of his work. In outlining one discontent of "civilized" life, Freud asks: "How can we expect people who are under the dominance of *prohibitions of thought* to attain the psychological ideal, the primacy of the intelligence?" (21:48, my emphasis). If the double-sense of the bind of the members to the group is primary – as both a perversion of love and a rationalization of hate – how does identification, and self-conception in terms of identity, lead to a condition that has not always been a specifically political concern and yet central to psychoanalysis? Although the idea of freedom has been pre-eminent for any *political* philosophy, as has another kind of love (the "love of wisdom" of philosophy, as well as the two kinds of erotic love – the procreation of the sexually differentiated body and the procreation of the psyche as affirmations of life and creativity expressed in Plato's *Symposium* by Diotima, a woman[5]) Freud's additional *symptom* of the compromise of intelligence can be singled out – most especially when the ability to think, to be discerning, to be reflective, is linked, as Freud does, to regression and to the psychical conditions of the infantile and primitive which has led to contemporaneity of a *primitive present*. His classical reconstruction of the origins of civilization in *Totem and*

Taboo – the primal horde, to the herd, to the collective of a society – are not (for us) simply speculative historical developments. Any anthropological verification, in the nature of a historical event, is irrelevant. The infantile and the primitive: Freud does not have our anthropological circumspection about a definition of the latter. He allows us, today, to avoid merely *academic* considerations, which have become both intrusive and categorical; censorship and suppression have not been reluctant to be invoked as necessities and during a time when the university has been determined by exacting moral principles and by an increasing control of public discourse. Prohibitions and imperatives have become simultaneous realities; the complicity between theory and morality has been detrimental to free thought, free speech, and free writing. The character, and influence of groups, was even noticed in a therapeutic situation. The experiences of subsequent psychoanalytic writers would confirm Freud's first findings. Working specifically with groups in a therapeutic setting, W. R. Bion remarked that

> judged by ordinary standards of social intercourse, the performance of the group is almost devoid of intellectual content. Furthermore, if we note how assumptions pass unchallenged as statements of fact, and are accepted as such, it seems that critical judgment is almost entirely absent.[6]

The lessening of intelligence in the group can be re-affirmed; but Freud's developments of group psychology is going to make him unique in his observations since his inquiry into the reality of regression would have more extreme consequences for our political understanding of liberalism.

How Freud, as a doctor, a thinker, and a humanist, creates an analysis of our contemporary situation by first recognizing the power of myths (classical ones and then, remarkably, one of his own in *Totem and Taboo*) will be central in the psychopolitical essay to follow. The creation of myths is, for him, a decisive event historically and *personally*. A few brief reminders of Freud's beginnings brings us first to a comment that he made in the 1894 "The Neuro-Psychoses of Defense," on a requirement, that is, the "psychical analysis of intelligent patients."[7] A patient (that is, to be a patient capable of analysis) one had to be intelligent and in a way that can be more specifically identified; cognition, much less a numerical "quotient," does not approximate the requirements of listening to oneself, while being heard, and with attention to linguistic meanings and affects. In the ur-case of psychoanalysis, Anna O., Breuer and Freud tell us that "she was markedly intelligent."[8] The sensitivity of an analysand is not superfluous for reading Freud. If we had to choose one, and only one attribute of the intelligent analysand, an essential one would have to be the ability to differentiate a perception in its immediacy (as, simply, seemingly true because obvious to the ego), and the possibility of it being illusory, a distortion, and a projection. *Analytic* intelligence has the ability to suspend immediate impressions and to expose oneself to several reappraisals and interpretations. An analysand, much more than an academic theorist who may be motivated by one ideology or another as it concerns the world (but rarely himself), must be capable of recognizing his misperception and a number of other impressions believed to be true, persuasive, and convincing. How did Freud first witness one of the many ways in which intelligence could regress and the whole personality suffer – *made* to suffer – because of the distortions of conscience and the debility of a *politically induced* guilt for history and civilization. The psychopolitics of mourning and depression have led the individual to "an extraordinary diminution in his self-regard, an *impoverishment* of his ego on a grand scale" (SE 14:246, my emphasis). Freud's emphatic language should not be overlooked; the vocabulary is extensive and repeated. When the relation of mourning and melancholia are affects for understanding one aspect of group psychology, the analysis of our present begins to be more recognizable. How did theological-political neuroses, as essentially moral, alter, and diminish, so much of the substance of the human – in self-regard, intelligence, freedom, and the ability to love?

In an essay on "the antinomy of morality," Dan Merkur makes two related observations: "Identifications with group members with each other are regressive processes."[9] When the identification and regression has specifically *moral* consequences, as they do today, a psychoanalytic inquiry is called for and one in support of the individual of psychoanalysis. The following essay is also, and primarily, a defense of the ego against the overwhelming initiatives of an all-purpose reality. The individual will be supported no differently than in a clinical situation; the principle will be to sustain, not criticize or undermine – and, ultimately, to therapeutically enhance the ego. In the Clark lectures, Freud told his university audience that

> the flight from unsatisfactory reality into what… … we call illness (though it is never without an immediate yield of pleasure to the patient) takes place along the path of involution, of regression… … The deeper you penetrate into the pathogenesis of nervous illness, the more you will find revealed the connection between the neuroses and other productions of the human mind, including the most valuable. You will be taught that we humans, with *the high standards of civilization* and under the pressure of our internal repressions, find reality unsatisfying quite generally, and for that reason entertain a life of phantasy in which we like to make up for the insufficiencies of reality by the production of wish-fulfillments… … If there is persistent rebellion against the real world… … it is almost inevitable that the libido, keeping up the sources of the phantasies, will follow the path of regression, and will revive infantile wishes and end in neurosis.
>
> (SE 11:49–50, my emphasis)

The lectures direct us towards Freud's interests in social life and how "the high standards of civilization" – what he will several times call the "categorical imperative," after the moral philosophy of Immanuel Kant – lead to the discontent, the unhappiness, he will outline in a number of ways. The opening decades of the 21st century have been clearer in terms of revealing a connection between the "rebellion against the real world" and a psychical regression that has found its consolation in the primitive and the infantile and with the creation of super-ego morality – and, more seriously, the force of the death drive – that may very well be unprecedented in liberal democracies. How do we take the theory of regression (as, in part, the revival of childhood experiences in fantasy – both omnipotent and anxious ones and thus already *split*) to better understand the *moralizing* social and political movements of today? If regression remains fixated on a past experience or fantasy which makes *development* impossible, as Winnicott argued,[10] how are Freud's important relations between the loss of freedom and diminishing intelligence serve as one of our first arguments for the understanding of the group today?

Due to the nature of his project in *Group Psychology*, Freud sets out with not a little reservation; he is under no illusion about the extent of the disparate ideas and how they will have to be organized into a whole and with contributions extending well beyond the ones well known at the time.[11] The presentation of the intricate parts will require him the better part of a decade to bring to completion; only the future (our own present) would be able to confirm how far-reaching his analysis would turn out to be. In Lecture XXIII of his *Introductory Lectures*, in the process of explaining "psychical (or psychogenic) symptoms and psychical illness," Freud goes on to stress how

> the main damage they do resides in the mental expenditure which they themselves involve in the further expenditure that becomes necessary for fighting against them. When there is an extensive formation of symptoms, these two sorts of expenditure can result in an extraordinary *impoverishment* of the subject in regard to the mental energy available to him.
>
> (SE 16:358)

His personal cross-references can be noted. What happens when the "mental expenditure" by the *individual* subject once it is over-used and the formations are made worse within the order of the group? Weakness is inevitable, as is susceptibility to influence. Freud's therapeutic preoccupations are evident in the systematic expression of his language; we should see his innumerable references and, once more, to "extraordinary *impoverishment*" which we can connect to *depletion* and all the other prior references. We have not always recognized Freud for his compassion and empathy for the needless suffering of an individual; or the noticeable worry for the character of an ill society. Following his insights, we can ask: how has the absolute devotion to one idea (the moral) led to the regression of an entire society – and with signs, noticeable especially among young adults, of psychical fatigue, depression, anxiety, and other *new* symptoms, many of them a direct cause of a psychical split between two irreconcilable drives: prohibition and permissiveness? The vigor needed for everyday self-determination has been severely blocked. We are going to have to be attentive to the nature of psychical conflict and its many-faceted forms of expression; the symptoms are so exhausting as to make thoughtfulness, for many, virtually impossible. Reflection has been replaced by illusory absolutes and neurotic ideations.

The intimacy of love-hate has been mentioned first. We can make one more observation so as to firmly separate Freud from the limits of his historical period and from other social "critics." The "historical perspective," for one, is no longer sufficient when we think about psychoanalytic thought for our present. "From a historical perspective," Stephen Jonsson writes, "there is no doubt that Freud's book crossed a threshold as it presented a theory that shed light on all the new ways in which masses and collectives were analyzed in interwar European culture."[12] In *Group Psychology*, Freud can no longer be regarded as an analyst of his own time and reduced to a *historicist* context. He was not, one-dimensionally, analyzing European culture in the aftermath of the First World War, for example, not unless we ignore his capacity for the perception of psychical alterations in history. A diagnostician develops a two-way relation to time, one in finding causes and tracing effects, the other in anticipating inevitable turn-outs and possibly altering them. Freud's ability to see into the temporal changes of the psyche led him to the conclusion that a coming period would begin to exemplify the very worst characteristics of the super-ego and its associated death drive, the latter to be interpreted not so much in its classical formulation and the tendency to constancy, to *feeling* nothing at all, but today as the drive towards the obliteration of history and what Nietzsche identified as the coming nihilism of Western civilization. Can we better identify the nature of this nihilism once psychoanalysis defines its many symptoms? The theme of haunting can be mentioned again. Ghosts are going to re-appear and remain with us.

In a chapter entitled "Populism and the Spectre of Democracy," Benjamin Arditi writes: "As an internal periphery of democratic politics, populism can be a dimension of representation, a mode of participation lodged in the rougher edges of democracy, but also something more disturbing given that it can thrive in political democracies while it morphs into something that can become its *nemesis*."[13] How do the most valued of our ideals lead, potentially, to their exact opposite? How does the desire for justice turn into Nemesis, the Greek goddess of vengeance? The worry, by social and political thinkers, has been expressed. Freud's depth-psychological inquiries promise to take us further than previous critiques; the primitive, as a condition of being, is no longer confined to the past.

> It would appear as though we were on the right road towards an explanation of the principal phenomenon of group psychology – the individual's *lack of freedom* in a group. If each individual is bound in two directions by such an intense emotional tie, we shall find no difficulty in attributing to that circumstance the alteration and limitation which have been observed in his personality.
>
> (18:95)

The many kinds of "limitation" will involve an an-going study in order to more completely unify the concepts of psychoanalysis as they pertain to the understanding of groups. More seriously, however, is Freud's identification of a set of phenomena that are leading him towards the identification of a unique "agency" that has particular effects on the self. Since the intimations of the super-ego are found in "Mourning and Melancholia," their relation is, for us, doubly important and we can again emphasize how its original discussion had several implications for a theological-political thesis. "We shall come upon evidence to show that it [the "agency," which acts alone] can become diseased on its own account" (SE 14:247). Has the super-ego morality of our contemporary liberal societies made many people *sick*? Can the illness be acknowledged as such; or will the characteristics of our psychical splitting continue to be more securely suppressed and disavowed? Freud's presentation aims at such a possibility; his writing, as a transference, aims at clarifying our perception. The sense of the super-ego, and its connection to an ego-ideal, prepares us for the argument to come. Ultimately, the theological-political resurrection of the dead will clarify the ubiquity of spectral metaphors.

After a scholarly introduction and reference to Gustave Le Bon's 1895 *Psychologies des foules* (that is, *foules* as crowds, implying a gathering of people in a place, which is distinct from a group organized around an identity and an accompanying set of ideas[14]), Freud isolates the four consensus characteristics of what he called *Massenpsychologie*[15] – among others, contagion, imitation, suggestibility, and the one most associated with libidinal ties, the social concept of identification that would be defined, more acutely, by the diagnosis of *hysteria*.[16] Once he recognized the relationship between *hysterical identification*, introjection, and projection, the understanding of group psychology would be better unified and capable of being systematically explained. Still, Freud was well aware of the work ahead. The tripartite structure of the psyche had to be presented and, with it, the force of the death drive. In the meantime, he continued, slowly and methodically. "Although group psychology is only in its infancy, it embraces an immense number of separate issues and offers to investigators countless problems which have hitherto not even been properly distinguished from one another… … Only a few points chosen from the whole material are to be dealt with here" (SE 18:71).[17] There were other issues that would only be more fully examined, both in the work to come on the unconscious of groups, and in future writings after 1921 and in *The Ego and the Id*. Before turning to one of the concepts of most interest to us and its development into the contemporary form of hysterical identification, introjection, and projection, there is one other *relation* which has not received sufficient attention. Emphasizing this one reality of the individual who is firmly imbedded in the identity of a group will be one of the obligations to come. Although Freud mentions both, he did not (at least explicitly) bring them together – in part because at the outset he was preoccupied with offering an analysis that others, like one of his interlocutors, William McDougall, author of the 1920 *The Group Mind*, had either missed completely or failed to mention. Freud writes: "We will try our fortune, then, with the supposition that love relationship (or, to use a more neutral expression, emotional ties) also constitute the essence of the group mind. At *first*, the essence are emotional ties. Let us remember that the authorities make no mention of any such relations" (18:91). *At first*: the italics force us to anticipate an addition. "Love" is not all; the emotion, moreover, will not be primary and will have to include its opposite. The intense ambivalence of the love-hate relation within the group would lead to further and even more complicated ideas – of which the masochism-sadism bind would be one. The inter-connection would require time to identify.

The presence of "love relationships" within groups and as an affect is accompanied by one other that further changes the nature of identification and makes the debility of contemporary politics more exposed. A supplement will soon be provided by one of the pre-eminent concerns of psychoanalysis as a therapeutic art of interpretation and medical science. If "love" has been introduced as an essential characteristic of group psychology, there was also another one that makes his work essential for our interpretations ahead. Once Freud moves beyond the appearance of the love of a group and its identification both with its own members and *with certain others in history* who have become symbolically revived, he could develop this emerging social observations without restraint. The essence of emotional ties had consequences both for the inability to think perceptively, and above all, self-critically – unless, as we shall see, acted out in the context of a masochist-sadistic projection. A double-identification has taken place: with each member of the group and with others, in history, who serve as models. Eros and Thanatos have already been anticipated once the uniqueness of *a specific other* is identified and analyzed for the rationalization of a perpetual mourning and melancholia. The dead of history will not be commemorated; they will be introjected, with nihilistic consequences once they are revitalized and acting in their capacity as moral legislators. This *depression*, as one symptom of being estranged from society, historical reality, and civilization, will prove to be decisive for our later inquiry as will its relation to a politicized *moral inferiority* and the sense of a permanent *self-reproach* that turns conscience into something far more sinister. The enforcement of a *cultural culpability* (that is, the imposition of guilt on Western civilization) will then make the super-ego and the death drive collaborative and unforgiving in their ability to make absolute judgments and to serve, as is claimed, the ends of justice.

In the opening of Chapter IV, "Suggestion and Libido," Freud brings the relation of love and intelligence into the closest proximity. The individual in a group undergoes "a profound alteration in his mental activity. His liability to affect becomes extraordinarily intensified, while his intellectual ability is markedly reduced" (18: 88). *Affect and intellect*, emotion and intelligence: for Freud, group psychology creates a simultaneous *eros/psyche* transformation that will perpetuate an original self-conflict; the libidinal and the intellectual confront each other, unconsciously, and intensely so, each vying for supremacy and yet perpetually tied in a circular deadlock. A dual process specifically occurs in the *politicized* individual whose identity depends on sympathetic like-mindedness with certain others; antipathy must also follow in the jagged symmetry of love-hate, Eros and Thanatos, with the drive of emotional aggression that reduces the intelligence of the individual while deviating it into political enthusiasm and feelings. Reason, as such, does not adequately explain the condition; intelligence, as conceived by Freud, is a sign of the individual being autonomous enough to be *creative* and *original*, instead of dependent, and not to submit to influence as a way to be accepted by others. The personal ideal of courage, for Freud, will not be insignificant. The free individual, who has a self-determined interiority that is not susceptible to the various impressions from the external world, and the imperatives of others, can remain psychically steadfast. The free, creative, and psychologically healthy individual does not have *peers*; he has, first of all, a healthy ego, a healthy sense of self, a healthy individuality, and he has *friends* who respect personal integrity and who, together, avoid the mimicry of conformism. The people in groups are intensely, single-mindedly in love with an idea, a cause, an ideal (and with those who share mutually recognized characteristics) and at the expense of a balanced assessment of reality. Is an extreme regression, a kind of psychical paralysis (understood temporally) much deeper than the cognitive, reminiscent of Freud's very early description of quasi-hypnoid states and a present *neurasthenia of consciousness*? Has our human phenomenological acuity been severely undermined by the regressions of groups and their influence on social reality and resulted in the "dwindling of the conscious individual personality?" (18:122). His descriptions are many and cumulative.

In addition to the examples of those who were classically the subjects of his analysis of diminished intelligence – children as well as primitives – the one modern subject to be added is the *political* "lover." The modern *activist*, to give him a contemporary definition (along with another, social justice *warrior*), has regressed to a peculiar state of mind. Children, primitives, the political activist: the trio unified by psychoanalytic perception is unlikely to be met with much approval, at least from those who regard themselves as the epitome of morality and who are actively working towards (fighting for) the ideal transformation of liberal democracy. Our modern sensibilities are under significant pressure from Freud. Due to group libido, he adds, "the conscious personality has entirely vanished; will and discernment are lost" (18:76). The "vanishing" of the personality, or the suppression of the "I," has resulted from a particular kind of political/moral sensibility. The ego, that is, the individual sustained by psychoanalytic thought – who is not the liberally produced subject of our times – will be given support instead of being subjected to moral instruction and orthodox requirements; because if the super-ego and the death drive have become the dominant psychical forces of the present, it was Freud who, uniquely, offered us both an analysis and a variety of remedies to restore the inherent possibilities of the human being, in and out of the clinical situation and for the sake of love, freedom, intelligence, creativity, and psychological health.

An earlier observation on love, in the Introduction, can be brought forward and given a wider scope. Everything in the nature of the ego in group psychology, as depleted and emptied, impoverished and weakened, has been anticipated by Freud. One *cure* towards the fulfillment of the ego occurs in the experience of love that is not politically motivated. "Self-regard appears to us to be an expression of the ego"; that is, the way the self perceives its own identity comes, when healthy, as an internal disposition rather than an external necessity. Self-regard cannot come from, or be created by, others. In *On Narcissism* (a work, parenthetically, that can also be stressed for its defense of the ego), Freud continues and adds: "The realization of impotence, of one's own inability to love, in consequence of mental or physical disorder, has an exceedingly lowering effect upon self-regard." Ego and love mutually sustain each other. Does the group, because its love is misplaced – to itself and its ego-ideal – suffer from a process that reduces its vitality and creates the permanence of a depressive state? The ability to love has been forfeited because of the super-ego imperatives that make social critique a fundamental motivation in order to take masochistic pleasure in suffering and, simultaneously, sadistically causing pain for others. The distortions of love occur when the pleasure of masochism and sadism become a guiding principle, further splitting the political psyche. The lowering of self-regard is compensated by a different kind of power and one forced, with impunity, on others. The super-ego, which is already present in Freud's discussion of narcissism, has a devastating effect on the individual and in relation to the impulsiveness of a new ego-ideal, an internalized presence that, as we will soon see, has been transformed from the *leader* to a curious subject of history who represents the appearances of specters and ghosts. "So long as he suffers, he ceases to love" (SE 14:82). So long as the experience of pain is primary, and an indulgence, he suffers more because of the phantasmatic nature of his traumatism; he can then justify the worst tendencies of the super-ego, including aggression, persecution, and moral sadism. Once we recollect Freud's analysis of both the loss of the inability to love and a lowering of self-regard, then our principal themes are unified into a better understanding of the theological-political neurotic who has been engineered in the contemporary liberal order.

In *Group Psychology*, Freud does not hesitate to repeat himself, as if he was not entirely sure his arguments would be noticed with the full force of their presentation. "The fundamental fact of group psychology – the two theses as to the intensification of affects and the inhibition of the intellect in primitive groups" (18:88). One foundation has been repeated. The entire edifice will be built slowly, methodically, each addition serving to add to the whole and committed to the permanent perception of a way of being, individually and socially. The "intensification of affects" now can be more precisely defined: the convolutions of love-hate and the loss of intelligence are inter-related. If Freud has been the consummate therapist – that is, someone serving the psychological health of his patients – the work of the 1920s is marked by a more comprehensive ambition: to provide a depth-psychological assessment of an entire culture while, always, addressing himself to one individual who has become conscious of the negative effects on life in its everydayness. Freud begins to consider whether the therapy of an individual may be extended to society. Is it possible, with sufficient analysis, to raise the *collective intelligence* of an entire society once its neuroses have been identified and, perhaps, treated? Can the regressive to the infantile and the primitive be altered and so initiate a new maturity, a new freedom and intelligence and love? Love, freedom, intelligence: Freud recognized how psychoanalysis would have to dedicate itself to their enhancement. "There was a humanistic side of Freud's temperament well-suited to the exploration of the meaning of freedom to human health and well-being."[18] This should not be a difficult axiom to accept: *psychological* freedom and well-being was one ideal of the psychoanalytic task. In the years to come, the relation of *love and happiness* would become central to Freud's aspirations as a therapist and a thinker: to increase the aesthetic appreciation of life and so begin to *feel* and think differently. On the way to making these two human pursuits a psychoanalytic ideal in *Civilization and its Discontents*, Freud had considerable work to do: the after-effects of regression soon brought him to other psychical mechanism and how they increasingly determined everyday life by paralyzing individual development.

"At quite an early stage problems of human phylogenesis arose. It became quite clear that the *pathological function* was often nothing more than a regression to an earlier stage of development of normal function."[19] The relation of regression to pathology, while significant for its our understanding of phylogenesis – and let us emphasize that the Greek *phylon* refers to a "tribe," hence the idea of the primal horde from *Totem and Taboo* – is here equally important ontogenetically, for the individual. The regression will turn into a simultaneous infantile and primitive state, fundamentally one of incoherent conflict, producing anxiety and vulnerability and transformed, as an acutely defensive formation, into a number of projective reactions. The diagnosis of pathology has been established; the observation of an illness leads in two directions, to its cause and, if possible, its remedy, partial or total. To prepare for Freud's explanatory model (of Eros and Thanatos) we can turn now to some of the most well-known characteristics of group psychology. Contagion, suggestibility, and imitation could all be analyzed separately. However, in order to pursue the neglected inter-relation of love, intelligence, and freedom, the implications of Freud's thinking will be followed insofar as the three united themes of *Group Psychology* provide us with an intimation of the explicit definition of the super-ego and, ultimately, the place of the death-drive in our liberal democracies. There will be several opportunities to isolate the most important concepts from this and the other writings of my essay. Development has not simply been stunted; the regression forces a return to a kind of ground zero before any growth has taken place. The psychical tensions are too inchoate for any one direction to be open. In whatever way we define one of the most overt symptoms of our age – as a group, tribe, and one coalescing around a politics of identity – it will be incumbent on us to provide as clear an explanation as possible of our contemporary situation as outlined by Freud a century ago. Some political commentaries have been perceptive; they have also been incomplete. We will add to the analysis of regression by following up on the three psychical processes that are much more specific and beyond the limited rationality of political analyses. The deepest of unconscious processes are the grounds, for Freud, of any understanding of social and political life. A new phenomenon, in terms of a hysterical identification, introjection, and projection will be the focus of the next section. In the meantime, a few explicitly political comments contribute to the argument as a whole; they are partial. The political, on its own, can only give us *one sense* of the problem.

While "ideology critique" has been the occupation of the traditional Left, there are now many reasons to substitute ideology for a better term: propaganda. One of Jacques Ellul's definitions of propaganda will serve us well in the examination to come. His sense of the character of an "organized group" is consistent with Freud's evaluation and most especially in terms of "psychological manipulation." Ellul writes:

> Propaganda feels, develops, and spreads the system of false claims – lies aimed at the complete transformation of minds, judgements, values, and actions (and constituting a frame of reference for systematic falsification) … … Having analyzed these traits, we can now advance a definition of propaganda – not an exhaustive definition, unique and exclusive of all

> others, but at least a partial one: *Propaganda is a set of methods employed by an organized group that wants to bring about the active or passive participation in its actions of a mass of individuals, sychologically unified through psychological manipulation and incorporated into an organization.*[20]

Ellul's terminology, and the analysis of a social process carried out by an "organized group," complements *Group Psychology*. The various groups, however disparate they may be, are intent on unifying and incorporating as many people as possible and with the effective strategies of psychological manipulation.

Freud's chapter, "Being in Love and Hypnosis," furthers a series of connections. He will have occasion to be sceptical about our most basic assumptions, most especially when it comes to our finer social feelings – of solicitude and compassion for that subject of late 20th-century consciousness: "the other" who, today, has been given additional titles and *acknowledgment*. His comments on justice, equality, and rights will be unsettling, to say the least, for those who have been one-dimensionally committed to the implementation of moral ideals but without recognizing their archaic origins or unconscious effects. He does not hesitate to expose the illusion of a morally inspired love. "It gives the name of 'love' to a great many kinds of emotional relationship which we too group together theoretically as love; but then again it feels doubt whether this love is real, true, actual love" (18:111). *Real, true, actual*: Freud has placed the three together. From now on, love (as claimed by the political activist) will no longer have the same resonance. Freud shares his scepticism on whether the emotional ties of a group can be called love at all or if a much different assessment will be given to its split character – expressed, fiercely, but in distorted and incommensurable ways. The privilege we give ourselves for our moral feelings may not be as secure as we would like to believe, especially when the pathos of heightened feeling, enthusiasm, fanaticism, and moral high-mindedness, stands in for love as its representative. Freud's continued analysis of groups, highly relevant in our time for understanding the claims made by clusters of identities, is uniquely able to expose all the ways in which people have been led by propaganda to accept a set of absolutist principles.

Did Freud augment the earlier theory of the *repression of sexuality* with the sense that love, as conceived and transformed in liberal democracies, was as impoverished as human intelligence and was suppressed as a feeling because, if true, would interfere with the aggression of the super-ego and the more negative impulses of the death drive? Was our intellectual deficiency inseparable from out inability to understand, and to *feel*, the full extent of love and its foundations for other forms of thought – the fully erotic, for one, or on the other hand the sexuality today becoming ever more moribund, fragmented into multiple selves and supported by capital advertisement, as if a product was being sold to everyone? Once the identification of the "love" shared among members of a group is analyzed in the context of a *hysterical identification* with the new object of solicitude, a different interpretation can be offered. While we can make an accurate political statement such as "the dogmatic order is impelled by a censoring ethos"[21] and trace the dogma/censorship bind as the creation of a way of life, Freud was motivated to find the depth-psychological causes for an orthodoxy that made the distortion of love and the loss of intelligence necessary to its social and political scheme. Although we can understand the loss of will and discernment, the specific effect on the intellect is an interest that also has not been fully explained. Our political sensibilities are, in many cases, deeply uncomfortable with the examples of a century ago and the lack noticed in "the mental life of primitive people and of children" (18:77). The conjunction of the primitive and the infantile, as a contemporary phenomenon, is not going to be met with approval from anyone who believes themselves to be acting in the best interest of all and for the sake of cultural equality, which can only be sustained, *de facto*, by deliberate illusion and by one grand excuse of the times – relativism; and yet, once we present one recent and specific example, we should be left dumbfounded by the extent of the moral drive and one that is inseparable from an increasingly dangerous death drive. The influence of our contemporary "ideals" will become evident when the moral re-ordering of society by the super-ego is complemented by an equally nihilistic aggressiveness towards Western civilization.

A term first used by Habermas in 1968 has been revived and taken its place with others. One other haunting reference (to *the phantom* of "Left Fascism") has been recalled by Samir Gandesha, who, in addition, has written about "the raw exercise of power relative to moral conduct, afoot in certain quarters of the Left both in the contemporary university and beyond it."[22] How we are being passive and silent in the face of initiatives that can only be understood as pathological (and, which are being supported by a complacent university administration bowing to the excessive demands of determined groups) is one more recent indication of a delusional culture. The mounting attack on the creative output of Western civilization (that is, its writing, its books, its libraries – the most important places on a campus, *pace* laboratories) is only one of the more troubling symptoms of our age. Once the infantile and the primitive were understood to be perpetually recoverable as affects and then projected into the world with life-altering consequences for individuals and society, it was only a matter of time before Freud uncovered the mechanism of the process: the transformation of the ego-ideal (from the individual political leader well known to us from history) was one more insight necessary for the development of his analysis. Today, our situation has changed: in his time and after, during an epoch of the individual *dictator* – in Latin, the *one who speaks* and declares with ultimatums– was a sole representative. The opposite of a dictator might be offered: the analysand is also someone who speaks, but not with declarations made from raised podiums or balconies, but with a free association capable of recognizing the difference between the perceptions of a personal psyche and reality. As we prepare to turn to our next topic and the transformation of a traditional ego-ideal, we can re-read a letter to Fliess, in the same year as the publication of *The Interpretation of Dreams*, to anticipate how far Freud's personal interests would be extended. The startling analysis of the rise of a "delusional insanity" from the most intense of opposites gives us one indication of the symptoms Freud will present more completely 20 years later. "Not only dreams are wish fulfillments, so are hysterical attacks. This is true of hysterical symptoms, but probably applies to every product of neurosis, for I recognized it long ago in acute delusional insanity. Reality – wish fulfillment – it is from these opposites that our mental life springs."[23] When such a delusion can be the outcome of an ego-ideal (and one, moreover, that appears to be responsible for the supposed benefit of our moral improvement) we are placed in a position by Freud that is not, for political enthusiasts, a welcome prospect. His analysis does not indulge or appease. Our ego-ideal gives us a sense of a pathology that will involve a three-part analysis of hysterical identification, introjection, and projection, inter-related mechanisms that Freud recognized as one of the consequences in the change in our ego-ideal from an individual political leader to a much more powerful *dead victim* of history who will be perpetually mourned and, because of the process, fail to resolve an active infantile and primitive conflict in the frenetic core of the super-ego.

(b) The 21st-Century Transformation of an Ego-Ideal

Freud's analysis of group psychology established three of its primary characteristics: after the libidinal ties of love-hate, the lessening of intelligence, and the loss of freedom, he began to outline more exacting details, beginning with two examples of social groups who, in different but compatible ways, served as historical models for the unity of their organization as well as the hierarchies of their order. The army and the church are representatives of an institutionalized social relationship; individuals in both are attached to each other, in identification, common beliefs, and shared purpose. Virtues, as such, are not lacking. The church and the army are, moreover, psychically intertwined in unexpected ways: although it would be understandable to associate the church with the morality of the super-ego and the army with the death drive, psychoanalysis does not allow us to easily categorize them separately. Each does not have a separate domain. Their shared psychical realities permeate how each group views itself as a unity; much smaller and politically motivated groups are not essentially different from the church and the army and, in many ways, much more powerful than either because they elude institutional definition.

In *Group Psychology*, when viewed from soon-to-be created tripartite structure of the psyche, Freud identified two main groups to carry on his discussion of extra-individual psychology and to provide perhaps the most obvious examples of a group which portrayed the authority of the super-ego and the power of the death drive. The army and the church are, however, soon put aside due to Freud's widening interest in the nature of less institutional groups. There are other, more numerous, and almost private groups whose "membership" depends exclusively on one identity or another; they are, today, exclusively politicized according to various motivations and methods of self-promotion. Our theme of the theological-political begins to be more discernible, and more privately than as an expression of the state and the church, the two separate forms defining traditional secularity as a structure, the either/or of church and civil society in a democracy. Our religious *illusion* (to use Freud's precise word), thought to be overcome, remains psychically effective, more so when disavowed as a presumed conscious choice and so more easily, and surreptitiously, displaced. Although it would be understandable to remain focused on the army and the church as primary examples of groups in society, they are not at all the main interest of Freud's analysis and where his argument, overall, is heading. His two examples are preliminary insofar as they represent a centuries-old *relation* of church and state; both, independently or bound together, will be ignored as Freud continues to think about the context of the development of a self-conscious secularity and the function of its new ego-ideal. The connections he soon makes are politically innovative when we pay closer attention to his intermittent but repeated and always informative comments on the Soviets and the consequences of the Russian revolution – which essentially *outlawed* religion from the state in order to give itself absolute power. One form of secularism, as organized by communism, can be studied. In *Group Psychology*, the intimations are left to be developed at a later time when the discontents of civilization are to be more elaborately presented. The Soviets will re-appear several times as an object of psychoanalytic interest for Freud when the political and the religious become psychically entangled. His political acumen on the psychological consequences of the Russian revolution has not often been noted; his psychoanalysis of the Soviet super-ego has been neglected, as has an insidious transference when the theological was introjected into the post-revolutionary politics of the state. Once he made it possible for the reader to notice the nature of the transference between the theological and the political, he shifts his attention. Another focus comes into view.

Freud begins by addressing the traditional role of the leader in the psychology of groups and how his meaning, classically evident in terms of personal authority, power, and influence, is overcome in a liberal society. The theological-political unconscious of liberalism has created the conditions for the abolition of the individual leader. The phantasmatic substitute, who will be created through the process of hysterical identification, introjection, and projection, will become the single most-powerful object of history and as the one instrument to both enforce the morality of the super-ego and the destruction by a now ideologically limitless death drive. Our initial theme of ghosts and specters and phantasms can soon be given an illustration beyond their allegorical meaning; a psychical resurrection has recently occurred and as a reflection of both a moral and political ideology whose concern has been, above all, dedicated to a certain victim of history and who will be the subject of an extreme ambivalence – the love-hate affects of being envied and despised as representatives of a certain historical *reminiscence*. The psychoanalytic dictum of hysteria and reminiscence is most prominent today. The subsequent development of psychoanalytic concepts and its vision, which describe the particular traits of theological-political groups lead Freud towards a new, enhanced direction. During a historical time in Europe when it would have been straightforward to concentrate on the presence of the political leader and his supreme authority in determining the makeup of society, Freud's unique turn leads him towards a much less obvious phenomenon. He begins to sense the transformation of the ego-ideal from the individual leader towards a new historical subject; only when he suspends the role of the leader as a historical phenomenon and instead reflects on the less obvious role of *small* group psychology does he begin to sense how *the future* may present an array of unprecedented problems. They will be unique; they are our own. The presence of the authoritarian leader is suspended in order to analyze a much more powerful psychical phenomenon that emerges at the same time as the development of the manifest secularity of liberal democracies. For him to pursue his growing psychoanalytic intimations, and the sense of a new important subject (which is not an individual *per se*), Freud begins to relate one other set of specific characteristics of group psychology. For the time being, another issue needs attention to prepare for what will follow. If Freud's opening of group psychology led him to review the literature of the time and then add his own findings on the inter-relations of libidinal ties, diminished intelligence, and the loss of freedom, his unique psychoanalytic contributions would become much deeper because they were historically anticipatory.

Although we could single out many political theorists for the analysis of the authoritarian *personality*, in the form of an individual leader, Freud moves beyond his initial conclusions and, by doing so, informs us about our own predicament. One individual is no longer the problem. Freud does not add to the traditional and well-known interpretations and critique because, above all, he was focused on the force of psychical reality, which in many ways remained hidden by the overt manifestation of a political consciousness. Theodor Adorno, for example, writes how "the leaders' appropriation of mass psychology, the streamlining of their technique, has enabled them to collectivize the hypnotic spell."[24] Adorno, the Frankfurt School, and a broad tradition of critical theory can be mentioned for their attempt to adopt Freud and fit psychoanalysis into a Marxist interpretation. Shaul Bar-Haim points out how writers "turned him [Freud] into a political figure, namely a *signifier* for the possibility of a *radical* social change."[25] It may be necessary to remember the intellectual currents of the 20th century while at the same time recognizing how the conditions today (in liberal democracies, not *overtly* fascist societies) require a different form of analysis, a *strictly* Freudian one. The individual leader, despite any recent burlesque appearances, is merely a distraction to the more insidious realities in liberal democracies and those promoted, and made real, by a number of groups whose influence has become all too noticeable.

The concept of identification and ego-ideal have historically changed in our century. Freud will give us all the concepts for us to more readily analyze our times and focus less on historical precedents, whether the "fasces" of imperial Rome and their symbol of authority, or the various expressions of totalitarian politics. He did not easily give up this one idea at first; one can understand his uncertainty. History was overwhelming; to get beyond the facts and the appearance of a totalizing society was a difficult undertaking. He wavered as to its significance in *Group Psychology*; eventually, his conclusions will be relevant for us. The leader will be superseded as an idea and as an organizing principle of a group. At first, he writes: "We already begin to divine that the mutual tie between members of a group is in the nature of an identification of this kind, based upon an important emotional common quality; and we may suspect that this common quality lies in the nature of the tie with the leader" (18:108). Although he initially defined this "emotion" in common as empathy, there are contemporary reasons for changing emphasis – as Freud did with the all-purpose idea of "love and libidinal ties" which he augmented, for his discussion, with a much more in-depth analysis. One significant change in the nature of identification can be described, in part, as a shift away from the identification with a leader as an ego-ideal. One characteristic of the identity politics of the present makes it structurally necessary to overcome the singular presence of the leader as an organizing force and maintain the adulation within the group itself, because of their particular social status and moral self-determination. Belonging to one or more of these groups is proving to be highly attractive; the young are, as always, the most susceptible. The impoverished ego finds immediate fulfillment in identifying and belonging, even as the desire is based in fantasy. Any previous marginalization in society gives the group legitimacy for their political initiatives to change society and for their *recognition*; one can understand the attraction, most especially for the immature, who are tempted by an identity when it so fiercely defended and promoted by the *status quo*. Stephen Reicher adds to this by calling it "validation" within the group itself, though when "validation and solidarity, social being and agency,"[26] is a privilege adopted for oneself, it must be denied for any others who are deemed to be incompatible to the group.

The group's identification with an individual ego-ideal, a human being – with a formidable presence of power, including control of the army and the ability to declare war, on states and people, has been substituted by a much more powerful psychical symbol. Postponing the identity of this object beyond a first reference in the previous section (as a particular dead victim of history) will allow for an examination of Freud's thought-process. Before doing so, a reference to H. Shmuel Erlich's ideas around the "paranoia genesis in groups" is relevant for the individual in a politically motivated association and as a psychoanalytic supplement to Guntrip's earlier description of schizoid identities. The noticeable and much-vaunted identities of groups have led to severe pathologies; they are, today, completely unrecognized in the social sphere because they are infinitely validated.

> Such individuals can rarely be defined as clinically paranoid or psychotic, because their *paranoia is contained and supported by a group matrix* and identity that provides consensual validation. Their paranoia is a much more difficult kind to define and cope with. It takes refuge in commonly held opinions and well-known political positions.[27]

These kinds of insights are, it seems to me, unique to psychoanalytic perception and therefore alert us the considerable danger of groups who, because of the consensus of "political positions," can appear to be both sensible, reasonable, and right beyond dispute.

Reaching one of our first junctures of the religious, the moral, and the political as a new unity for Freud's theological-political argument, the work of the translator and editor has proven to be invaluable since the decision was made to allow the German original to stand in one particular passage. The individual who has experienced the powers from the group – influence, suggestibility, imitation – has an additional one and as a remnant from ancient history. The *biological* metaphor of contagion has a more instructive *metaphysical* one. The individual in the group must demonstrate himself to be capable of leading his new life "*ihnen zu Liebe*." Freud's original can be variously translated, but to do justice to "for their sake" or "for the love of them," one other almost concealed meaning is required. The individual must show himself capable and willing to *sacrifice* himself – that is, to give himself up for a supposedly "higher" cause, one that makes the individual expendable. If we now return to the argument made in the Introduction and the theological-political nature of the super-ego, we can begin to more securely establish another point. Far from being a straightforward critic of religion, his emerging ideas bring together the relation between the psychical and the metaphysical as a preliminary way to explain the foundations of a future theological-political society. The individual can and will be sacrificed for the greater good; he will do so either through eventual submission or, if the conditions are right, through a self-destructive act whereby the ego becomes an object of contempt. The ego, in any case, is utilized and treated as a serviceable object. The masochistic-sadistic bind, as a political category, will soon be supplemented by Freud's many-leveled interpretation of the group. If we recall his analysis of the transformation of archaic religious rituals into modern obsessional acting-out, we can anticipate how sacrifice has once again become current and essential to our primitive present. Far from being post-modern, as has been so often repeated since the approach to the end of the 20th century, Freud gives us no comfort in our supposed modernity and instead analyzes us as psychologically regressed, infantile and primitive, acting out allegorical rituals of sacrifice and exactly as in the temples of antiquity when there was *no difference between the state and religion.* The regressive psychology of groups of the present has revived the ancient phenomenon of sacrifice. The unconscious drive of the super-ego, characterized by a fundamentally theocratic imperative and impelled by the certitude in the absoluteness of a moral ideal, is more than willing (as the religious-political imagination always has) to sacrifice the individual in order of the whole to be *made sacred* and because of its extra-legal judgments and redemptive aspirations. Indeed, today we have resurrected an ego-ideal who is both an object of veneration and who serves as the justification for the most determined judgments on those who are pronounced guilty by virtue of their relationship to a specific civilization. The sacrificial intentions are indicative of our highest values; dispensing death, in different forms, including *virtually*, confirms our perverted desire for the sacred. To make the world metaphorically sacred is one way to redeem the past and to transform the present with, when necessary or convenient, the cruelty towards a sacrificial scapegoat. Individuals are, as always, dispensable when ideals have to be established for the supposed good of all. When René Girard began *Violence and the Sacred* and wrote that "sacrifice still waits its proper interpretation,"[28] his historical and anthropological interests were (as his dialogue with Freud would show) much more directed towards our present and our sacrificial propensities. They have become, in our time, more egregious. The psychopolitical dynamics of modern liberal democracies are showing all the pathologies of archaic theological-political doctrines and rituals – but given the illusion of secularism, they have yet to be fully perceived except by the thinkers who, for some time, have traced the unfolding of culture towards a self-destructive nihilism. Nietzsche's readers will have long drawn certain conclusions about the drive of culture and who is sacrificed today by different means that are far less obvious but perhaps more effective because they are never spectacular except as represented on the screens of social media "platforms." Jean-Gerard Burzstein gives us one of our most important commitments: the analysand will not be sacrificed under any condition. "As its fundamental philosophy and practical theory, psychoanalysis refuses to sacrifice the interest of the individual who carries the function of subject."[29] To restore the individuality of the subject takes us to the unconscious function of religious traces, in affects, in thoughts, in acts. The depth-psychological analysis of a displacement, of the theological into the political, results in a noticeable shift. "The ceremonials and prohibitions of obsessional neurotics drive us to suppose that they have created a private religion of their own."[30] Today, the ceremonials are no longer liturgical; they are bureaucratic and based on observances, of certain historical truths and their demands for acknowledgment. How rituals and taboos are converging today, as bureaucratic and moral displacements, both to better regulate our character and social life, in ourselves and with others, are appearing to have determined results.

One well-known political theorist, with an interest in Freud and the super-ego, can read *Group Psychology* and simply write that Freud "took as an object of investigation the Christian relationship of the individual to what he call the "mass" (*die Masse*)."[31] In my estimate, this interpretation of *Group Psychology* by Étienne Balibar is one-dimensional and inadequate; the connection is much too patent and, for Freud, misleading. One argument can be made here and to anticipate the more developed one from *The Future of an Illusion*: as long as we continue to see Freud as, simplistically, reductively, a critic of religion and of the Judeo-Christian tradition in particular, we will barely remain at the manifest level of his complex thinking and therefore fail to recognize the depth of his analysis, which anticipated the possible developments of liberal democracies well beyond his own time. The tie between mass psychology and religion is much too predictable, especially for the political philosopher, who, in this instance, adds to a significant symptom of unconscious disavowal. Secularity does not assure either intelligence or freedom; such an admission – of a simultaneous lack and illusion – would be, however, a prerequisite.

Only the self-conscious and autonomously motivated individual can, through a concentrated life-experience of reflection and analysis, cope with the pressures of conformism and herd security association. We can first realize that "in failing to understand the psychodynamics of large group behavior, we fail to protect our freedom."[32] In the opening of the essay on the contemporary super-ego, how freedom is obliterated can be witnessed by the propaganda of *any* group that, so convinced of its own truths, it will not spare others to achieve their objectives. The intolerance to independent views is discredited with prejudice. The modern political sensibility has affirmed sacrifice at the expense of freedom and ideals of restitution (in the form of vengeance) rather than the slow, drawn-out and dialogic work of an entire community. The *cognitive knowledge* of our condition is, however, not enough; all the critiques of ideology have not contributed to giving us an authentic sense of life except by making us more accustomed to the negative, in the world and *in ourselves*, and often with the rhetoric of accusation, like the all-purpose *phobia*. Freud is no ordinary political thinker. What he presents is a comprehensive set of ideas and psychoanalytic concepts that leads his readers to new responsibilities, as individuals and as citizens who are obligated to reflect on themselves, first, and on the nature of society and how it has reached an intolerable set of super-moral demands. Guilt and shame are distributed with insistence. Freud's examples should strike us with more clarity; they are not reducible to history (that is, to a particular time), but rather to a perennial condition that because of the tripartite structure of the psyche, can exhibit the most intense of impulses, compulsion, and obsessions. The pathological extremes of the schizoid and the paranoid are not so easily recognizable because they are confirmed by a greater number of people and groups. The ideal of "inclusivity," appearing so moral, so universal, can also stand for the worst kind of contagion and group identification; *incorporation* has become, for some (especially the young) the only choice possible to avoid being isolated or feeling unimportant in comparison to the *images* in their lives. The ubiquity of signs is one more piece of exclusive propaganda. Symbols have become iconographic, even as they multiply and morph into more disparate wholes and as part of a collective identification. The self-promotion, however, does not conceal unconscious desires and motives. They are well known to psychoanalysis and, to be precise, from a *tragic* source. The singular example of Oedipus is as meaningful as ever.

The ideas of "Family Romances" are transformed as only the fantasies of the infantile and primitive super-ego could. Thomas Ogden writes: "The impact of the Oedipus complex in the formation of psychological structure is determined by the child's method of attempting to resolve the conflict of subjective desire."[33] The implications for a personal *failure* are more serious when the results are projected into political ambitions.

> *The liberation of an individual*, as he grows up, from the authority of his parents is one of the most necessary though one of the most painful results brought about by the course of his development. It is quite essential that *liberation* should occur and it may be presumed that is has been to some extent reached a normal state. Indeed, the whole progress of society rests upon the opposition between successive generations. On the other hand, there is a class of neurotics whose condition is recognizably determined by their having failed in this task.[34]

The twice-mentioned liberation is no small matter. It once again points to Freud's commitment to the individual's psychical freedom. If we then follow his sense that one class of neurotics has come about because of their inability to deal with the pain and difficulty of this independence and instead regressed to an infantile condition of antipathy, discontent, and rebellion, then we may begin to wonder about certain groups of people who have re-imagined their relationship to the history of civilization and, more immediately, to their mothers and fathers as *their origin*, which they unconsciously resent.

For the first time in *Group Psychology*, Freud makes the connection between the religious and the political that should, from here forward, be kept continuously in mind so as to better recognize his repetitions in other writings; they are numerous and should be seen as one of his most important contributions to the analysis of culture. When the connection is made, he will refer to this one phenomenon for the rest of the decade with an array of examples.

"If another group tie takes the place of the religious one – and the socialistic ties seems to be succeeding in doing so – then there will be the same intolerance towards outsiders as in the age of the Wars of Religion" (18:99). *The religious and the socialistic*: the first transference has been stated. *Taking the place of*: the displacement, from the religious *into* the political, will now be a constant preoccupation. While political philosophers have recognized the intimate tie (to be specific) between the thought of Karl Marx and Christianity – for one, in terms of its salvific and redemptive aspirations; or, if one prefers, for their messianism – Freud's analysis goes, as it were, in the opposite direction. No idealism here. Once Freud recognizes the bind between the religious and the socialistic, what he has done in effect is to expand the limits of categories, and of social life, to show how the commonality between religious and political drives can criss-cross each other and psychologically merge. Are the complications of *politicized* sexuality and gender today indicative of a most unusual desire: to become *angels* and in preparation for an unconscious apocalypticism of culture? Is the angelic a political aspiration?

There are, it seems, very few if any thinkers who took Freud seriously enough to consider his recognition of the extraordinary tie between the religious and the socialistic and how the effects of one on the other could, in principle, be far worse in combination than alone. The theological-political has become a powerful unity and potentially without any adversaries strong, or self-possessed enough, to oppose its omnipotence. The assumption that Freud is heading towards a deepening critique of religion would be to completely overlook the far more in-depth argument of his inquiry. There have been simply too many insights on the condition of being in the present epoch for us to acknowledge them and then move on as if they were not urgent or did not have an overwhelming effect on our everyday lives – in ways that, for a psychoanalyst, should be pre-eminent, that is, first and foremost about the psychological health of individuals. Christopher Bollas uses a term that allows us to see a wider historical and psychological perspective and so gives our present context all the more poignancy. The psychoanalysis of our finer moral feelings has once again become necessary in order to expose its other sides; they are not as beneficial as they are portrayed. Bollas defines it as "the Puritan mentality" and characterizes it as "the idealized self aiming to *save the world* through display of exemplary being."[35] *Save the world*: my emphasis. We are in a dire situation when those who pretend to be our "saviours" are going about their business with the tactics of composed bureaucrats. The force of security has become pronounced. *Exemplary being*: that one must also become both an affirmation for the self and a social spectacle is part of the exhibitionism of the times, one that can be understood as the insistence of the super-ego categorical imperative and, with even a more daunting consequence, its association to aggression becoming culturally destructive and according to the worst tendencies of the death drive. Franco De Masi writes: "promising *salvation* at the cost of perverting the perception of human reality, the perverse superego becomes what can only be described as a pathological organization."[36] The forms of expression, by psychoanalysts, are not incidental. Contemporary politics, so self-possessed and sure of itself, has assumed the role of being *salvific*. Misperceptions have not been slight. The well-known symptoms of certain pathologies and perversions are going to be transferred from their initial understanding, in *sexuality*, for example, and towards a wider array to *erotic* desires, fantasies, and delusions. One classical word, "deviation," can be interpreted from the stand-point of a regression and then a shift towards something other than development. While we have been long-accustomed to the accepted idea in "the stunting effect of civilized conditions"[37] due – to an exaggerated degree, to the over-valued assumptions of sexual morality – there are aspects of inhibitions that have other, more archaic origins and are fare more noxious than any merely sexual restraint. We should have, by now, lost any naïve belief in "sexual liberation" as a pre-condition for a *healthier* society. There are different forms of freedom; not all of them are beneficial.

Our contemporary situation reveals how the conscious dissolution of the religious has not abolished particular psychical drives but has simply transferred them, unconsciously, from one domain to the other. The religious unconscious has determined the power of the socialistic. Timothy Snyder has called the process "eternity politics." "Like all immorality, eternity politics begins by making an exception for itself. All else in creation might be evil, but I and my group are good."[38] The connection will be, to some, polemical or simply geo-political; and yet one can hardly avoid the overwhelming sense of our moral pretensions in liberal democracies and who has made them a priority. One thinker who, in another time, was a representative of social conscience, can be recalled today. Albert Camus writes: "Politics is not a religion, or if it is, it is nothing but the Inquisition."[39] Immorality, evil, the Inquisition; these are severe judgments. They are no longer safely referenced for a distant time when, for example, the nature of Stalinism showed itself to all in trials, exile, and executions. The fundamental difference between the fascism of Freud's era and the characteristics of our own theological-political present comes down to a question that, once he forced himself to answer, led to a host of analytic findings. After the doubt – "the question would also arise whether a leader is really indispensable to the essence of a group" (18:100) – the implications of his analysis of group psychology could be elaborated.

The leader has been superseded in the fervour of our liberal democratic ideas. In the place of one individual, who represented power and, in part, charismatically, made identification alluring, a new phenomenon has taken place. Once the living and present leader was no longer sufficient for psychological purposes (for identification) finding an *infinite* substitute became one more imperative. Group psychology has led to a regression and a specific kind of hysterical identification. The modern political activist has phantasmatically regressed to both an infantile and a historical period where he can be the helpless victim, which in turn allows the subsequent projection to be driven by the aim of *reparation*, a concept that Melanie Klein has made relatable especially to "love." In *Love, Guilt, and Reparation*, she brings together several of our interests. This capacity for identification with another person is a most

> important element in human relationships in general, and is also a condition for real and strong feelings of love. We are only able to disregard or to some extent *sacrifice* our own feelings and desires, and thus for a time to put the other person's interests and emotions first, if we have the capacity to identify ourselves with the loved person.[40]

We can, with Klein, agree that healthy identification with others is important; but once we return to Freud's arguments in *Group Psychology* and in the years to follow, the one who loves for political reasons does not "sacrifice" himself (masochistically, or others, sadistically) for purely idealistic reasons; on the contrary, he has committed himself to sacrificing himself as well as anyone who is deemed, in any way, to be responsible for the immorality of history and so perverts the process in its entirety. Otto Kernberg's analysis of individuals who were, because of different psychical difficulties, unable to love, confirms a prior analysis. His definition of "limitations to the capacity to love,"[41] which is one more impression to add to the others in the ongoing debilitation of the present-day individual in terms of a political condition, is relevant for us insofar as the conscious affirmation of the love of the political actor is, in fact, not love at all but a set of psychical affects that can only be fully analyzed more fully in sections to come.

The ending of section (V) on the church and the army introduces a discussion of the nature of religious belief and, in particular, the effects of love and hate expressed by the group – for each other, and for others outside the group. If the theological-political argument presented in the Introduction can be furthered, then Freud's observations are not to be restricted to a religious group but extends to a political one as well – because they essentially share psychical traits which *preceded* their social existence. Freud invented all the analytical concepts for us to understand the nature of our predicament now. Substituting the political for the theological introduces us to a topic that will be one of his increasing preoccupations; in many of the writings to follow, the word *religion* is a condensation of a much wider psychical relation. Religion cannot stand alone as a supposed unity; in Freud's writing, the term functions on two levels simultaneously. The manifest appearance should not lead to a partial and incomplete vision. My supplement, in brackets, will hopefully not be intrusive. "A religion [politics], even if it calls itself the religion [politics] of love, must be hard and unloving to those who do not belong to it" (18:98). One of the consequences of identity politics, and most especially those motivated by the of ideals of emancipation, justice, equality – historically, that is, ideals created by philosophy and religion – is by all appearances supposed to be motivated by empathy and love for those who suffer from these social ills. All indications point to an opposite situation; love, in any case, cannot be defended as a *political* emotion because of its inseparable ties to other, far less amiable feelings of hostility and aggression. Again, the brackets are mine; the transference, if permitted, will be more clarified by Freud himself. "Fundamentally indeed every religion [politics] in in this same way a religion [politics] of love for all those whom it embraces; while cruelty and intolerance towards those who do not belong to it are natural to every religion [politics]" (18:98). The statements can be an important turning point and as a graphic transference. On the face of it, the statement seems straightforward. The great majority of readers have been more than satisfied with its manifest meaning – and, because of our complacency, Freud's consciousness, as a thinker, as a writer, has been overlooked. My supplement, of the religious and the political as transferred into a shared set of characteristics, makes his arguments throughout the 1920s a programmatic endeavour. Once the connection is made, the theological-political as a psychical relation can better inform us about our situation and, more importantly, how *our being* is transformed by less than beneficial goals. If we begin with one statement and then pursue the possible meaning of "spirit" (as opposed to the manifest law, to use one metaphorical distinction) can we begin to understand how psychoanalysis may have reached an unprecedented level of significance for us today? "The spirit of Freud's writings should not be missed."[42] The historical transformation from the religion of love to the politics of the perverted and pathological libido leads necessarily to intolerance – one of the most obvious characteristics of today's identity groups despite their obsessive need (as a reaction-formation) for tolerance and with three others that have become slogans: equality, diversity, inclusivity.

One wonders at what different points Freud began to realize, not without increased interest if also some apprehension, finally with certainty, how his view of religious groups was equally true of political ones; when the emergence of secular culture became much more prominent (to give one date for us, the 1960s) then the apparent supersession of religion should have allowed the religious sentiments of antipathy for others to subside. The opposite has occurred. Religion did not create the narcissism of minor differences; they were not abolished with the transition to secularism. Without religion, the psychical drives formerly evident in religion could now be expressed more completely and without limits in politics, with equal if not more severe consequences. Freud has already made the first of his most important breakthroughs in relation to his social analysis, one that will make previous intimations essential to the understanding of the dynamics of the psyche and their effects on everyday life. Several additional factors are needed to bring together both the discovery of the super-ego, as part of his more precise terminology, and how previous insights can be better unified into a comprehensive set of ideas. Identification with the ego-ideal, once disassociated from the individual leader, will lead to the social and political reality we can readily witness today.

The purpose of opening with an interpretation of *Group Psychology and the Analysis of the Ego* has been motivated by a few inter-related concerns. One stands out: the work is "a platform for Freud's initial deliberations about his structural theory by elaborating on the concept of an ego ideal which later evolved into the superego."[43] If the work on group psychology anticipates some of the more explicitly political arguments made in later publications (and we can therefore anticipate an interpretation of *The Future of an Illusion* as a *theological-political* work), Freud's ideas on the nature of culture were already on the way to being fully formed. Scheidlinger believes that Freud's concept of the super-ego "evolved." Any such development is not for us essential except insofar as it leads to the comprehensive ideas and the manner in which the hysterical identification and introjection of the ego ideal became consistent with the power of the super-ego. "The idea of one's *home group* can become extreme, the holders excited by their revelation and by their own identification with these unquestionable truths."[44] The word "revelation" is, in this instance, more than appropriate since it recalls one of the foundations of the divine as manifested in the world for those with conviction and therefore indisputable because metaphysically understood as an epiphany. An "eternity politics" also requires its own revelations of truth. Freud's most original contribution to our understanding of social and political life makes it no longer possible to be naïve about ideals, their origins, and the methods used to implement them by both propaganda and institutional policies. *Group Psychology* can take us from the sketch of two traditional associations – each, in their own way, representative of two distinct powers, the earthly and the heavenly – to the consideration of the role of the leader and how he has been replaced by a subject of infinitely greater power. One significant change in the nature of identification can be better described and, in part, as a process of the shift away from the identification with a leader as an ego-ideal. The leader will be substituted by a historical reality and a reminiscence that will be specific and, also, indicative of a precise kind of identification. One of the most unique developments of late 20th-century politics has only increased in the ensuing decades and led to the creation of a new ego-ideal. The group's identification with an individual ego-ideal (a human being in the present – with a formidable presence of power, over life and death) has been substituted by a much more powerful symbol. The ethical concern for the "other" was not compulsive enough. A much more formidable one had to be invented. The theological-political group of the present is under psychological duress – which, in part, explains how vociferous and demanding (that is, authoritarian) they have become. The obsessive "love" for the victims of civilization will involve more than symmetrical hatred for the past history and present reality of that civilization: a biological death drive has come into evidence that has a much different sense that Freud's early formulation and the principle of constancy. The connection has been made: are we at a historical moment when the morality of the super-ego and the destructive sadism of the death drive will attempt to abolish, in fantasy, the reality of civilization while at the same time eradicating a certain difference and so deny our cultural and terrestrial origins as a biological species?

(c) Hysterical Identification and Its Aftermath

To suspend any prior certainty in the leader as an ego-ideal could not have been without its lingering doubts; the historical evidence of individuals was unquestionable, more so when they were called "fathers" of the nation and/or authoritarian. And yet, once Freud made the decision to consider another interpretation of a *psychical* reality as opposed to a historical one, whether the powerful figure was associated with either the church or the state, a different understanding occurred to him. Not only did he re-think the nature of identification, as such, he made it possible for us to look elsewhere than the leader as a *living person*. Well into *Group Psychology*, the structural theory of the psyche, the reality of the super-ego and the more dangerous death drive, was already operative. The connections were many and far-reaching: for one, the idea of a *hysterical* identification could provide an explanation for two other related afflictions; one, the double-condition of mourning and melancholia of the *political* neurotic; and, two, the three-part process that would define the anti-developmental aspect of regression for the individual, the group, and to an entire society that turned against itself and its historical accomplishments to obsess, instead, about its moral failings.

Freud's first definition of identification, including its associated ambivalence, leads to other ones as he develops them from the idea of the child-parent relationship: "identification endeavours to mould a person's own ego after the fashion of the one that has been taken as a model" (18:106). Initially, we can remain with the standard model as exemplified by children and parents: the identification with the father and the libidinal attraction to the mother (or vice versa) and the binding structure of the Oedipus complex. However, to that first foundation, we can follow Freud's thinking on the formation, the "molding," (as well as the "taking," that is, the introjection) of the ego. The models, today, are no longer bindingly parental, nor is the process grounded in a certain social education – of a moderate *conscience*, for example, which remains a necessary aspect of a healthy, non-pathological psyche. The knowledge of a classical reality has been altered; previous conceptions of identification (with parents, a leader, social mores, or God) may have to be, in large part, revised to reflect a new psychical reality. Otto Rank could write that "the ego ideal is really a representative of inner demands and claims, which have, however, already assimilated the external demands of society."[45] Can we still maintain that the "external demands" (of society) are primary? Are there not more original mechanisms that occur, on many infantile and primitive levels, prior to "assimilation"? Once we add a characteristic of identification specifically in terms of hysteria, which has internal and the earliest of infantile roots, the presentation of my psychopolitical essay will have to expand towards this one inquiry. In his analysis of a *hysterical identification*, Freud noted how the desire to *be* the object of identification was inseparable from a peculiar kind of jealousy and envy. Siegfried Zepf writes that "in Freud's understanding, the motive for hysterical identification is envy."[46] Initially determined by the Oedipus complex, the explanation has been well-founded and traditional. The rivalry (between son and father, or child and parent) intensifies at the same time as it is compounded. Once we identify a displacement – from a family identification to a hysterical one, which is deeper and more archaic – the traditional form of the psychical process has been substantially altered from the familial. The modification has a more intense unconscious goal: the hysterical identification is not only a replacement (of the father *and* mother as representatives of society) recent and entirely new social symptoms have disparaged them and perversely attempted to *eradicate* both of them as the living reality of civilization. At the deepest levels of the machinations of the death drive, the destruction is aimed at ending the proper line of the successions of generations. The death drive has become much more pathological and megalomaniacal than the mere desire for constancy; its irrepressible fantasies are tending towards apocalyptic fantasies and *ex nihilo* inaugurations.

Freud augments all prior knowledge of hysteria going back to the earliest days of psychoanalysis by giving us a particular example of "the complete mechanism of the structure of a hysterical symptom" (18:106); that is, in this one case, the mimetic adoption of a mother's unhealthy condition (a cough[47]) by her daughter as the attempt to take her place and *be* her. We can begin to better identify the object of a new hysterical process: the affects of mourning are not separated from the fantasy of a full-fledged resurrection. The political neurotic hysterically identifies with the same fantasy-anguish – of the *trauma* of historical civilizations that are overwhelmed by others, from other cultures – that he suffered as an infant prior to socialization and during the primary contact with reality and its objects. Freud adds that "the symptom may the same as that of the person who is loved" (18:106). We are, here, at one other decisive transitional point in our understanding of hysterical identification and the death drive as an unconscious attempt to *nullify origins* (one's parents, individually, and civilization, universally) and replace them with a new object of identification who is *dead* and, moreover, was forced to assimilate *to* Western culture *from* a supposedly pristine state of nature. A hysterical identification with someone who is "loved" leads us firmly away from both the mother and father as well as the living leader to an object of history who is dead and who can, in addition to being infinitely preserved, perpetuate a simultaneous state of mourning counteracted by a resurrection that is, also, a vindication. Once the dead object of history is introjected as a permanent aspect of the super-ego, while at the same time protected with utmost security and aggression, the political neurotic achieves unparalleled moral status – one that will have to be defended with obsessive conviction since he has become saviour, protector, and redeemer. The hysterical identification and introjection creates a quasi-sacred self who, as *chosen*, by virtue of a special identity, strengthened even more if fantasies of persecution are also connected, can stand apart from the profanity of the world. One immediate benefit, among others, can be noted: the political neurotic is "relentlessly demanding attention – to be loved – while freely entitled to disregard the Other";[48] that is, everyone else who has not been included in a prior list of candidates. Being loved is deserved – much more than anyone – because the introjected object is now protected, shown "love," and serving as the redemption that will be exhibited, through projection, with systematic efficiency. The implications of the identification and introjection for a political fantasy are immeasurable, both for redeeming the past with a total interpretation of the historical events (in, for example, the construction of history according to the limited perspective of the "post-colonial" theorist) and for the vision of a now imminent future. We can refer to Chasseguet-Smirgel's profound insights into the political fantasy of a "utopia" and its beginning with a *tabula rasa* – which leads her to stress a reminder for us as we continue to trace how civilization and the body are being denigrated to the point of a fantasy-extinction. The *apparent* simplicity of the comment is extremely suggestive; and for reasons later to be supplemented with even more startling observations on her part. "Our personal conflicts may cause us to forget that we are all children of men and women."[49]

Another of the noticeable transformations of the contemporary psyche can be analyzed in terms of both the understanding of initial identification with parents and the fantasy of a "family romance." In the past, the child fantasized about *different* parents – for example, wealthier, more distinguished ones; today the "romance" unconsciously fantasizes about a completely different origin or, more extremely, none at all and that makes it possible to repudiate two simultaneous origins, the parental and the cultural, biology and civilization both becoming objects of scorn to be repudiated. Once we begin, and then move on, from Freud's impression of "the later stage in the development of the neurotic's estrangement from his parents,"[50] we can then re-trace the process of regression to the primitive self and how it has exhibited new symptoms of social and political life. The outcome appears much more severe than "estrangement." We are ever closer to the nihilistic repudiation of parents as the sexual origin of the individual as well as the representatives of history of civilization. If we take one example of the development of psychoanalysis, Sandor Ferenczi can be recalled for a comment for our times and how the theological-political obsession has found one of its determinants in hysterical identification. "The well known impressionability also of many neurotics, their capacity to feel in the most intense way for the experience of others, to put themselves in the place of that person, finds its explanation in hysterical identification."[51] Once we now add the important analysis of a hysterical identification as a form of replacement, the political group can exploit the undisciplined affect of their mourning to justify rage and persecution. The "place" they take corresponds to (in fantasy) one outside and prior to civilization since the present-day has overwhelmed the primordial, autochthonous, and indigenous. The revival of Rousseau-like idealisms about nature is one more anomalous feature of the theological-political reality of the day. Has human life *in nature* ever been ideal?

Complementing Ferenczi's idea of hysterical identification with Melanie Klein's projective identification – which, in her 1946 "Notes on Some Schizoid Mechanisms," presented what can be described as a perceptual dislocation in the ego in part caused by paranoia – the *political* reality of analytic concepts are ever more informative. One of Klein's many ideas on the matter can be briefly mentioned and to add to my impressions that the introjection of the ideal is, from the beginning, ambivalent – good because a victim, bad because dead. One loves the victim for the benefits it will provide; one hates the victim for being a copy of the primitive infant and a historical reminiscence of an anguishing experience. In states of frustration or increased anxiety, the infant is driven to

> take flight to his internal idealized object as a means of escaping from persecutors. From this mechanism various serious disturbances may result: when persecutory fear is too strong, the flight to the object becomes excessive, and this severely hampers ego development and disturbs object-relations. As a result the ego may be felt to be entirely subservient to and dependent on the internal object—only a shell for it. With an unassimilated idealized object there goes a feeling that *the ego has no life* and no value of its own.[52]

My main preoccupation with the severe weakening of the ego due to the social and political initiatives of the 21st century is made evident by Klein. The ego is unconsciously disparaged by the introjected ideal who begins to activate all kinds of affects from within the masochistic-sadistic power of the super-ego. The ego is not only made to feel that it has no "life" of its own; life is regarded as unworthy and undeserving from the judgment of the super-ego that begins to exert unlimited power of vengeance and retribution for the mere existence of life. The conditions of the political neurotic of the present has made it necessary to take refuge in the internalized ego ideal and, because of the fantasy of persecutors in the external world, made it a matter of a co-related process to ultimately project the ideal back into the world in the form of aggression and moralizing sadism. In *Instinct and their Vicissitudes*, Freud completed the three-part process: identification and introjection led, necessarily, to projection. "In so far as the objects which are presented are sources of pleasure, it takes them into itself, 'introjects' them… … and, on the other hand, it expels them whatever within itself becomes a cause of unpleasure." (14:136) As soon as Freud identifies an ambivalence of feeling, love and hate, envy and pity, pleasure and unpleasure, the negative aspect of projection soon takes up the political neurotic's relationship to the reality he has now determined to *both* drastically change according to the highest of moral standards and destroy in order to envision a new reality. The process, however, "hampers ego development" and maintains the ego in a state of unmoving stasis; the regression has reached its terminal point in the fantasies of the infantile, the primitive, and the dead.

How can the idea of hysterical identification be made central to our on-going discussion once the ego-ideal is identified as the victim of history (of, for example, "colonialism" or any other historical events in the unfolding of our world civilization, which has always involved migrations, conquests, and displacements) and, more particularly, someone who was overwhelmed by the development of any civilization as a whole? How we are forgetting, intentionally, our origins? Ivan Sherick tells us that "hysterical identification" is a "clinical concept that currently appears to be almost absent in the psychoanalytic literature."[53] If that is indeed the case (in the clinic), can we, justifiably and as Sherick believes, return to the concept of hysterical identification as a productive concept for the understanding of psychopolitical symptoms? Not only can we do so to further clarify our conditions in liberalism and its psychical origins in the primitive state of the infant, at the same time we can see hysterical identification being part of a three-part process – projection completing a cycle towards the transformation of the real.

The three-part process of a new ego-ideal, and the moralizing obsessions of our times, can be reconstructed and as the necessary foundations for our understanding of Freud's imminent creation of the *über-Ich* – which will stand (as it does today), formidably, over everyone who is not conscious of its debilitating effects. If an original diagnosis began from one experience during the analysis of patients leading up to *Studies on Hysteria* ("*Hysterical patients suffer from incompletely abreacted psychical traumas*") the modern form of hysterical identification will be a dual and displaced process: the fantasy of a psychical trauma suffered by someone else, historically, and its intimate displacement of an infantile experience of helplessness and vulnerability. The explanatory power of both the processes of hysterical identification and introjection led Freud to the understanding of the psychical dynamic capable of the most excessive kind of morality. When we then become aware of the implications of introjecting a *dead* ego-ideal, for the *political* effects of mourning, and then projecting it back into reality, he was then fully prepared to introduce the concept of the super-ego as a moral agency compelled by one irrepressible drive, one that would be characterized by an obsessive purpose: to transform the history of civilization. Where did such an obsession come from? How did it arise? More importantly for us, how was its appearance inseparable from the nature of the super-ego and the death drive during the most primitive stages of its formation?

Freud added significantly to our understanding of group psychology when he traced an internal agency capable of inflicting specifically moral pain on the ego. He does not waver from his fundamental concern as a therapist: what makes the ego suffer. "A leading characteristic of these causes [of suffering] is a cruel self-depreciation of the ego combined with relentless self-criticism and bitter self-reproaches" (18:109). Now defining his first impressions of the individual in a group, Freud notices a relentless but unconscious "self-depreciation of the ego," one to be countered, defensively, by a super-moral criticism of the world. The impoverishment has to be counteracted. A new relation comes into view and well beyond its merely sexual expression. The *moral* masochism aimed at the ego is also projected as sadism into the world. The masochistic attack on the self, as the repeatable experience of childhood, can only be resisted, defensively, by a countermeasure towards what is outside the self and what is judged to be "bad" and deserving of both criticism and judgment. The group has solidified its identity by relieving itself of any self-evaluation through the absoluteness of its moral sentiments. The psychopolitics of our contemporary situation allows the individual in a motivated group to divest himself of self-criticism and project it outwards with incredible force, thereby simultaneously protecting himself and judging all others who are perceived to be in any way responsible for the moral failings of the world and, above all, for the death of the victim of history and uniquely attributable to Western oppression and violence. Despite the projection into the world and all the attempts made to alter reality, the psychological process is destined for failure because the *interior conditions* cannot be changed by any alteration in the "objective" world. "They show us the ego divided, fallen apart into two pieces, one which rages against the second" (18:109). The desperate and obsessive focus on the conditions of the world is one of the signs of a complete lack of self-regard. Whether "divided," and characterized by a peculiar kind of splitting, or fragmented, the emotion felt is visceral. Freud's word is *rages*: the intensity of the psychical conflict cannot be passed over quickly and so can be mentioned once more. The relentless division of the ego, worse if fragmented by the many different and competing psychical processes, can only preserve itself by a constant, if ultimately futile and destructive, acting out, in thought and speech; and with one fatal structure: it must, on no account, relieve itself of the perceptions it has projected into the world since the construction of reality justifies the process. The dissatisfaction must be chronic and perpetuated so as to rationalize the psychical conditions of rage and its politically instrumental reactions. Freud's insights into hysteria, evident in 1893 when connected to splitting, reaches one of its conclusions later. In his obituary for Jean-Martin Charcot, he wrote: "No one should object that the theory of splitting of consciousness as a solution to the riddle of hysteria is much too remote to impress and unbiassed and untrained observer."[54] The splitting, in our analysis, is more specific than in consciousness: the super-ego is split between its morality and its nihilism.

When Janet Miller tells us about "the development of introjection and identification as mechanisms of defense,"[55] the whole of the process is compulsive, originating in the vulnerability of the infantile ego and expelled from its interiority in order to be able to deal with it in a much larger and uncontained field – that is, reality. The scope extends well beyond its effects. Jacqueline Schaeffer adds that "the introjection-projection cycle is infinite."[56] And infinite for psychically structural and historical reasons. The political neurotic, who has initially regressed to the vulnerable state of the infant and the primitive, and who has become immature and sickly, identifies hysterically with the victims of history and, most especially, those who were expediently used in the creation of civilization – that is, the world as we have known of it historically since its human beginnings, with extending earthly boundaries of geography and culture. The moral re-evaluation of human history will serve no positive purpose except to ensure that later historians – and the persistence of our civilization – will look back and wonder at the extent of a hybris so complete it could give itself the privilege of being an absolute judge of history from one discreet time and place. The process of hysterically identifying with the victim of history allows the political neurotic to re-direct a simultaneous mourning and melancholia towards the objective world in the form of an intense projection from the super-ego. The substitution of the individual leader as an ego-ideal by the dead historical victim has led, first, to the encrypted security of the dead through introjection. The dead victim is a displacement of the helpless child; defending the victim is the attempt to protect the remnant of the infantile in its earlies struggles *to be*. The mechanism can be analyzed in terms of the most extreme manifestation of the psyche: in its desperation to be (to live – and to love) it has obsessively turned towards the most destructive impulses imaginable: the hatred of life and the political idolatry of the dead.

The victim of Western violence represents the most overwhelming political object since he can now be instrumentally used to justify the ends and means of a new moral relation which, as it appears socially and politically, does not reveal its psychological origins nor its theological-political bind. The morality of history effectively conceals the grounds of a new personality of our times. With *Group Psychology*, Freud begins an unprecedented number of writings that, by the end of the decade, will be a contribution most especially relevant for our understanding of contemporary phenomena. His analysis can at least make it possible for those who remain steadfastly committed to Freud and psychoanalysis to offer the possibility of a much-needed discussion and one that has been thus far denied and suppressed. We are motivated, psychoanalytically, to oppose the moral coercions of the times and doing so by emphasizing the need to re-think our relation to fundamental human possibilities of love, freedom, intelligence, creativity, and psychological health. By hysterically identifying with a real or imagined victim from the historical past, one takes their symbolic place – with the results being highly charged and useful in the domination of others. One can, in the name of the victim, and with the personal affect of infantile helplessness, rage against the world with full justification and persecute anyone deemed to be in any way responsible. “The concept that crowds, or even entire societies, can imprison themselves in their own illusion of victimage”[57] has been one of the predominant ideologies of our times. To identify with the victim gives one enormous privileges. We will also see how the concept of “narcissistic perversion,” manifested as a moral/political symptom, will further develop Freud’s foundational three-part character of the group. “Narcissistic perversion is characterized for an individual by the predominant need to assert, and the pleasure of asserting, oneself at someone else's expense. It is a specific pleasure… … This pleasure is secured by manipulation and behaviour pragmatically organized at the expense of real people."[58] The envy of the victim is instrumentally used (unconsciously, to serve oneself and the group) to be able to assert the highest of moral principles – like justice – but in order to more effectively manipulate everyone without any resistance. The form of *pleasure* will be soon explained. The narcissistic perversion of the political neurotic leads to the consequences we have now witnessed increasing in the first decades of our era; they are as sadistic as they are driven by a perverse desire for the annihilation of the accomplishments of civilization.

Once we suspend the ubiquitous presence of the leader in group identification and substitute *him* with a modern consideration, then the figure of an individual has been set aside. How has he been replaced since the group depends on their identification not only with each other but, also, an ego-ideal? The answer gives us an impression on the transformation of the times and how previous strength, force, and power of one individual (let's even attach a name or two – i.e., Stalin or Mao) has today been substituted by a most peculiar opposite, and in more than ways than one. Today, the group psychology dominated by an identity is formed by identifying with an ethical imperative shared among the members – they who are striving for the good since they themselves *are* good – and for an ego-ideal in the past who has been a victim.

At the end of VIII, "Being in Love and Hypnosis," Freud writes. "*A primary group of this kind is a number of individuals who have put one and the same object in their place of their ego ideal and have consequently identified themselves with one another in their ego*" (18:116). The placement of the ego ideal in themselves and through the process of introjection serves different purposes simultaneously. It will become more evident that the new ego ideal of liberalism has been introjected into the super-ego and to allow the group to become a dominant presence in society; by doing so, it has given itself the sacred privileges of a priestly class and to rationalize their sacrifices of others.

This first conclusion gives us the opportunity to recollect and reconstruct how Freud arrived at the possibility of a change in a previous certainty. The shift in Freud's emphasis from the leader to the introjected object provides us with a revealing description of our present psychopolitical situation and the place of the victim in our modern sensibility.

> Contemporaneously with this 'devotion' of the ego to the object, which is no longer to be distinguished from a sublimated devotion to an abstract idea, the functions allotted to the ego ideal entirely cease to operate. The criticism exercised by that agency is silent; everything that the object does and asks for is right and blameless. Conscience has no application to anything that is done for the sake of the object; in the blindness of love remorselessly carried

to the pitch of a crime. The whole situation can be summarized in a formula: *The object has been put in the place of the ego ideal.*

(18:113)

One should carefully note Freud's assessment: once the ego-ideal has been introjected as a victim, it allows the dynamic of the super-ego to come immediately into effect and without any restraints. *Anything* can be done for the sake of the victim. Morality makes everything done in the name of the good permissible – "in the blindness of love carried to the pitch of a crime." Contemporary events are evidence of the force of the psyche Freud predicted and how the conjunction between morality and *criminality* was an ultimate logic of its drive.

The introjected ego-ideal and the victim of history is an event of the greatest importance if the psychopolitics of the present are to be accurately diagnosed. We can, for the last time in this context, mention hysterical identification to understand the force of the present drives and how they are both remorseless and potentially *criminal*, to now give one sense of Sighele's *delinquente*. The group can become *criminal* if given sufficient permission. For the sake of the victim, anything can be done; the petty and severe denunciations on social media, for example, are part and parcel of a persecutory society. In the past, individuals were murdered; today they are obliterated in a new and ingenious way, virtually, in the frenetic and uncontrollable back-and-forth of social media. Liberal morality does not need to shed any blood. Technology has made it possible to destroy human beings and without so much as any evidence of their disappearance – until such time as they re-assert themselves and their ego in opposition to those who will be, unavoidably, considered enemies.

The group can, under the right circumstances, become criminal – and in a manner that can be historically verified: they have put themselves in the place of the law and can exercise the persecution of the perceived guilty at will and (with graver consequences) with the full cooperation of the media and institutions, who are more than self-satisfied to give themselves the same judicial prerogatives and disguised with the justified pursuit of "rights," a concept soon to receive Freud's far from idealistic attention. The work of the 1920s alerts us to the danger of a perverted psychopolitics – *prima facie* appearing as the moral improvement of liberal democracies but concealing many inter-related unconscious factors that are far from beneficial. What are the particular features of criminality of the group and its super-ego? It has been able, in many instances, to circumvent the law and the state and to give itself both the power to publicly denounce individuals and to condemn them with extra-judicial methods. The accused has no recourse to *justice*; the law, as an institution, has been bypassed. Ongoing trials are conducted by prosecutors who need not concern themselves with defenses; they are excluded and rendered moot (and mute) by the clamour of moral denunciations.

The movement between the introjection and the projection leads to a perpetual condition of chronic dissatisfaction – both with the self and the world. For all the claims for the care and solicitude and love for the victim, there is much more evidence for the stronger impulses of persecution and judgment. Our first three categories – love-hate, diminished intelligence, loss of freedom – can continue to be evaluated. Each of them, independently and together, have long been abandoned as *felt* since the now destitute ego acts within the limits of a tightly coordinated identity – one perpetually under internal threat and appeased only because of its relationships to others who are equally suffering and who are unified in their pursuit of the "emancipation" they themselves have made impossible. Freud begins to reach his conclusion to the work when, recollecting earlier observations in *Totem and Taboo*, he brings his arguments together, many of them which have not always been sufficiently recognized for their humanism and his personal commitments, as a doctor, as a therapist. Freud's findings move back to grounding archaicism: the horde and the herd. He does so to outline the entire range of his argument and one of *his ideals*: the attempt, against all odds, to heal the human individual. Our final remarks on the preliminary identification of the super-ego before its definitive creation in *The Ego and the Id* has served to highlight several of the most important historical developments in the history of social and political life. The previous relation of the psychology of the group to a leader – whose origins, for Freud, rcturned us to the primal horde – has been transformed in present liberal democracies. The leader has been eclipsed by the three processes of hysterical identification, introjection, and projection. Final remarks will take us to the work where the super-ego is more specifically defined and as the single most-important agency for our psychopolitical essay.

(d) The Primal Horde and the Individual Now

Before arriving at the single most-important argument of *Group Psychology*, which comes as an appendix in the "Postscript" and to re-state Freud's psychoanalytic ideals of individual freedom, intelligence, creativity, and love, a reconstruction of a phylogenetic process can be summarized so as to recall my definition of a primitive present. If, at the outset of *Group Psychology*, Freud had concentrated on the group's libidinal ties and the lessening of intelligence while also tending towards the essence of the group and what he called the individual's "lack of independence," the foundation of his social analysis began to be more systematically and completely outlined. He saved his most penetrating analysis for last, referring to the added notes as "a number of side-paths." Needless to say, the "side-paths" were not at all peripheral. The "Postscript" to *Group Psychology* is a culmination of the whole of his argument and for re-connecting himself to *Totem and Taboo* in order to present a response, and a revitalization, of mythic meaning for our self-understanding. "There was so much that offered us promises of insight" (18:134), Freud writes, almost casually if not for the previous note to the reader. The introduction is an understatement. One does wonder how the arguments of the "Postscript" (and the far from idealistic assessment of justice, equality, and rights – today among our most revered ideals) have been so neglected.

Since the beginning of psychoanalysis and not so differently today, Freud has been the object of highly charged reactions; one, apparently, has been missed. He is on certain occasions an *anti-moralist* insofar as the excessive moral demands, those beyond the measure of a proper conscience, made on the individual are for him antithetical to psychological health. Although the specific date is not crucial (we can set it slightly earlier), Gilles Ribaut writes: "praise of moral values is not to be found in all of Freud's texts. To be now specific, Freud develops the opinion chiefly after 1923–1924, when the Oedipus complex is becoming the core of the psychic history and eventually the main foundations of the civilized man."[59] The morality of the super-ego has been detrimental to health following the murder of the primal father (when authority and submission was put in place, for reasons of security) no less today when Western civilization is attempting to deal with the new reality following the announced death of God. Psychoanalysis could not be separated from its therapeutic aims, even as Freud moved from the individual to society; freedom from the limits of *some* excessive constraints was an ideal for the ego as it was, in principle, for society. The three processes of hysterical identification, introjection, and projection have led us to a reconsideration of the dynamics of today's psychopolitics. The dead are making extraordinary claims on the living. The Introduction highlighted the metaphors of specters, ghosts, and phantasms to explain the supposed phenomenon of the return of the religious. Freud's "Postscript" relieves us of any naivete or ideological distortions – or our secure illusions – by explaining the origins of morality and the methods of ordering specific values for social life. When he then offers us a model for how transformations occur, at any time and under a variety of historical circumstances, as reactions or revolutions, we can then witness how the present-day individual can be reduced to a condition of being in the primal horde and, therefore, in an infantile and primitive moral present. To return to our Introduction and the aspirations *to* modernity, our contemporary situation does not mean the failure has been total; from the perspective of a future work towards its accomplishment, modernity has been stalled and because of a primary social and political regression.

Freud gives us a psychological chronology, tracing the shifts from the primal horde toward the moral herd once the archaic leader has been "murdered," (and today in the displaced repetition of the murder of the God of monotheism) and finally to the individual and the pressures to conform to the group within a highly sophisticated society that has organized its moral imperative around systematic subjugation – of thought, of speech, of life, with a compulsion only possible by a highly co-ordinated bureaucracy. Horde, herd, society: we should have no illusions about our present as substantially different from our archaic selves since our psychological development, always so susceptible to changes, has shown itself to be capable of adopting restrictive safety measures when feeling most threatened, whether the dangers are real, effects of a paranoia, or resulting from the attempt to re-order the nature of reality at the symbolic and practical level. The diagnosis of perversion for organizations,[60] which will be a working concept for us introduced by Susan Long, is extending well into the social sphere as a whole. The substitution of the leader, who has been effectively removed from power by a new band (of brothers *and* sisters, who have banded together despite highly ambivalent feelings for each other), takes place with the same repercussions as the murder of the primal father did in Freud's primal horde. Re-emphasizing the myth in *Totem and Taboo* allowed him to set himself towards considering the substance, and origins, of our most deeply held ideals. One of Richard Rorty's hermeneutics of psychoanalysis is central to the argument to come. "Freud's discoveries of unconscious mechanisms endanger the notions of morality and rationality."[61] Freud does indeed make *morality* vulnerable; because he differentiates the power exerted by morality, to the detriment of individual intelligence and freedom, and the kind of thought and acts necessary for civilization to prosper at all levels of the human. In order for morality to be healthy and productive, it must be tempered by the moderation of conscience; any excessive movements towards the realization of high ideals can have dangerous outcomes for the individual and society. Illness can be produced and aggravated and lead to a number of disabilities. Freud's mythic reconstruction of three historical movements are evident, *simultaneously*, at the present time. The horde, the herd, and the identity-group are psychically unified. His analysis may be subtle and intentionally understated; but it shows Freud at his most creative when he points to the impoverished state of the modern individual who is given all kinds of false impressions about his freedom despite the enduring limits of being and according to the most "progressive" of institutional initiatives. The widely shared belief in the progress of society, with all its confidence in moral uprightness and growth towards complete attainment if not perfection, has been driven by a psychical regression and with many characteristics that Freud will have to outline in greater detail in the works that he writes in subsequent years. Far from the analytic idea of the free individual, the political neurotic "creates his own world of the imagination for himself, his own religion, his own system of delusions, and thus recapitulates the institutions of humanity in a distorted way" (18:142). *His own religion*: but also, to the detriment of everyone else's choice of "faith," of a personal belief in any number of human interests (not just the theological) that are distorted for everyone. How distortions will be analyzed as masochistic-sadistic perversions, in 1924, will be one more supplement to Freud's heightening awareness of different factors at work, all of them dynamically inter-active. He has already begun the investigation into the psychical repercussions of religion once society has proclaimed itself secular and yet, despite its confidence, without fully understanding the meaning of such a momentous shift in worldview and *being*. In the "Postscript," Freud's psychoanalysis of morality can only be compared to Nietzsche's own genealogy, both for outlining its origins (which were established, for Freud, in *Totem and Taboo*) but more importantly for us, for their organization as can be clearly witnessed today. As for Nietzsche, his historically prior genealogy can be brought forward into Freud's work for a formidable one-two combination for our times and beginning with the sense of what is the meaning of a "moral prejudice." On the question of morals, Nietzsche asks: "have they hitherto hindered or furthered human prosperity? Are they signs of distress, of *impoverishment*, of the degeneration of life? Or is there revealed in them, on the contrary, the plenitude, force, and will of life, its courage, certainty, future?"[62] The word *impoverishment* should echo for us. How have the excesses of morality depleted the ego of its possible freedom, intelligence, creativity, and love? The psychically regressive and degenerative are not, however, synonymous. Regression, because it is fundamentally temporal, does not mean the condition is permanent.

Nietzsche and Freud have made high-minded moralists understandably uncomfortable; *political* commentators have been quick to make judgments and doing so with the simplistic labeling of, for example, conservatism or the anxiety about anti-democratic values. Due to the systematic creation of a weak culture (that is, individuals with a number of afflictions and who, in many cases, are made to be so since the gain from illness has become a quasi-virtue), Freud relies on a classical value when a difficult truth has to be confronted. From the many impressions he leaves us with as our responsibility, echoing Nietzsche, the need for "personal courage" is one to be promoted again as an antidote to the degeneration of human life.

> We are reminded of how many of these phenomena of dependence are part of the normal constitution of human society, of how little originality and personal courage are to be found in it, of how much every individual is ruled by those attitudes of the group mind which exhibit themselves in such forms as racial characteristics, class prejudices, public opinion, etc.
>
> (18:117)

Prejudice and public opinion: they are social obstacles intentionally created to make it more difficult for the individual to be either original or have the moral courage to avoid being susceptible to mimetic contagion. When the explanatory story of the primal horde is recalled in order to provide a psychological analogy to the present, all the negative characteristics of the group, the ones he had identified at the very beginning and in support of previous researchers, i.e., Le Bon – imitation, suggestibility, contagion – is now greatly expanded when "we admit that it is exercised not only by the leader, but by every individual upon every other individual" (18:117–118). Every individual who has been duped by morality is pressured not only to conform; he has been adopted into the regulations and goals of the group to create absolute and unquestioned consensus. The pressure of groups in liberal democracies has exceeded, if with different methods, the role of the authoritarian leader. One characteristic stands out from the others in the individual within the herd: feelings of shame and guilt and the need for, if not exoneration, a kind of contractual pardon, one granted only if certain conditions are met. Freud does not yet explain the psychological function of guilt and its relation to time and history. He merely mentions *Schuld,* which Nietzsche had alerted us to its sense of both *guilt* and *debt*, as if saving its complex impact, of morality and the *economics of the psyche*, for another time and another context – that is, in the conclusion of *Civilization and its Discontents*. What should not be forgotten is the understated ideals he presents as necessary *character virtues*, for the individual to be courageous and original.

One begins to speculate, in the interim, if the coming revised structure of the psyche in *The Ego and the Id* is already being prepared, making an analysis of guilt and its role in the function of the super-ego necessary for his continuing examination. That he specifically uses the Aristotelian term *zoon politikon*, the "political animal," serves to make Freud's thinking reliant on the classical virtues of the ancient Greeks, and for reasons soon to be made, remarkably, unequivocal when the mythic poet stands out as the first and most exemplary individual. Is the political, paradoxically, the one human activity returning us more decisively to our animal selves and the trepidation of insecurity and exposure to the uncertainties of the world, thus making safety, and order, a prime imperative – which ultimately also explains the absoluteness of today's morality as *reactionary*? Have we created an animal morality for the protection of the amorphous herd and, by so doing, neglected the reality of the individual who has been prohibited from being discerning and partial? The regression-thesis of *Group Psychology* is, in a sense, anthropologically complete when Freud returns us to our animal origins. Once he introduces the concept of reaction-formation (more exactly, the *relation* of social justice and rights to *Reaktionsbildung*) an especially apt diagnosis of our modern predicament can be added to the rest. Our *Bildung*, our "formation" and education, is taking place with increasing imperatives of domination. The comments of 1921, while not entirely new, are emphasized here because of their contemporary relevance, that is, for us today and most especially for anyone who believes themselves to be personally more moral than anyone else; and if so, how and why. Free of any and all idealism, Freud essentially prepares us for a very uncomfortable realization: far from being a testimony of our "goodness" or our moral developments as a species and society, the pillars of social morality (justice and equality and rights) are not as pure as they would like to be; the personal incentives are considerable, as is moral self-interest. Their motives are hardly unconditional. Justice and rights have been developed as essential in a liberal democracy; they are not, however, without complications that make their reality a burden and one in excess of certain acceptable limits. Being *too good* is unhealthy; the *desire* to be good, to appear good to everyone else, has begun to exhibit peculiar characteristics.

Owing to the process of socialization – exemplified, in one way, by the momentous transition from the private household and the family to school – the child has no choice but to relinquish his feelings of exclusivity, for attention and love, and accept the regulations of a reasoned (if not always demonstrable) *equality*. Freud's first statement will have to resound for us the rest of the way. The educational context is doubly important. Freud has been culturally neglected on this matter, and understandably so; we can add one more reason for Freud's cultural significance and how a place of prominence may once again be reserved for him – for *his* courage and originality. When "school" is understood to be, also, the contemporary university, Freud's arguments should leave *academic moralists* with some much-needed thought; if not them, at least some of their more sceptical colleagues who are less than impressed, and far from persuaded, by the ceaseless promotion of the good by a highly determined bureaucracy that has become *professionalized*. Is there not a conflict of interest between professional moralizing and the wages attached to the aims of dissemination?

Freud continues with an argument that, it seems to me, addresses us directly. "The first demand made by this reaction-formation is for justice, for equal treatment for all. We all know how loudly and implacably this claim is put forward at school" (18:120). The consequences of such an ideal, in educational institutions, can hardly be overestimated; from preschool to the university, educators (who, today, perceive themselves as moral instructors who *profess* the good, by critiquing the bad and the evil), have placed morality above the fundamental grounds of learning and education. The child will, for the rest of his life, necessarily think about the discrepancy between a stated ideal that in *some cases* has been beneficial, and in others tries impossibly to cover over the mendacity of an equal society and the rights for all, which is everywhere declared and barely evident in the real world. The initial impressions are, for some, not easily given up. After all, children immediately recognize (in the schoolyard if not in the strictly supervised classroom) the differences of every child but himself – who is, of course, the subject of comparison and, sometimes, of rivalry and the deepest of antipathies. How Freud states a fact of life in school for children is instructive. "Social justice means that we deny ourselves many things so that others may have to do without them as well" (18:121). Justice is expressed negatively, as a form of a privation. *Social justice*: when it is founded on an unconscious reaction-formation, Freud reveals one overlooked element to the force of the current drive for justice and equality. Are we obliged to conclude that our psychopolitical activism is regressive and infantile and ultimately founded on a social contract between members who are the most vulnerable, who *perceive themselves* to be weak and therefore seek to make everyone equally so, reducing everyone to an equal state of impoverishment? If the model of the child is also carried over to the consistent comparison with the primitive within the primal horde, then Freud's return to archaic beginnings of human society and from the provocative theories of *Totem and Taboo* continues to show the lasting effects of social regression. The primal horde and the political animal are contemporary phenomena. His attitude is almost one of resignation, if not for the conviction that psychoanalysis as a way of thinking, a therapy, and a way of life, can contribute to an enhanced awareness.

The response of an analysand to Freud's transference, much more than a theoretical argument, is no small matter. The *positive* transference, as a counter-suggestion to hysterical identification, introjection, and projection, proves to be a singular moment in our analysis. The consciousness of being manipulated by the categorical imperatives of the day, once they are exposed for their possible distortions and as the propaganda of a new theological-political reality, allow for a decision to be made. Freud's therapeutic questions are not to be taken for granted; his support for his psychoanalytic ideals, which we will continue to emphasize, can be done only when we are fully conscious of the social forces acting against the individual. Freud has rightly been viewed as sober-minded and eminently rational. Have we missed some of his impassioned declarations?

> Each individual is a component part of numerous groups, he is bound by ties of identification in many directions, and he has built up his ego ideal upon the most various models. Each individual therefore has a share in numerous group minds – those of his race, of his class, of his creed, of his nationality, etc. – and he can raise himself above them to the extent of have a scrap of independence and originality.
>
> (18:129)

Independence and originality: his ego-ideals are going to be repeated. Freud begins his conclusion and prepares his "Postscript" with one affirmation he has been saving from the beginning, for its unambiguous support of the individual against all the moral pretensions of the group. Psychoanalysis, among its other goals, is the practice of respecting the inviolability of the individual and assisting in the development of independence and *originality*, that is, his ability not to simply be an emulation of everyone else. The ending of *Group Psychology*, upon repeated readings, seems to be one part of a long thread; its weave will continue into a much bigger, better recognizable pattern in the decade ahead. Psychoanalysis can be defined as a classical humanism since it makes every conceivable attempt to secure the freedom and intelligence of the individual against all the incursions it endures from society and, today, from the exacting moral demands of identity groups who have given themselves the prerogatives of a new kind of social engineering.

Before turning to *The Ego and the Id*, Postscript B can summarize how Freud views the unfolding of human history from the primal horde to the collective organization of the herd (society) and its culmination in the emergence of the individual, which requires, for one, a distinct self-inspiration. Only the individual, first, can begin to progress towards a maturity that would transcend the condition of being both a political animal and a member of a primal horde, a herd, a group, a collective. For reasons he will present over a decade of work, the almost-modern world has been forced into a regressive epoch; the individual has been coerced back into the limited structures of the horde and its anxious insecurity. The return to the primal horde and the imagined murder of the father by the sons created the conditions of an expected freedom; as has been the case – indeed, from time immemorial – the plan of committing a murder and the consequences are entirely separate. The expected freedom resulting from the murder created an impasse. The attempt to overcome an Oedipal relation, stated otherwise, only served to install it all the more more securely. None of the brothers could be free; none of the *siblings* are free and, moreover, have become increasingly suspicious of each other and, in many cases, entrenched in mutual hostility, visceral or unconscious as the case may be. Misanthropy has been institutionalized. Ideologies are exacerbating an already fractious relationship. As a substitute – to prevent anyone from claiming any privilege for his individuality – they created the concept of a community, "all with equal rights" (18:135). Equal rights, which were historically created very late in Western society, much later than the idea of justice, which extends to the beginning of human communities, entailed a reduction of individuality. "There were a number of fathers and each one was limited by the rights of others" (18:135). One could, at this point, turn to the relation of "fathers" and "mothers" (that is, the contemporaneity of brothers and sisters) in modern society and their intense conflict, but the issue would involve a considerable digression. The ideological antagonism between men and women is ongoing and its end cannot yet be anticipated; some of the realities produced by the struggle are, however, already apparent and are tending towards the opposite of any manageable reconciliation; like so many other liberal antagonisms, they are more acute because more dogmatic.

Freud's myth, at the end, introduces a momentous event that, strictly speaking, was not social or political in nature; antecedent causes were psychical and formed during the primal experience within the super-ego. The justice and rights of a herd or society, capable of suppressing its origin, could be perpetuated both within a system of moral sentiments and the domain of *the law*. There was, however, one way for the individual to recognize the rationalization of a herd society and respond. The theological-political foundations of the herd would have to contend, consciously or with indifference, with an *aesthetic disposition*. Freud's comments have not always received the attention due to them. Myths, like taboos, were not simply archaic; they were perpetually present as psychical realities. Today, then, there has been an analogous murder of the primal father. Brothers and sisters have unified in a collective undertaking to (in one model) supersede the leader – no different than the father of the family or, finally, God – and substitute the amorphous group as a new sovereign authority that has begun to not only become independent of the state; it has forced the state to adopt its "ideals" as well as its methods. Can we, with Freud, begin to envision a response to the moralism of the times that would not, necessarily, be agonistic and confrontational? Or are enemies inevitable? Does Freud rely on a distinction he also recollected from the ancient world and to counter the destructive elements of the super-ego with the creativity of the id/ego relation, thereby turning fantasy and the imagination into creative acts? Can a countermovement to morality be imagined *aesthetically* at the level of lived experience and not only in creative endeavours? Is one possible or foreseeable? In the momentous transition from the mythic to the classical (specifically, in ancient Greece) Freud thought so. To the ideals of love, freedom, and intelligence, he adds one more. Human creativity remains the one spirited expression – in an attitude to life, not simply its work and product in an artistic act – as an antidote to the mounting pressure of morality and the death drive.

The aesthetic creation of the poet was the first inkling of the *revelatory power* of the individual insofar as he could inherit the mythical reality of the past, of the primal horde, and re-write it for the purpose of the present, thereby making it possible for the influence of the horde to be, if not abolished, superseded in thought and for individual lives. The nature of the desire of the imagination was essential to the process. "It was then, perhaps, that some individual, in the exigency of his longing, may have been moved to free himself from the group" (18:136). But how could such *an individual* accomplish this feat, alone, when his entire collective had been organized to prevent such *an act* from being carried out? Are human beings not self-determined by a personal ethos than can avoid conformism, even when the pressure is substantial? The alternative can be called, simply, creativity, the act by someone who by virtue of his independence of spirit and freedom from libidinal ties with the group can remain impervious to the contagion of diminished intelligence and the supposed benefits of the horde, the herd, and collective identification. This has been, and is, exceedingly difficult; it demands the individual to perceive the pathology and perversions of the group and therefore to separate himself – even when it means, as it does today, repudiating the supposedly moral aims of an entire society and to recognize it as the pathological social neurosis it has become. Freud does give us an option: to first understand the difference between the political neurotic of the present-day primal horde and the free, the intelligent, the creative individual who can remain autonomous.

Who fulfills the role of a courageous and original human being *first*? Freud's answer is also a testimony on *his* behalf. "He who did this was the first epic poet; and the advance was achieved in his imagination" (18:136). Freud's recollection of the origin of the psychology of the imagination and its subsequent aesthetic creation was momentous because the first epic poet (Hesiod, the author of the *Theogony*, is not one example among others, most especially because of his character Prometheus[63]) transformed not only the inherited narrative of his culture; he redefined the nature of the human and its possibilities. Freud adds. "He invented the heroic myth" (18:136), for example, the individual who was to remain virtually unique and revived symbolically in *European history* for his daring and courage. Is there a better example than Prometheus?[64] By showing the transition from the primal horde to the heroic individual and as an example for modernity, Freud was suggesting it was still possible (always would be possible) for the one to analyze the mythic realities of the past and understand their universal significance for the present. The single most-important argument Freud makes in the "Postscript" and maintains as the ideal of psychoanalysis as a whole is the striving for the achievement of human freedom against all the limits imposed in the world to impede its reach. "The poet who had taken this step and had in this way set himself free from the group" (18:136). *Freedom from the group*. The transition from the limits of the primal horde, including its "justice" and "equal rights," was accomplished by the poet who dared to re-write how the past was to be understood and therefore made it possible to envision a different future. As we continue to follow Freud's developments as an individual, as a therapist and a thinker, he places himself in the position of a founder who will give us the means to achieve personal freedom against the excessive impositions of reality – an experience that, for him personally, no doubt shaped the single-mindedness of his dedication and led him to devote himself to his next work, a project that made the recognition of the super-ego and the death drive indispensable for our deeper understanding of social and political life.

We cannot appreciate the extent of Freud's ideas in the "Postscript" if we simply confine this one momentous event in the history of civilization to the individuality of the poet and the creation of an art-form. The aesthetic has to become, as Nietzsche envisioned it, *ontological*, a matter of creating a form of being through the conscious recollection of a relation, because as we now know and has been many times confirmed, the dichotomy of myth and logos does not hold. Freud's *Totem and Taboo*, read in light of the "Postscript" and *together*, gives us a portrait we can now emphasize. We cannot separate, with any degree of certainty, either a historical or narrative difference between myth and the logos of philosophy. More importantly than the myth/logos relationship, and the perennial question of the so-called "quarrel" between poetry and philosophy, it is above all the individual who has expressed *muthos* and *logos* together and deserves to be recognized as one of the first individuals who by virtue of his inspiration and revelation raised himself above the group and reflected back to everyone an inherent human ability. Freud's recollection of mythic poetry is one enduring example of an individual being capable of countering the regression of a group and an entire society. *Totem and Taboo* was his modern response to the primitive present as well as a warning for the coming secularism of liberal democracies.

Freud is a thinker of the history of human freedom and intelligence and the therapist who has dedicated himself not only to freeing the neurotic patient from his or her pain; psychoanalysis became the thinking most committed to the freedom of the (potentially) modern subject. The transition to *The Ego and the Id* can now be more completely pursued for its psychopolitical implications. We will then move from the vision of the mythic poet as the individual representing the freedom to re-think the nature of reality and the function, today, of a highly dominating super-ego. We will see if we can come to one affirmative conclusion; avoiding being a "master," *about anything*, might be prudent. "The ego is no longer the slave of the superego and may actually become its master."[65] Before the aim of overcoming the power of the super-ego, or the perhaps overstated ambitions of becoming its "master," it may be more realistic to set out in what ways the psychical agency most representative of morality has developed, in our time, with such force and power. A personal note from Freud's *An Autobiographical Study* does not lose sight of the individual. We may, without idealism, emulate his own thinking as he confronted and defied the truths of the day. "It helped to rid me of another shred of the innocent faith in authority from which I was *not yet* free" (SE 20:16, my emphasis). Freud had to come to a personal realization about his former dependence on authority before he could devote himself more completely, more consciously, both to his freedom and to the freedom of others. His own awareness, and the development of his own intelligence, was in part made possible by a significant point made by Hans Blumemberg. "The boundary line between myth and logos is imaginary and does not obviate the need to inquire about the logos of myth in the process of working free of the absolutism of reality."[66] Is not *Totem and Taboo* precisely such an example of the logos of myth and with an even more startling perception of the causes of our present, in the murder of the primal father and its repetition with the announced death of God, that are further explained for their effects in *The Ego and the Id*?

Notes

1 Freud, Sigmund. "On Narcissism: An Introduction." SE 14:76.
2 Freud, Sigmund. "Mourning and Melancholia." SE 14:244.
3 Guntrip, Harry. *Schizoid Phenomena, Object Relations and the Self*. London: Karnac, 2001. He adds: "the libidinal quest for objects is the source of the capacity to love, and the maintenance of loving relationship is the major self-expression activity of the total self," 92. In many ways, the analysis is devastating: the political neurotic is unable to love because, for one, the regression to the infantile and primitive part of the self (and the machinations of the super-ego) make it impossible to relate authentically to external objects.
4 Ferenczi, Sandor. "Freud's 'Group Psychology and the Analysis of the Ego': Its Contribution to the Psychology of the Individual," *Final Contributions to the Problems and Methods of Psycho-analysis*. Ed. Michael Balint. Tr. Erich Mosbacher and others. London: Karnac, 1994, 371.
5 Plato's *Symposium* (Tr. Alexander Nehemas. Indianapolis: Hackett Publishing Company, 1989) can be cited here for one main reason: the dialogue on Eros as conceived by Diotima, who presented us with the two kinds of the human erotic, both in terms of their capacity to create – for procreation and the continuity of life (which is first affirmed sexually between a man and a woman) and for sustaining human creativity as an essential attribute of the human. Socrates' summation of Diotima's speech on *ta erōtika*, "the art of love" (270a) unifies, for us, two lived experiences and their unity, the aesthetic and the amorous. The ideals of art and love will be some of the most important of Freud's principles.
6 Bion, W.R. *Experience in Groups: and other papers*. London: Brunner-Routledge, 1989, 39.
7 Freud, Sigmund. "The Neuro-Psychoses of Defense." SE 3:47.
8 Breuer, Josef and Freud, Sigmund. *Studies on Hysteria*. SE 2:21.
9 Merkur, Dan. "The Antinomy of Morality in Freud," in *Ethics of Evil: Psychoanalytic Investigations*. Ed. Jon Mills and Ronald C. Naso. London: Karnac, 2016, 60.
10 D.W. Winnicott. "Metapsychological and Clinical Aspects of Regression with the Psychoanalytical Set-Up," 16–26, *International Journal of Psycho-Analysis*, 1955.
11 For a historical inquiry into group psychology as a problem and how it was variously analyzed prior to Freud, see Jaap Van Ginneken's "The Killing of the Father: The Background of Freud's Group Psychology," 391–414 *Political Psychology*, Vol. 5, No. 3 (Sep., 1984).
12 Jonsson, Stephen. *Crowds and Democracy: The Idea and Image of the Masses from Revolution to Fascism*. New York: Columbia University Press, 2013, 121.
13 Arditi, Benamin. *Politics on the Edge of Liberalism: Difference, Populism, Revolution, Agitation*. Edinburgh: Edinburgh University Press, 2007, 53, my emphasis. A nemesis can also be defined as an enemy, a figure who will receive considerable attention in a later chapter and due to Freud's utter distrust in the ideal of "the love of the neighbour."
14 The development of a 19th century "crowd theory," as presented by Urs Stäheli (In "Seducing the Crowd: The Leader in Crowd Psychology. Tr. Erich Saroth.

New German Critique, 63–77, No. 114 (Fall 2011) is not ultimately relevant for Freud's analysis and, more precisely, the *ideas* (and ideals) of a *politically* motivated group whose main focus is, additionally, moral. Freud is much less concerned with the spontaneous acting out of a crowd, say, during a demonstration or a riot or even an insurrection, than with the systematic ordering of a society according to the leading ideas of a group and what they are capable of organizing.

15 To be distinguished from *Volkerpsychologie*. Freud was not focused on any nationalist psychology.

16 Each of these characteristics were outlined, as Freud acknowledges, in the work of Scipio Sighele in his 1891 *La folla delinquente*. A recent translation has appeared in a collection of Sighele's writings with the title *The Criminal Crowd and Other Writings*. Edited, with an Introduction and Notes, by Nicoletta Pireddu. Translated by Nicoletta Pireddu and Andrew Robbins. With a Foreword by Tom Huhn. Toronto: University of Toronto Press, 2018. Sighele's concept of "delinquenza," once associated more tightly with criminality, increases our problem considerably. Have *some* of today's groups edged closer towards a *criminal* disposition? The question, from the perspective of institutional manipulation, should not be hyperbolic. We should neither be surprised nor shocked in unifying the potential for moral and the criminal. 20th century politics should have relieved us of any naivete.

17 This is an aspect of his methodical procedure. He recognized, very early, how complicated the manifestations of the psyche could in fact be. The atemporality of the psyche made its recognition an arduous and multi-level task. To give one example of his thought-process and his scientific principles, the lecture he presented as "The Aetiology of Hysteria" led him to say: "the real examples are all incomparably more complicated: to relate a single one of them in detail would occupy the whole period of the lecture. The chain of associations always has more than two links; and the traumatic scenes do not form a simple row, like a string of pearls, but ramify and are interconnected like genealogical trees," SE 3:196.

18 Viney, Wayne and Parker, Elizabeth. "Necessity as a Nightmare or a Pathway to Freedom: Freud's Dilemma, A Human Dilemma," 299–311 *Psychoanalytic Psychology*, Vol. 33, No. 2, 2016, 305.

19 Freud, Sigmund. "Two Encyclopedia Articles." SE 18:253, my emphasis. The reference is found in (A) "Psycho-Analysis."

20 Ellul, Jacques. *Propaganda: The Formation of Man's Attitudes*. Tr. Konrad Kellen and Jean Lerner. New York: Vintage Books, 1965, 61.

21 Voruz, Véronique. "Culpability and the Politics of Love," 205–226 *Law and Critique*, Vol. 22, No. 3 (Nov. 2011), 208.

22 Gandesha, Samir. "The "Authoritarian Personality" Reconsidered: the Phantom of "Left Fascism"," 601–624 *American Journal of Psychoanalysis*, Vol. 79, No. 4, 2019, 602.

23 Freud, Sigmund. *The Complete Letters of Sigmund Freud to Wilhelm Fliess, 1887–1904*. Tr. And Ed. Jeffrey Moussaieff Masson. Cambridge: The Belknap Press of Harvard University Press, 1985, 345.

24 Adorno, Theodor. "Freudian Theory and the Pattern of Fascist Propaganda," 118–137 *The Essential Frankfurt School*. Ed. Andrew Arato and Elke Gerhardt. London: Continuum, 1982, 137.

25 Bar-Haim, Shaul. "The return of the Political Freud? Some notes on the new historiography of Psychoanalysis," 121–139 *History of the Human Sciences*, Vol. 32, No. 2.

26 Reicher, Stephen. "Crowds, Agency and Passion: Reconsidering the Roots of the Social Bond," 67–85 *The Psychology and Politics of the Collective: Groups, Crowds and Mass Identification*. Ed. Ruth Perkin-Gounelas. London: Routledge, 2012, 80.

27 Shmuel Erlich, H. *The Couch in the Marketplace: Psychoanalysis and Social Reality*. London: Karnac, 2013, 124, my emphasis.
28 Girard, René. *Violence and the Sacred*. Tr. Patrick Gregory. Baltimore: The Johns Hopkins University Press, 1977, 90.
29 Burzstein, Jean-Gerard. *The Topological Transformation of Freud's Theory*. Tr. Marie-Laure Bromley-Davenport. London: Karnac, 2016, 32.
30 Freud, Sigmund. "Preface to Reik's Ritual: Psycho-Analytic Studies." SE 17:261.
31 Balibar, Étienne. "Construction, and Deconstruction of the Universal," Tr. Melissa McMahon, 21–43 *Critical Horizons*, 7:1 (2006), 39–40. That Balibar equates the "suspension of domination" with the "liberation from illusion" is telling. Which has to come first? Because if domination has been suspended but we continue to be led by the ideals of our illusions, then Freud becomes ever more necessary. The reliance on many of the old and exhausted critiques are no longer adequate in understanding our social conditions today.
32 Covington, Coline. "Populism and the Danger of Illusion," 250–265, *Contemporary Psychoanalysis*, Vol. 54, No. 2, 2018, 251.
33 Ogden, Thomas H. *The Matrix of the Mind: Object Relations and the Psychoanalytic Dialogue*. London: Karnac, 1992, 95.
34 Freud, Sigmund. "Family Romances." SE 9:237, my emphasis.
35 Bollas, Christopher. "Psychoanalysis in the Age of Bewilderment: On the return of the oppressed," 535–551 *International Journal of Psychoanalysis*, Vol. 96, No. 3 (2015), 536.
36 De Masi, Franco. "The perverse and psychotic superego," 735–739 *International Journal of Psychoanalysis*, Vol. 101, No. 4, 2020, 737, my emphasis of the word "salvation." He adds that "the superego tends to destroy life in every hyper-moral system," 737. Once again it seems to me that only psychoanalysts have been able to identify one of the problems of our contemporary world: morality and its destruction of life.
37 Freud, Sigmund. *Three Essays on the Theory of Sexuality*. SE 7:151.
38 Snyder, Timothy. *The Road to Unfreedom: Russia, Europe, America*. New York: Tim Duggan Books, 2018, 22.
39 Camus, Albert. *The Rebel: An Essay on Man in Revolt*. New York: Vintage Books, 1956, 301. His statement is close to the conclusion of the chapter entitled "Nihilism."
40 Klein, Melanie. *Love, Guilt and Reparation and other works, 1921,1945*. London: Virago Press, 1988, 311, my emphasis of *sacrifice*.
41 Kernberg, Otto F. "Limitations to the Capacity to Love," 1501–1515 *International Journal of Psychoanalysis*, 92, 2011.
42 Appel, S. "Freud on Civilization," 625–645 *Human Relations*, Vol. 48, No. 6 (Jun 1995), 643. He adds: "Freud's psychological and sociological writings warrant re-reading." We could pass over the comment and think nothing of it. Or we could take it with utmost seriousness and re-commit ourselves to re-reading Freud with the acute sense of what he has to tell us about our present condition. Moreover, only when we come to *The Future of an Illusion* will we able to more firmly notice how his intricate thinking and writing has been far less one-dimensional than has been supposed. Is Freud really the critic of religion we have more or less accepted as true? Or did he have a much more extensive psychoanalytic purpose?
43 Scheidlinger, Saul. "Group Psychology Revisited: An Opportunity Missed," 389–392, *Psychoanalytic Psychology*, Vol. 20, No. 2 (2003), 390.
44 Hinshelwood, R.D. "Ideology and Identity: A psychoanalytic investigation of a social phenomenon," 131–148 *Psychoanalysis, Culture & Society*, Vol. 14, No. 2 (Jul. 2009), 136, my emphasis. The use of the word "revelation" should not be read as simply a rhetorical choice. Once Freud's explicit writings on group psychology

use the language of religion, we should be immediately prepared to shift the emphasis from the theological to the political and to recognize a momentous transition in the complexity of his thinking.

45 Rank, Otto. *Don Juan Legend.* Ed. Tr, with an Introduction by David G. Winter. Princeton: Princeton University Press, 2015, 53.

46 Zepf, Siegfried. "Modes of Identification: Freud's Concepts Reorganized," 44–55 in *The Scandinavian Psychoanalytic Review*, 32:1, 46.

47 The symptom of "*tussis nervosa*" goes back to the case of Anna O. SE 3:23.

48 Pieszanski, Alberto. "Hysteria, A Century Later: Post-Kleinian Theory and Techniques," 102–111 *Psychoanalytic Inquiry*, Vol. 37, No. 2 (2017), 104.

49 Chasseguet-Smirgel, Janine. *Sexuality and Mind: The Role of the Mother and Father in the Psyche.* London: Karnac, 1989, 3–4. She has been one of the more astute of psychoanalytic writers for so clearly exposing the ambitions of past political ideologues (for, example, during the Chinese "Cultural Revolution" and, more sanguinary, the events in Cambodia under the Khmer Rouge) and how they have been extremely hostile to civilization. The topographical changes have not altered the psychological conditions. The "social justice warriors" of liberal democracies may not have *peasants* to idolize (that is, people who were rural and worked on the land – ideologically, who were one with *nature*) but in some cases they have a more enduring object of history who was inseparable from the natural world. In North America, the indigenous has come to represent the revered object of history and as the justification for a nihilistic attitude towards social reality.

50 Freud, Sigmund. "Family Romances." SE 9:238.

51 Ferenczi, Sandor. *First Contributions to Psychoanalysis.* Tr. Ernest Jones. London: Karnac, 1994, 37. The essay is "Introjection and Transference." 199.

52 Klein, Melanie. "Notes on Some Schizoid Mechanism," 1–24 *Envy and Gratitude and Other Works, 1946–1963.* London: Virago Press, 1988, 9, my emphasis. Klein's observations are more extreme than Freud's diagnoses of the impoverished and depleted self because in her investigations of the primitive psyche of the infant, she recognized how utterly destructive the impulses could become, most especially if they were retained in the form of defenses and deployed during adult life. *The ego has no life.* The theological-political impulse of our times has led to an increasing sense of psychical suicide as a mandatory desire.

53 Sherick, Ivan. "Hysterical Identification in an Eleven-Year Old Girl," 675- in *Psychoanalytic Review*, Vol. 101, No. 5 (Oct. 2014), 675.

54 Freud, Sigmund. "Charcot," SE 3:20.

55 Miller, Janet. "The Enemy Inside: An exploration of the defensive processes of introjecting and identifying with the aggressor," 55–70 *Psychodynamic counseling*, Vol. 4, No. 1 (1998), 59.

56 Schaeffer, Jacqueline. *The Universal Refusal: Psychoanalytic Exploration of the Feminine Sphere and its Repudiation.* Tr. David Alcorn. London: Karnac, 2011, 186.

57 Girard, René. *The Scapegoat.* Tr. Yvonne Freccero. Baltimore: The Johns Hopkins University Press, 1986, 41.

58 Racamier, Paul-Claude. "On Narcissistic Perversion," 119–132 *International Journal of Psychoanalysis*, 95 (2014), 119.

59 Ribaut, Gilles. "The Two Sources of Morality in Freud's Work," 135–141 *Psychoanalysis, Monotheism, and Morality: The Sigmund Freud Symposia, 2009–2011.* Ed. Wolfgang Müller Funk, Inge Scholz Strasser and Herman Westerink. Leuven: Leuven University Press, 2013, 135. One addition will be taken up at a later point. Ribaut raises the possibility of "a society free from the superego," 141. We will see how the idea is not possible and not desirable since the

proper function of the superego, to regulate a moderate conscience, remains a social necessity.

60 See Susan Long's *The Perverse Organization and its Deadly Sins.* London: Routledge, 2008. The theological concept of "sin" allows us to slightly shift the emphasis and return the idea not so much to its Judeo-Christian origins (as a moral problem, and one ultimately to be *judged*) but to its Greek context, especially in its literary and philosophical tradition, to define *hamartia* not as a moral problem but as an existential and psychological condition of being incomplete and self-divided.

61 Rorty, Richard. "Freud, Morality, Hermeneutics," 177–185 *New Literary History*, Vol. 12, No. 1 (Autumn 1980), 185.

62 Nietzsche, Friedrich. *On the Genealogy of Morals: A Polemic.* Tr. Walter Kaufmann and R.J. Hollingdale. New York: Vintage Books, 1989, 17.

63 My interpretation can be found in *Animal Sacrifice and the Death Penalty*. Eugene: Wipf & Stock, 2022.

64 In *The Psychoanalysis of Fire.* Tr. Alan C.M. Ross. Boston: Beacon Press, 1964), Gaston Bachelard gives the name of the "the Prometheus Complex" to the inherent desire of the unique individual who gives himself the task, solitary if need be, to introduce a new possibility into the world. In his Preface, Northrop Frye writes: "Bachelard does not explicitly say that mythology, considered as a body of stories, is potential literature, but the whole trend of his book is towards that principle," vii. We have perhaps no better example than Frye to remind us that myth is a structural principle of literature and, therefore, for us, that Freud's myth of *Totem and Taboo* and its self-reflection in the "Postscript," exemplify his own ideal.

65 Ross, Nathaniel. "Man's struggle for freedom: A psychoanalytical inquiry into the individual and social dimensions of human autonomy," 209–221 *Bulletin of the Menninger Clinic* 38, 1974, 218.

66 Blumenberg, Hans. *Work on Myth.* Tr. Robert M. Wallace. Cambridge, Massachusetts: The MIT Press, 1985, 12.

2

THE POWERS OF THE SUPER-EGO AND THE DEATH DRIVE

> Psycho-analysis is an instrument to enable the ego to achieve a progressive conquest of the id. From the other point of view, however, we see this same ego as a poor creature owing service to three masters and consequently menaced by three dangers: from the external world, from the libido of the id, and from the severity of the super-ego.
>
> *The Ego and the Id*

(e) From the Psychology of Groups to Their Super-ego Pathologies

The previous discussion of some of the most identifiable aspects of group psychology can now be supplemented, as Freud did, with a description of the new structure of the psyche and, in particular, the elaboration of the super-ego and its relation to the death drive. The "severity" of the super-ego is but one of its definitions; when Freud several times mentions a "menacing danger," how the super-ego and the death drive become collaborative (and antithetical in aims and method) demands particular attention for the consequences it has for the social and political sphere. *Pathology* is the most widely used and recurring diagnosis. A psychical reality has been the cause of a set of different illnesses that together can be described as severe pathological dangers. The inter-related processes of hysterical identification, introjection, and projection can be further explained by interpreting how Freud's *The Ego and the Id* outlines the characteristics of both an excessive morality and a dynamic towards a peculiar kind of death drive. Identifying two contemporary obsessions will be primary.

DOI: 10.4324/9781003410911-3

The moral and the nihilistic are unconsciously complicit. The process of regression remains operative and perpetual as one of the effects separating what Annie Reiner has called a "mature conscience,"[1] which for her is a human potential to be realized and lived, and the pathologies of the super-ego. Conscience (and *personal* ethics, which psychoanalysis supports for the individual) have been ideologically superseded by the increasing propaganda of an unlimited morality. Readers will have to make their own sense, as an analytic interjection, of what Donald Carveth has called a "still small voice," one we can associate with a certain kind of call and that is alert to "the morally objectionable internalised sociocultural ideologies of which the superego is compromised and that are reflected in its normative, never mind pathological expressions."[2] As someone who has recognized psychical realities in society, he reminds us of our susceptibilities; the internalization of pathologies – our "sociocultural ideologies," as opposed to a healthy conscience – is one of many that Freud will present in *The Ego and the Id.*

Unlike other individuals working in the field of psychology who, remarkably, have resisted the concept of the super-ego and suggested it could be disregarded, conceptually or clinically, there can be no question of having the slightest doubt about its presence in group psychology and society at the present time; nor can the death drive, even more so, be separated from its force and its proximity. The analysis of the theological-political nature of our times can be provisionally explained only by relying on Freud's theory of a sinister complicity between a back-and-forth relationship, binding in the relation of a perverse love-hate. A dualistic theory, between the comprehensively erotic and the nihilistic impulse, presents no obstacles, nor can the idea of a constitutive and agonistic relation between a *conception* of love and hate, life and death, Eros and Thanatos. The libidinal ties of the group and its identity were inseparable from the hate they necessarily express towards others who are in any way suspected of being unlike, different, or in disagreement. The psychology of the "we" in contradistinction to all others is necessary for the maintenance of a tenuous identity. Some surprise has to be expressed for anyone who seems skeptical about the existence of super-ego. The perspective from a clinical psychologist stands out, as does his ambivalence. Elliot Jurist writes: "the superego has receded and cannot be salvaged, but neither can we really live without it."[3] The emergence of secularism and therefore one aspect of the super-ego has "receded" (in terms of a viable conscience), while at the same time taking account of what the process has consequently created and with more substantial force – the previously mentioned "super-morality." Jurist's rhetoric can be noted: for him, the super-ego cannot be "resurrected" and yet he admits to its persistence. Our phantasms continue to appear, along with specifically theological metaphors.

Freud's systematic presentation will have to be brought together in order to realize how the process, with its many parts, functions together. One other impression, from a psychoanalyst, can be stated for the sake of comparison. R. D. Hinshelwood writes: "It is unusual for the super-ego to be challenged or debated now."[4] A conflict of interpretations, owing to either a relation to Freud and psychoanalysis or the new directions taken by various psychological theories, continues. One attempt at explaining the psychoanalytic divisions about the super-ego cannot be sustained. Dan Merkur writes: "psychoanalysts' failure to develop a consensus regarding the super-ego may ultimately be traced to Freud's limited interest in the psychology of morality."[5] The statement comes as a surprise, of a different sort than denial. The "limited interest" is, on the contrary, intense and concentrated. How can it be missed? Not only did Freud acknowledge morality as an unavoidable dilemma of human life, and "super-morality" more so; how morality governed society was inseparable from the discontent of civilization he himself diagnosed.

Freud's impression of "pathological outcomes" and the super-ego are standard. "If they [the ego's object-identifications] obtain the upper hand and become too numerous, and unduly powerful and incompatible with one another, a pathological outcome will not be far off" (SE 19:30). Once the identification has become hysterical, a new pathology comes about. The dead victims are "unduly powerful" (the most powerful of all objects since they are now displaced from the past and introjected into the super-ego to become phantasmatic in their effects) and established to exert the most influence. Above all, Freud has given us a most profound sense of the split in the super-ego and how its impulses are incompatible. Luc Donnet tells us, "the distinctive ambiguities of the work of culture can be found in the agency of the Superego."[6] Our analysis will have to identify, precisely, how the "ambiguities" are projected into the world.

Freud also emphasizes how *too many* ideals are hazardous because, today, their representation by different and competing groups are each vying for recognition and legitimacy to the exclusion of anyone else who does not matter as a subject of concern; if they are "too numerous," they can lead to a psychical imbalance between the demands of the moral imagination and what reality (that is, others who do not identify with any one group) can accommodate and *tolerate*; moral demands can become insupportable. When too many ideals are the outcome of an unrecognized pathology, the force of reality becomes morally overbearing; for the time being, there is a certain complacency, a certain acquiescence, to the moral demands of society. The majority is enduring, that is, putting up with the demands. The lack of independence, or the courage to respond, has made ideological forces both enabled and entitled; any opposition serves to exacerbate their identity and hostility. One wonders if the increase in moral imperatives, which shows no sign of a slow-down or moderation, will reach a point of saturation and an understandable reaction is a possible future outcome. Moderation has been marginalized almost to the point of non-existence and irrelevance. Too much goodness cannot be easily accommodated; not everyone has the need (or the desire) to appear self-righteous or, ultimately, to devote themselves to the *specific* collective moral goals of society. There are many more ways to be "good" than according to moral standards. The ideal of moral "perfection" can only lead to the kind of expectations that have sometimes ended up as the human catastrophes of political movements.

The introduction of only a few of the characteristics of the superego will be a preparation for a more detailed analysis and in relation to a drive that is masochistic-sadistic. The psychopathological can be repeatedly heard. "It will appear that the superego becomes the source of the problem of psychopathology primarily when the ego is not strong enough to ensure a realistic superego reaction or to contain an unrealistic one."[7] The pressures exerted on the ego (the individual) are considerable; the increasing strength of the superego leads to the further debility of the individual who is forced into a tightening middle. How has this particular phenomenon become prevalent; how has the 21st-century superego become pathological and can we better account for its unique ability to shape public opinion? How has a frenetic moralism passed unnoticed and, apparently, been so widely accepted? We can again stress a first position: the correlation between the super-ego and specific forms of neurotic illness. "In addition to representing that which is higher in human nature, the superego is also implicated in a variety of pathological conditions."[8] We are faced with a dilemma, morally and otherwise: the superego does indeed stand for what is "higher" in ourselves. On one level, our moral sense and the development of virtues, for example, empathy and compassion and authentic concern for the welfare of others, is an important element of a healthy civilization. Conscience has been necessary. Liberal democracies can be given credit for the historical attempt to make life, in a collective, more healthy. And yet the part of ourselves most associated with our humanity has also been susceptible to the worst kind of excesses. *Politically*, the manipulation of morality has led to evident examples of our individual and collective overextension. Are we now approaching the severe danger that Freud warned us about? Although there is no need, for the time being, to examine how super-ego omnipotence can lead to the *extreme* experiences of certain forms of *functional* psychosis[9] – though paranoid and schizoid projections have been mentioned, the theological-political nature of morality can lead to a systematic persecution of others, known to us, as one example, from a so-called "cultural" revolution from the last century. Freud's historical examples will be exact: the Soviet and the theological-political, together, will recur in his psychoanalysis of the politically manifest and in a more than verifiable history. To continue to build on the argument, Karen Horney presents us with one of the potential effects of the super-ego, politically. "Descriptions of the super-ego are revealing because, in every case, they are at once psychological and associated with the worst kind of political regimes."[10] The super-ego and political *regimes* have an attraction and relation; when they are, as in our time, theological-political, the force of the super-ego is multiplied exponentially. Later episodes, such as the "penitence" of the Gulag, confirmed Freud's evaluation of the prospects of a political revolution. "In our analyses we discover that there are people in whom the faculties of self-criticism and conscience – mental activities, that is, that rank as extremely high ones – are unconscious and unconsciously produce effects of the greatest importance" (19:26). Conscience is, of course, desirable for the order of any community and society. When, however, the previous reality of "self-criticism" has been conveniently displaced by a defensive condemnation of others, the previous high values have turned into their opposites. Freud's differentiation has already been taken into account as have arguments by later analysts and others. Donald Carveth has reminded us more than once not to conflate conscience with the super-ego.[11] Their qualities and psychical demands are very different. Psychoanalysts who are treating patients are right to defend the super-ego and its conscience function; they are, however, in a position to be able to moderate its demands and, most importantly, influence the ego and protect it from undue cruelty. The exorbitant desires of the super-ego can be modified in a clinical setting, not so in everyday reality when the contagion of groups has made self-reflection undesirable. The privacy of the clinic cannot be underestimated; nor can the one-to-one relation that is established, first of all, on trust and a common purpose – of interpretation, understanding, and healing.

The psychical difficulties Freud identified were not slight; because if we consider some of our most well-promoted ideals of the present as inseparable from their pathology, our social and political situation is precarious and, as he stressed, dangerous. Are our ideals leading us to further regressions and causing a malaise in society, one also experienced when the theoretically *critical* and the *negative* are overwhelming? Are we thereby forced to take nothing for granted, most especially the clamor of our "goodness," and analyze our ideals as inseparable from reaction formations? Are the regressions and pathologies signs of a specific kind of "corruptibility"?[12]

Freud continues with his presentation and, returning to re-examine well-established principles, writes: "The super-ego is, however, not simply a residue of the earliest object-choices of the id; it also represents an energetic reaction formation against those choices" (19:34). Our super-ego has been severely modified, and intensified, by the historical developments of our liberal societies. The traditional understanding of the super-ego can no longer be identified as it used to be. We can now wonder at the possible transformation of the psyche in history once the traditional is first acknowledged. "The super-ego is ultimately an internalization of family values and social/cultural values."[13] While the *beginning* of such an internalization is demonstrable for the socialized child, there are now many more indications for considering in what specific ways the super-ego departs from these "values" and is instead made, and characterized, by many more complicated aspects that are socially evident in phenomena that have been, for the most part, ignored. The foundations for the development of our contemporary super-ego has led us to one provisional and transitional point vis-à-vis the nature of the three-part process of identification, introjection, and projection. The argument to be presented requires us to show how the now virtually unrestrained power of the super-ego has been able to repudiate both the influence of religious sensibility, its conscience, and the role of parents and culture in socialization. Early socialization may be undone, revised, corrupted; the process of regression may be so profound as to lead the individual and groups back to a primitive super-ego that has been unconsciously connected to the fantasies of a pre-civilization condition in nature. The drive of the present appears to be more phantasmatic and absolute as it attempts to annihilate the idea of the real, as it did in infancy with its proximate objects.

An early essay, in 1926, by Ernest Jones, can be recalled. "The genesis of the super-ego is certainly connected with the passing of the Oedipus complex."[14] If Jones means "passing" as its overcoming (or resolution) the situation today leads us to an entirely different argument: the passing has been mired in an unresolved conflict. Due to the *new* and altered antagonism with the Oedipus complex – a change in the child's relationship to the mother and father as *antecedents*, the super-ego has also become perverse in unexpected ways. We can recollect the beginning of the discussion on regression and now make additional observations. The individual of our present psychopolitics has a number of characteristics that can be added to the previous ones: being fundamentally unable to reconcile himself to the Oedipus complex – acknowledging, necessarily, the chronology of generations and the meaning of tradition – the pathological super-ego sets itself toward an impossible task: the fantasy of a genetic inauguration and to alter the nature of terrestrial reality.

Taking note of "some effects of the primitive superego," André Green writes about the "paralysing superego, impeding a positive evolution."[15] The superego has been paralyzed, but not only in the present of time; the condition revives a primitive state of psychical being in the infant. The neurotic has regressed to the primitive superego and, in the most enigmatic recesses of the unknown, created a strange osmosis with a fantasy existence, in nature, *prior* to Western civilization. The social production of an overbearing sense of guilt, for prior history (exemplified and most especially in the context of North America, by post-1492 fantasies of trauma and culpability) has led to a collective ambition to alter the reality of the past with a substitute paralysis of the present. Guilt is ubiquitous, as are spurious attempts to overcome the past with illusions of redemption and one ideal, a *reconciliation* which is psychically avoided since it would, in principle, bring about the overcoming of the original "trauma." The ideal is itself paralyzed; any possible achievement will be thwarted every step of the way since it must remain a *chronic* condition and never, under any condition, be overcome. Ideological traumatism, which will later be described as a theological-political form of "gain from illness," depends on its perpetuity. As an *ism* of our time, trauma has become infinitely exploitable.

Our liberal society has begun to exhibit a fundamentally new development both in its self-understanding and in the irrepressible drive of a super-ego that has been universally forced to confront one perceived reality. Freud prepares the reader for the argument to come: he seeks to identify the "source" and, with it, a remedy. "I shall presently bring forward a suggestion about the source of its [the super-ego] power to dominate and in this way – the source, that is, of its compulsive character which manifests itself in the form of a categorical imperative" (19:35). The categorical imperative could not be more precise *for us*. Dominating and compulsive, the super-ego presents its projections in the form of highly moral directives. The super-ego has shown itself to be compelled by a new moralism that has exceeded the normal function of the super-ego, as moderate conscience, and begun to exhibit all the worst tendencies of the authoritarian imagination. The super-ego has been persecutory and judgmental, but without the slightest restraint, for example, in the form of forgiveness or mercy. Any conscious religious ideals have been rejected. Along with dogma and orthodoxy, sensibilities have also been eroded. We are now witnesses to the perfidy of the moral and to what Freud calls the "dictatorial Thou shalt" of our theological-political present. Being aware of the vocabulary is, again, noteworthy: the power and domination of the superego is compulsive and culminates with the "categorical imperative," that is, a moral and ethical *thou shall*, and *thou shall not*, that will present individuals with considerable duress – both from its most enthusiastic adherents and from others who sense the excessive demand to be "good" while also recognizing its manipulation. A prior note can be repeated: the conjunction of the morality of the super-ego and the function of the state/capital relation can no longer be separated. They have now established a joint venture whose proportions are not entirely new, but whose context in a world of global domination (of the moral good and the goods of the market) are soon going to be indistinguishable. Attention to media images and projections is filled with all kinds of marketing of the moral, as if the methods of capital and the super-ego have formed an unconscious alliance of influence and where the moral good and consumer goods are unconsciously intertwined. Capital has found its most legitimate ally, understandable given a propaganda conception of the human. One other contemporary issue can also be mentioned by Freud and with observations of utmost relevance for us.

> The differentiation of the super-ego from the ego is no matter of chance; it represents the most important characteristics of the development both of the individual and of the species; indeed, by giving permanent expression to the influence of the parents, it perpetuates the existence of factors to which it owes its origin.
>
> (SE 19:35)

The noticeable contradiction of our contemporary political situation can be better presented when Freud gives us the dynamic involved: at the same time as the super-ego is determined by one of its origins, it also sets itself towards completely re-framing the status of the real according to its new ideals; and yet, because it can never recognize the source of its compulsions, the results are increasingly pathological. The individual and the species are, to use prior definitions of the super-ego, corruptible, perverted, and worse of all, persecutory. Freud's conjunction of the individual and the species once again requires a comment, in part, because of its newness. The *radical* super-ego of our times exhibits one highly omnipotent desire: it does not acknowledge either of its origins (parents and society) because it has determined to begin from an existential and biological *tabula rasa*, as Chasseguet-Smirgel has so persuasively argued. If the entire process laid out by Freud in terms of the child's biography vis-à-vis his parents can no longer be sustained, is it possible to speculate on how mothers and fathers have been displaced and their functions for identification has been, if not completely eliminated, severely altered? Is the Oedipus complex, as a traditional structure, less relevant than it used to be in part because one identification (with parents and society) is being replaced by a number of other fantasies and most especially the identification with our main political subjects – indeed, two together: the dead object of history and the fantasy of re-imagining the human body?

Freud has been no stranger to controversy, in his lifetime and long after. In "On the History of the Psychoanalytic Movement," he gave voice to a prevalent experience; not much has changed. He writes: "I have long recognized that to stir up contradiction and arouse bitterness is the inevitable fate of psycho-analysis" (SE 14:8). It would seem that the present allows us to further this situation and to present Freud's discoveries of a century ago and their utmost relevance for today. If we recall his support for the individual against all social pressures, his own self-evaluation is not without importance. Note the reference to *moral courage*.

> Since, however, my conviction and general accuracy of observations and conclusions grew stronger, and since neither my confidence in my own judgment or my moral courage were precisely small, the outcome of the situation could not be in doubt. I made up my mind to believe that it had been my fortune to discover some particularly important facts and

> connections, and I was prepared to accept the fate that sometimes accompanies such discoveries.
>
> (14:22)

The sense of his own accomplishment can be affirmed. More important that his personal intellectual satisfaction and his discoveries, we can at the present time add to a form of thinking that may not be self-evident: his discoveries and connections have *matured* and need to be presented in light of our current historical conditions. The analysis of a century ago have, today, become stark; the courage to confront them has also become more decisive. Freud's character ideals, courage and originality (both all-important in being independent from public opinion), are re-affirmed and during those moments in his arguments when they are most necessary.

In addition to both the unlimited expressions of the desire and the pathological controls of the super-ego, Freud also makes sure to again to emphasize our "higher nature," that is, the ego-ideals represented first of all by the parents and how we "took them into ourselves" (19:36). Far from being one-sided, he presents psychoanalysis as comprehensively as possible and as the description of the human, with all its vagaries. The "aberrations" he presented in the 1905 work on human, and especially infantile, sexuality, were to be transferred from one libidinal expression to another. As he approaches the end of III, "The Ego and the Super-Ego," he moves on and forward towards what will increasingly become the knowledge of an intense conflict between the ego and its ideal, "between what is real and what is psychical, between the external world and the internal world" (19:36). The terrible source of conflict for the human being (and most especially for the psychology of the political neurotic) will play itself out in the compulsive drive of the super-ego as it projects its ideal into the world in order to transform it through moral exactitude and a fierce projective imposition. The frequent references to religion are going to be more and more prevalent as Freud moves towards the writing of *The Future of an Illusion* and as the recognition of the psychology of religion being essential in an unconscious political disposition. The theological-political center of his argument, once the focus takes up our attention, proves to clarify a number of situations, for the individual and for society.

As we begin to think more about the pathology of the super-ego and its place in contemporary political sentiments, it is necessary to account for the process by which it exceeds its healthy function. For example, as many have stated and to differentiate the normal from the pathological superego: "it is only in severe pathological states that the superego perversely turns against itself."[16] How can we begin to examine these "severe" states; and when do they become *perverse* – soon to be discussed in the bind between masochism and sadism and therefore turned *both* against the self and against others? We are here forced to deal with a considerable problem: we can, with some optimism, believe in the pursuit of such ideals as justice, equality, and rights, just as we can commend all individuals who are led by their mature conscience. But we have reached a situation where the moderate expectations of individual conscience has become perverse and we are led to examine in what ways "pathological figurations of the super-ego"[17] become analyzable. The question to be specifically addressed, after the super-ego and the death drive are connected, will be on the specific nature of their relation and how they are manifested in political situations. "When we speak of the pathologic superego, in all probability we are imputing the occurrence of pathologic projective identifications onto a normal superego."[18] If the initial and many-times repeated ideas are correct, then it would seem that the transformation of the conscious aversion to religion, and the secular turn of liberal democracies, has been evident in the form of the present-day superego as a theological-political phenomenon. A "projective identification" is preceded by an introjection that will have long-lasting consequences.

Mentioning one of the processes of the super-ego, Freud outlines the normal chronology of its formation: "mastering the Oedipus complex itself, and social feeling through the necessity for overcoming the rivalry that then remained between the members of the younger generation" (19:37). While Freud has outlined a traditional resolution, the purpose of the analysis to come involves an examination of how the contemporary super-ego has been transformed due to the (at least) *partial* failure of dealing with the Oedipus complex and the relationships exhibited by the younger generation. In both cases, two failures have become more noticeable: on the one hand, a change in the nature of the Oedipus complex and in many cases an intense ambivalence towards both parents – with unconscious hate outweighing love (or respect) – and on the other hand a much more complicated rivalry now involving the social body of different groups who, each together and collectively are mounting an absolute opposition to the external world and to the reality of Western civilization. One symptom can be added to others. Individuals are now *re-naming themselves* as one characteristic of a displacement; they are, in other words, repudiating their origins and denying the reality of their mothers and fathers as *name-givers*. These are entirely genetic fantasies and privileges (in history) possible only for the divine and for the theological nature of revelation. The Greek word *hybris* comes to mind; its meaning, as form of "arrogance," is inadequate. We may well be seeing glimpses of the absolute narcissism of a primitive and infantile super-ego and its fantasy internalization of a possibility reserved exclusively for the divine and inaugural human beings – such as the man and woman whose names were *changed*, in Genesis, to Abraham and Sarah and who became founders of peoples. Have liberal activists gone as far as to presume, as part of an unconscious fantasy, to be mothers and fathers of *the arche* – a new beginning? The repudiation of a biological constant of the human is but one symptom of our times. The biology of the death drive has, ironically, asserted itself in a different (but not unrelated) way – not by aiming at constancy, but in sadistically destroying its being and compelled by a metaphysical desire to renew the human world of history and the body. We are witnessing the development of unprecedented social phenomena. Are we now in an epoch that will annihilate, in theory, both God and Darwin? Is the pathologically moral compelled by an unconscious fantasy to nullify both metaphysics and biology?

The traditional super-ego, developed in part on the introjection of a parental ideal and on the beneficial restraints of morality and regard for social life, has become self-possessed and unregulated by any standards. In part because of the shift towards an ever more determined secularism, the previous limits of religion have been consciously rejected, only to become much more effective as unconscious projections. Since, as Freud notes, "the ideal itself can to a great extent remain unconscious and inaccessible to the ego" (19:39), we now have the analytic insight to be able to trace how, because it remains unconscious, the ego-ideal can become relentless in its most adverse effects. The introduction of the death-drive will be one more component in the unfolding of Freud's social ideas.

It is all the more urgent to return to the relation between the super-ego and the death drive and to begin to recognize a highly ambivalent social and political situation now underway: at the same time as the politically motivated superego of groups is, from all appearances, committed to advancing social ideals, they are at the same time moving towards an unconsciously nihilistic goal. From the earliest days, the death drive has not been a welcome concept in psychoanalysis. The tendency has been to minimize its reality, in and out of the clinic. Does Freud indirectly ask us, today, to reconsider its role and, indeed, its centrality in social and political life? One distinction can serve us well. The section can conclude with a repetition: the sense of a mature conscience as opposed to the increasing tendencies of our contemporary morality. Throughout this section, only a few of the more outstanding examples were used by Freud – on the features of inordinate *number* of super-ego ideals and their *intensity*. Present-day psychoanalysts introduced a most difficult illness and one more severe than neuroses. Together, ideals could lead to a psychotic condition. Omnipotence and megalomania are effects that do not work in moderate conscience. "The normal superego can be distinguished from the pathological superego in the following way: it is concerned with nuanced moral judgment which takes reality and human consideration into account, rather than delivering absolute moral condemnation."[19] Judgment can be discerning; condemnation is absolute. The proper perception of reality is one condition of psychological health. One emerges from the work of a mature conscience; the other is projected as condemnation and to give itself the power of acting, against others, for its own benefit and to serve the ends of justice when, in appearance, it resembles retribution.

Stated otherwise, and to bring in Jacques Lacan during this transition, we can begin to frame one of our concerns in the following way: if the modern force of the super-ego morality is inseparable from its sadism, can we now provide *one interpretation* of Lacan's anticipatory conflict between "the ethics of psychoanalysis" and "the triumph of religion"? The conflict will be presented, as it has been from the beginning, as an unconscious religious drive displaced into the political sphere as a moral absolute and the work of psychoanalysis as the attempt to identify and, hopefully and eventually, bring the drive to conscious recognition. When Lacan, in the aptly named lecture "Discourse to Catholics," introduces "the difficulties psychoanalysis truly brings into play in ethics,"[20] we can further the overall point of the argument and, at and prior to any discussion of religion on its own, make the contentious claim that we can only come to the realization of the importance of the *ethics of psychoanalysis* when the malice of the super-ego and the death drive is identified and then *treated* as it should be. If we have recognized the power of the "destructive superego," should we not be focused on a project that makes the "emancipation from the superego"[21] our decisive goal? Ronald Britton has, in effect, aligned himself with Freud's project of human intelligence, freedom, creativity, and psychological well-being against two powerful forms of death-drive destruction, the cultural and the biological. How we can become free from a pathological and perverse super-ego and the increasing drive towards a cultural and biological destruction will remain our ongoing task. The question may not be, specifically, about how does one go about "subverting the superego"[22] but rather, in a classical dictum, how we can begin to think in a shift: "where the super-ego was." The option of a greater support for the ego may be preferrable as one way to contribute to growth instead of a regressive stasis.

As we anticipate a further examination of the death drive, Franco De Masi leaves us with a number of descriptions of a "difficult patient" who, for us, has become much more everyday and by being psychotic and functional. For the "über-moral" individual, a functional psychosis does not entail overwhelming incapacity since a different organization has taken place in the psyche.

> The superego's dependence on the destructive part of the personality impels the individual to embrace non life-affirming goals disguised as "moral" precepts. In this way, the pathological forces progressively dissolve the relationship with a human object, and construct in its place psychical structures – the psychopathological organization – that generate illusions in the patient, who is, thereby, seduced and captured by the promise of omnipotence.[23]

De Masi has been most insightful in making the connection between "non life-affirming" goals and their disguise as specifically moral precepts. The moral conceals the nihilistic; in turn, the psychopathological individual creates expedient illusions that only serve the overall sense of self-importance and, in its extreme form, the megalomaniacal omnipotence capable of making judgments that have all the force of phantasmatic theological verdicts. The death drive's involvement has been one of the factors that has made, in Freud's early formulation, severe and dangerous. How the death drive has become so overpowering can continue to be one aspect of the essay and to present it as doubled and aimed at the two objects we have so far identified.

If, Freud writes, "a perversion has the characteristics of exclusiveness and fixation – then we shall usually be justified in regarding it as a pathological symptom" (7:161). The immediate context of his observations, the section on "The Sexual Aberrations," should not mislead us and force us to restrict the field of our vision. The explicitly sexual is only one of the ramifications of how a perversion can be expressed. The most important factor, for us, comes in the sub-section of "the mental factor in the perversions." Once we can abstract ourselves from the early sexual context, then we can take one important statement that "the omnipotence of love is perhaps never more strongly proved that in such of its aberrations as these" (7:161). Omnipotence and aberrations of love. The consequences of this one recognition is as far reaching as the first intimations of a split psyche and its capacity for generating different levels of meaning. The *power* of love is so often, and idealistically, celebrated; psychoanalysis does not permit any indulgences in ideals. The perversions of love, when they are grounded in the psychical affects of the theological-political imagination, can turn into much worse than their mere opposite into hate. Once the aberrations of our capacity to love are transferred from the sexual to the theological-political, we have the making of a new understanding of Freud's outlook when it came to the social and political questions of the 1920s and for our situation today.

(f) The Double Death-Drive of Morality

Freud's elaboration of an entire system of depth-psychological thought has involved the creation of ideas that proved to be controversial both in his lifetime and after; among the most divisive (for both practicing psychoanalysts and others) has been the concept of the death drive at the same time as the new structural model of the psyche in *The Ego and the Id.* Dany Nobus, for example, describes the tripartite model of the psyche as an "infernal trinity."[24] *Infernal* brings us perilously close to a theological reference. Do theological metaphors indicate just how severe the super-ego can become? Could humanity be ultimately driven by two essential and inescapable characteristics – of life and death, of love and hate towards the ego and the objects of the world? Was it impossible to overcome a dualistic nature capable of compassion and aggression, often *at the same time*? Freud summed up how the place of the death drive in his "dualistic theory" had been received. Two instances are sufficient. In *Civilization and its Discontents*, he commented. "The assumption of the existence of an instinct of death or destruction has met with resistance even in analytic circles" (21:119). The word *resistance* is not chosen by chance. In a paper on technique, equally if not more importantly, he added: "I am well aware that the dualistic theory according to which an instinct for death or destruction or aggression claims equal rights as a partner with Eros as manifested in the libido, has found little sympathy and has not really been accepted even among psychoanalysts."[25] That psychoanalytic colleagues found the idea so difficult to accept must have led Freud to realize, not for the first time, just how unique his thinking, and discoveries, had always been; on this one issue, of a common relation between love and hate, Freud was beginning to reach another pinnacle in 1923. His power of observation, independence of mind, and creativity were as acute as ever. One senses no hesitation on *his* part. The responses, by others, have been innumerable and more intense than in the conflict about the role of the super-ego in the psychical reality of human beings as individuals, in a group, in society. Mentioning only a selected few gives us some idea of how the matter has not at all been settled; for my part, returning the death drive to a place of prominence is, today, a necessity despite the belief that, for some, "the death drive seems to have been killed, and long ago laid to rest, by North American psychoanalytic authors."[26] A euphemism is not a matter of indifference. Three deaths can be placed side by side: the primal father, the God of monotheism, the death drive – all of them killed and, apparently, "laid to rest," if not for Freud's reminders of remnants and how they persist all the more vigorously when they are presumed to be *resting*, in peace, or not, depending on attitude. The analysand and a reader continue to be conscious of each other, with and without metaphors. One cultural writer makes an intriguing connection. Anna Schaffner writes: "Freud's conceptualization of the death drive is the first great metaphysical theory of exhaustion."[27] We can add the German expression of *Weltschmerz*, a "world-weariness" that is inseparable from depression and an impoverished ego.

David Black's "Concluding Remarks" and his belief that "the death drive, as such, probably merits no future in psychoanalytic thinking"[28] seems, for him, final. However, the *as such* makes all the difference; because we are far from any consensus on how the death drive has been conceived and, for us, what its relevance may have most especially today. The opinions are many. "The theory of the death drive has met, *as we know*, with only very little success."[29] The "as we know" is too self-satisfied; and there are many ways to evaluate "success." One cannot expunge an idea from the whole out of discomfort or inability to consider what its implications may be in the long run.

Can "we" afford to ignore the death drive today? Our times makes the re-evaluation of the idea once again worthy of the most serious consideration, as long as a few arguments are first set out, starting with its *biological* foundation, which in itself is hard to reconcile with Freud's opening in *Beyond the Pleasure Principle* that "it is not advisable for us analysts to go into a problem further so long as our way is not pointed out by quite definite observations" (18:8). Jean Laplanche agrees: "to my mind, it [the clinical situation] is the yardstick for any theory of the drive."[30] The relationship in the analytic setting is more important than any speculations on their own; analytical free-associations and reflections are essential in the recognition of such a human drive prior to any attempt to provide a model for it, biological or otherwise, as essential or anomalous. The death drive was discovered, first of all, in the experiences of patients; neurotics showed (lived) the effects of Thanatos in their thoughts, in their perception, in their acts, to the detriment of their health and, it goes without saying, in the day-to-day life of those who experienced the affects firsthand, in the trying moment of personal relationships and a perpetual imbalance, of feelings and perceptions.

Despite this one obligation – to try to understand origins of the death drive for therapeutic reasons, and countering it with Eros, the psychoanalysis of love – the concept has, as Freud realized two decades later, met with perplexity. Claudia Frank's historical and conceptual evaluation leaves us with a responsibility; the definition of an "evil principle" is not hyperbole. "The concept of the death drive fostered and fosters misunderstandings."[31] Can some of our misunderstandings be overcome with a renewal of our effort in recognizing its effects and of minimizing its impact? Moderate or severe, there is no denying its force, first in the post-natal infant (as Melanie Klein showed with the graphic realism of fantasies) and for us today in society. In our case, with interests outside the clinical setting and with the emphasis on our social and political reality, the superego and the death drive will be considered for their complicity and, today, for their mutual (if seemingly) contradictory effects. A re-interpretation of the death drive can be attempted once the contemporary situation is perceived from a distinct perspective. The "dualism" and splitting could not be more stark: the categorical imperative of the super-ego, compelled by the loftiest of moral ambitions and the attempt to rectify the historical failings of civilization, are contributing to an intense form of aggression (that is both commanding and prohibitive) and a tendency towards a nihilist compulsion. Certain repetitions will be made again, for emphasis; some readers will be struck, in one way or another, that a highly moral epoch and an accompanying nihilism is difficult to accept as concurrent realities.

Assessing the literature on the death drive leads to one general position if not one decisive conclusion: far from any consensus on the existence or the practical outcome of the death drive, for its analytic power or its therapeutic relevance, the community seems to be irrevocably divided. The death drive cannot be consciously suppressed, just as it cannot be unconsciously repressed and be rid of. Amnesia will provide no comfort; consolations are not being offered and are not forthcoming. Before turning to the idea of the death drive as an explanation for many of our modern phenomena in the theological-politics of liberalism, a few comments to the detractors of the concept are going to be used as a starting point. Three reactions will be highlighted from many others. The death drive was first pronounced dead; it has also been called irrelevant and an unnecessary complication. One might perhaps be more analytic than usual and agree with the "antiquated nature" of the super-ego, but only because Freud had alerted us to its mythical origin among the collective of the primal horde. My earlier mention of the *primitive present* can be recollected. Our political groups appear to share many of the characteristics of the horde, the herd, and the present-day collective. "We wonder why a concept so central to the history of psychoanalytic theory and technique now seems be considered irrelevant."[32] Irrelevant by whom? The statement might be too one-sided and sweeping. One notable thinker who has made personal advances in the nature of religious origins in a dialogue with Freud, when asked about the death drive, answered curtly: "It's a good example of pointless complication. In my view the death drive exists, but it is entirely linked to mimetic rivalry."[33] The argument to come will respond to the dismissal of a "pointless complication" and show how the difficulty, for us, cannot be disavowed. The mimeticism and contagion of groups remains one observable grounding; in itself, rivalries are not enough to explain the issue, even as we first pointed out the relation between ego-ideal introjection and envy. While, as Freud has made clear, the rivalry is never absent (in part because of intense ambivalence towards the ego-ideal, as loved and hated, sacred as dead and profane in its decomposition), there are many other important factors that have to be presented within the whole range of the death drive's intrusion into reality. Rivalry is only one component of the whole. When the confrontation is specifically political and the contentious issue of "ideals," the death drive will take on considerable importance. Before doing so, a few more comments will not be in vain. Three further categories are necessary since they are, together, essential in working out of the problems of the concept and its meaning for us today. The strictly biological question is, understandably, first.

"Let us take the Freudian notion of the 'death-drive'. Of course, we have to abstract Freud's biologism: 'death-drive' is not a biological fact but a notion indicating that the human psychic apparatus is subordinated to a blind automatism of repetition," Slavoj Žižek writes.

> In this perspective, the 'death-drive', this dimension of radical negativity, cannot be reduced to an expression of alienated social conditions, it defines

> *la condition humaine* as such: there is no solution, no escape from it; the thing to do is not to 'overcome,' to 'abolish' it, but to come to terms with it, to learn to recognize it in its terrifying dimension, and then, on the basis of this fundamental recognition, to try to articulate a *modus vivendi* with it."[34]

A Freudian response has to immediately state the considerable difference between the idea of a constitutive death drive and its particular historical manifestation today. *The death drive is not historically constant*. It is impossible to consider the death drive's conditions as equal from one time to the next, from one epoch to another. The argument, here, is consistent with Freud's presentation: he has made it clear that, in the future, the super-ego and the death drive would begin to exhibit new and more intense characteristics. There is to be no *reconciliation* with today's death drive. The *modus vivendi* is impossible, as Žižek sees it, and because there are particular forces that are determining how life will be understood and lived. While we can, with Žižek, "learn to recognize its terrifying dimension," analytic work must then lead to both an individual response and, perhaps too, a modification of its effects and a lessening of its contemporary nihilistic tendencies. Otherwise, passivity and conformism becomes the rule. There can be no amicable relation between the ego and the imperious nature of the death drive. Once the drive has been separated from its biologism (but not from a re-interpretation of biology already alluded to) and Freud's ambition to align psychoanalysis with one view of science, we can begin to see its greater human relevance and the forms it takes as aggressive, destructive, and nihilistic. Freud's interest in social questions became more and more focused on the nature of human aggression and violence and a severe contradiction that should be one of our realizations from an especially political history: how do political ideals and utopian schemes so often lead to the most brutal kinds of events? How is the death drive towards the abolition of civilization merged into a total attack on the constancy of culture and nature?

"The introduction of the superego concept marked a substantial move away from a predominant interest in drive psychology and added a new dimension to the understanding of intrapsychic conflict."[35] Although the "intrapsychic conflict" can be emphasized, the equally important and still operative dynamic of the drives cannot be neglected. How has the relationship between the super-ego and the death drive allowed us to better understand the social and political symptoms of the times as they have organized a new (but not historically unknown) moral obsession? We can acknowledge the plan of *The Ego and the Id* as, *theoretically*, "an attempt at founding a scientific metapsychology"[36] while at the same time not forgetting Freud's motivations, which were not, simply, conceptual. We even have a suggestion of "the metaphysical drift of Freud,"[37] a correlation not to be easily dismissed since psychoanalysis is inseparable from "metaphysics" as an interpretation of human reality and from out of the conflicts of human interiority. The word metaphysics has become disreputable, in part because of certain preoccupations in late 20th-century philosophy. That one interpretation has not been, thankfully, conclusive, since an entire movement when the subject was denigrated almost to the point of extinction can be viewed, today, from the compulsions of its theoretical and destructive intentions, most especially when a certain malice against the ego (self-deceptively presented as an overcoming of René Descartes' subject) was psychological in nature. The omnipotence of philosophy was not averse to undermining itself as long as its theoretical power was confirmed and, more troubling, presumed to be "emancipatory." Rehabilitating the concept of the metaphysics, of *the ego*, is not out of the question *for* psychoanalysis since we could then recognize Freud for being a thinker of human reality and for alerting us, therapeutically (that is, for our psychological well-being) to the conditions we have ourselves devised. Our attempts to become free have had highly mixed results. We take the opportunity to once again make a distinction between the ego of psychoanalysis and the subject of society and its institutions, including the university. They are not the same. Metaphysicians are admittedly sophisticated; their theory has been, as the Greek *theoria* confirms, *spectacular*. Whether it has been illuminating (for the benefits of life) is an outstanding question. My deepening skepticism about the motivations of the university, as an increasingly moral institution, has not wavered. Freud, however, is incomparable for alerting us to the force of our unconscious and how projections can often transform the nature of reality – and ourselves in the process. One term, *jouissance*, has been a ruse. Academic *enjoyment* has come at a great expense. The price, in my estimate, has been much too high and mired in masochistic and sadistic imperatives. A re-thought metaphysics is an altogether appropriate concept to align, conceptually, with psychoanalysis since their mutual support will in principle make it possible to resist, as forcefully as possible, the movements of our society as they are now fatally committed to an impossible end. We can continue with the main argument and ask ourselves how the aggressive tendencies of the super-ego and the death drive have begun to reveal themselves in what, at first, should be utterly contradictory: why has the super-ego become so masochistic and sadistic precisely in the realm of morality and among the groups who are, apparently, so dedicated to the ideals of equality, justice, and rights? While they claim to be defending emancipation (*from what* and *for what* is not always clear despite their vociferous claims) the political groups of the day have created conditions antithetical to their intentions. The analysis at the moment then has to turn to how aggression and a not insignificant *psychical violence* has been operative for quite some time in Western culture and aimed at itself. The academic denigration of the subject opened an entire array of equally negative arguments in terms of perceiving the past; the groups clustered in this or that department is now an ideological *fait accompli*. The question of permanence will have to raised by those in and out of academic institutions.

Taking up one side of the equation, Uri Zilbersheid writes: "I wish to emphasize the fact that the activity of the super ego is the main activity of the destruction turned inwards."[38] The impulse towards destruction, however, does not remain limited to an internal process – against the ego. When Melanie Klein, in addition, said that "I have tried to show in various connections how destructive impulses, the expression of the death instinct, are first of all felt to be directed against the ego,"[39] the "first of all" does not end there. On the contrary, previous arguments have insisted on the ability of the specifically political neurotic to project the destructive drive toward the external world – which has been ideologically organized to be isolated and specific. Once the super-ego and the death-drive are brought together by Freud, the exclusive direction of the "turning" runs both ways, as the previous analysis of hysterical identification, introjection, and projection have shown. The drive moves back and forth and as needed. We notice, as a reaction to a masochistic trend, a destruction that is turned much more towards the external world, both to protect the introjected dead-object of the ego-ideal and to carry on the unsparing moral condemnation of reality. Otto Kernberg adds the second side of the equation and writes that "the unconscious formation of self-destructiveness is not simply destroying the self, but to destroy significant others as well."[40] Thc topic of masochism and sadism, which Freud would soon address in 1924, was conceptually necessary in order to understand the double-relation of the death drive.

It comes as somewhat a surprise, then, given Freud's presentation of aggression and the death drive and how it has been followed up to this point, that Jonathan Lear believes that "psychoanalysis lacks a *theory* of aggression."[41] The claim can be taken seriously only if the previous arguments, and the ones to come, are unsatisfactory; they may be, for some, incomplete, but they are not lacking. Lear's assertion is, for me, incomprehensible, more so when we realize how our contemporary situation has exemplified an excessive moral care with an equally pronounced aggression. A theory, if one is needed, can be framed from the realities of our times. The reality is demonstrable beyond any desire, or need, for a theoretical confirmation. Only Freud has allowed us to understand how moral aggression could be deceptively concealed and so missed almost entirely. The forms of aggression are, in any case, no longer hidden; neurotic thought and acting-out depends on being exhibitionistic at its core and intimidating, which morality can do without limits. Commenting on his early training as a psychoanalyst, in 1972, Howard Levine writes: "We were also taught that although aggression was one of two fundamental entities in the dual instinct theory, the death instinct was "only" a theoretical construct and did not have clinical applications of relevance."[42] A prevailing attitude was not without its source in Freud's own formulation;

the language of its reality was too closely associated with "instincts" and biology. The German *Todestrieb* can stand out. In order for aggression, the masochism-sadism relation, and the death drive to be explained in the context of a psychopolitical analysis, the references to biology have to be altered to reflect the conditions of our times. Any prior explanations now require some supplements. The prior allusion to metaphysics is not misplaced. Once the death drive is understood to be a metaphysical problem (that is, a total attempt to transform not only objective reality, but also the human body), its symptoms today can be more easily recognized; they are everywhere advertised with the greatest commitment, as if nothing less than freedom was at stake, with expectations for its fulfillment that are absolute. The current levels of anxiety, for example, can be explained in one way as the completely moribund projections of political groups who, one the one hand, make declarations about the most outlandish kinds of freedoms and, on the other, continue to add to the making of a super-moral society of prohibitions. The growing anxiety among the young can be understood more readily once we see how the morality of prohibitions and the ideals of "transgressions" are promoted side by side and with equal commitments. No one has yet pointed out their fatal contradiction, especially for the young who are forced to bear the force of ideological pressures and, due to the enthusiasm of elementary educators, forced to deal with promotional presentations. Our problems are not going to be surmounted by advertisements or liberal educational policies. Bureaucracies are busying themselves with the mere re-ordering of institutions, but "if one treats the discontent only with ideals, then the death drive and destructiveness will insidiously creep back."[43] The problem might, indeed, be far worse: treating perceived problems with ideals will, without a doubt, result in expected reactions. This is now the situation at hand. The ideals have roused the super-ego and the death drive with ever-increasing power.

The beginning of the elaboration of the death drive and "The Two Classes of Instincts" in *The Ego and the Id* can be called one of the more revolutionary advances in our knowledge of the human social animal and, for us more particularly, for our understanding of political life and the analysis of our *unbehagen*. The "instinct" of Eros, of sexuality and of life-affirmation, has long been central to psychoanalysis. "The second class of instincts was not so easy to point to; in the end we came to recognize sadism as its representative" (19:40). Our engagement with this most decisive of concepts for a psychopolitical essay will revolve around the *nature* of the death drive and how its "representative" cannot be limited to one manifestation, but rather comprises a masochistic-sadistic bind that will, when more fully examined, give us a sense both of its origins and, more importantly, a clearer view of the situation of the present. One obstacle will have to be overcome if Freud's developing ideas are to inform our contemporary situation. We can only fully understand the introduction of the super-ego and the death drive once the construction of the system is consciously unified so that, as a start, the preceding arguments on group psychology (on hysterical identification and its relations) are brought forward into the current discussion. The hysterical identification, introjection, and projection of the dead victim of history cannot be separated from the attempt to unconsciously repeat a prior historical epoch and the attempt to alter its reality, *then* and now. The futility of such an endeavor – to somehow overcome, as an example, the past of Western history – will only result in further suffering by everyone concerned and most especially by a trend that today has become a growing phenomenon, that is, the imposition of guilt on those deemed responsible: *everybody* whose origins are, in one way or another, connected to one geographical location.

A brief recollection of the concept of projection from *Beyond the Pleasure Principle* should be sufficient to give us a sense of Freud's ideas. Older impressions are sustained and given a place in the whole. In one of the discussions of the pleasure/unpleasure relation, he writes:

> First, the feelings of pleasure and unpleasure (which are an index to what is happening in the interior of the apparatus) predominate over all external stimuli. And secondly, a particular way is adopted of dealing with any internal excitations which produce too great an increase of unpleasure: there is a tendency to treat them as though they were acting, not from the inside, but from the outside, so that it may be possible to bring the shield against stimuli into operation as a means of defense against them. This is the origin of *projection*, which is destined to play such a large part in the causation of pathological processes.
>
> (18:29)

The connection between pathology and projection has to be considered from its affective condition of pleasure/unpleasure and from the prior discussion on the super-ego. The *Ego and the Id* is building a more systematic presentation based on that one relation. The pathology of the super-ego is not evident in the individual excesses of conscience but rather in the extreme moral demands of groups and, perhaps surprisingly, their success in so manipulating the self-consciousness of an entire society. The drive of the super-ego is sadistic and cruel and in proportion to the masochism of the political actor who, unable to tolerate incommensurable perceptions, determines the entire world to be morally unfit.

While the mechanism of the death drive has been in part alluded to, it is now necessary to be much more specific about its political implications. The identification, introjection, and projection, as long as it was masochistically experienced, was in a sense the building up of affective power in order to better project it into the reality of the world. How does the projection of the *politically manifest* neurotic conceal psychical characteristics that need to be more fully exposed? Finally, how are these traits, as pathological, put at the disposal of the most intense drive of all – the one towards, first, a masochistic-sadistic relation and, second, the drive towards aggression, psychological if not physical violence? Freud's formulation immediately puts us in a position of responding. "On the basis of theoretical considerations, supported by biology, we put forward [in *Beyond the Pleasure Principle*] the hypothesis of a death instinct, the task of which is to lead organic life back into the inanimate state" (19:40). Since the biological "support" has been set aside (because the death drive is an ontological and *metaphysical* problem) it is necessary to disconnect the death drive from any and all biological explanations unless they are explicitly related to a phenomenon that Freud himself could not consider, that is, the psychopolitical death drive of the biological body. Our earlier intimations of the unprecedented hostility towards the nature of the Oedipus complex is today more and more in evidence. Are a fraction of political neurotics so filled with self-loathing that they are pursuing the extraordinary desire of nullifying the reality of *their parents*? The death drive has reached its apotheosis. The forces of the theological-political, as apocalyptic, are compelled by an exclusive principle.

Freud's movement in the direction of a "physiological" explanation has no bearing on what is to follow; contemporary conditions, however, allow us to consider the biology of the death drive in a new way. All kinds of references, for example, to an instinct being active in "every particle of living substance" is much too speculative to be of any help in the analysis of psychopolitics whose reality needs no such biological description. While the first thesis is fully accepted – that Eros and Thanatos are inter-related in a perpetual conflict – *in politics* the relation has little if anything to do with biology except insofar as we are, indeed, a political animal today caught between two formidable realities. Our death drive is not biological insofar as it is grounded in the argument of constancy, but rather the anguished realization of the condition of our terrestrial existence – as human animals. How the two are to be conceived, for the future, remains a pressing issue. The recollection of projection from *Beyond the Pleasure Principle* gives us an immediate direction of thought; the force of an internal conflict, re-activated during regression and indicative of infantile and primitive impulses, has returned with effect. Freud realized that "the death instinct would thus seem to express itself – though probably only in part – as an instinct of destruction against the external world and other organism" (19:41). When Freud reaches this position, then it was a matter of time before the destruction turned inwards and outwards could be taken from its first intimation in the sexual sphere and applied to the conditions of social life. The perversions of sexual life could easily be turned towards social and political ends.

Freud's continued attempts to find a physiological explanation for the concurrent expressions of love and hate are, to stress the point, now modified in our psychopolitical essay. Once his interpretation of a death drive aimed at civilization, it became easier to concentrate on the presence of aggressiveness and violence in the psyche and in its projection into the external world. The present attitude towards history may be one of the most unprecedented symptoms of today's drive and one inseparable from the antipathy towards Western culture. One problem remains outstanding. At the moment, he acknowledges the sadistic elements within Eros. The aggression and sadism seem to reveal, as Freud admits, a fundamentally "dualistic point of view." How, then, can we account for the co-existence, and the mutual dependence, of Eros and the death drive when its relevance seems to be precise in the realm of society and its divided politics. The 1924 "The Economic Problem of Masochism" gives us one possible answer as well as preparing for other elaborations to appear, soon, in *The Future of an Illusion*.

It was impossible to fully realize the extent of the death drive during Freud's lifetime and even long after; but we are now in a position to understand just how much foresight he did have and how the biology of the death drive would be noticed only when a social movement aggressively attempting to repudiate the Oedipus complex would, inevitably, make its appearance in social life concurrently with a *super-morality*, a concept he once again uses in "The Economic Problem of Masochism." Freud analyzed the *coming* neuroses of culture. Adding one more component to the whole, the bind of masochism and sadism will give us an additional portrait of the political neurotic of our time and how his afflictions are increasingly contagious in liberal democracies. We will see how one impression of the sadistic impulse, what Freud calls "instinct for mastery" (SE 12:322), once its power comes into effect in the realm of the political, it soon exhibits all too well-known symptoms – that is to say, the pleasure of the cruelty inherent in the *control* over people's lives and, as Oscar Steinbach reminds us, the limits on their freedom – above all, of being able to express contrary views and unpopular ideas.[44] The expression "*beg* to differ" has become all-too real. So has the refusal. There are no psychopolitical alms to be had. We are, as can be expected, confronting the problem of *power* and from those who are weak and vulnerable and have made themselves into victims and therefore justifiably enraged and fully permitted to act out as they see necessary. Whether a new set of ideals can be introduced into the university and into the thought in general of entire societies is now more than ever necessary, for unless the psychoanalytic and the metaphysical ideals of freedom and intelligence, love and creativity and mental health are not, at least, restored as a human reality, the unfolding of the 21st century may prove to be filled with a set of destructive principles for our common human experience. Jeffrey Rubin has a reminder for us; coming halfway through the examination of *The Ego and the*

Id is appropriate given the difficult arguments to come on the bind of masochism and sadism. Once the symptoms are identified and the pathology of our current psychopolitical situation is presented, there will be more than sufficient opportunity to turn to Freud and to re-affirm the still active human values and the relation of "psychoanalysis and the good life."[45] The burden of our diagnosis has not precluded finding our way, by the end (close to our termination) at a much more open and free future. In the meantime, however, we have to continue to affirm our allegiance to the psychoanalytic project, as conceived by Freud, and to make his considerable work more relevant for our contemporary situation. "If psychoanalysis is destined to prosper and advance, it must be open to revisiting controversial ideas that gave it radical prominence to begin with."[46] Given my argument from the beginning and the sense of powerful initiatives well underway – which have been described as "the suicidal tendencies of the West"[47] – continuing with an interpretation of Freud's work in the 1920s may make it still possible to overcome the dual threat of the super-ego and the death drive and its expression in the impulses of masochism and sadism. The ethos of the analysand and the reader, conscious of positive transferences, remain essential in the reflections to come.

(g) The Masochistic-Sadistic Bind

The conclusion of "The Economic Problem of Masochism" sums up one of the three forms Freud analyzes and the one he concentrates on more than others – *moral* masochism. That he uses a term we have emphasized before as it exceeds the proper boundaries of conscience, the effect of an "ultra-morality" (19:169), takes us to one more development of his thinking during the 1920s. Isolating Freud's previously used word, *danger*, gives us an impression of a consistent argument.

> Moral masochism becomes a classical piece of evidence for the existence of fusion of instinct. Its danger lies in the fact that it originates from the death instinct and corresponds to the part of that instinct which has escaped being turned outwards as an instinct of destruction. But since, on the other hand, it has the significance of an erotic component, even the subject's destruction of himself cannot take place without libidinal satisfaction.
> (19:170)

The masochism-sadism relation, moving back and forth from the individual to the world as an unconscious projection, perpetuates a binding system (the "fusion") whereby the introjected ego-ideal induces pain and guilt while also making it possible, and expedient, to release the affect destructively in the form of retribution. Our earliest presentation of mourning and melancholia remain in effect; for as we continue to hold on to "the important relation between masochism and depression,"[48] the melancholia is also experienced by the individuals in groups whose conscience has not been atrophied to the point of non-effect. The economic explanation for a pleasurable masochism can be understood when the dead ego-ideal provides all the justification necessary for the unleashing of destructive aggression towards reality and others. The pleasure comes from moral power experienced in the social sphere. External judgment mitigates internal shame and guilt. One can inflict pain-free cruelty, without conscience and justified judiciously while at the same time attaining the status of moral superiority. "Masochism appears to us in the light of a great danger" (19:159), Freud writes, again using a language of an impending threat. The danger is not only to the self but to society as a whole; the greatest danger is for others since the regression can access the most archaic of impulses, including the most serious ones as weapons of power.

The previous discussion of the biologism of the death drive and the need to re-interpret its significance remains in effect in Freud's essay; for when he introduces the "Nirvana principle" and how it is "entirely in the service of the death instincts, whose aim is to conduct the restlessness of life into the stability of the inorganic state" (19:160), the prior introduction of a *metaphysical* principle is essential in understanding the ultimate desire of the group. The political neurotic is motivated by a death drive that would like to nullify the conditions of physical existence and therefore repudiate the facts of life – of the history of civilization and its continuity in the reproduction of tradition and by the succession of generations in history. While moral masochism *begins* with feelings of guilt and from the demands made by the dead super-ego ideal, the pleasure experienced by the release of moral retribution is felt to be libidinally satisfying as it produces the relation of legitimate judgment and a perpetual sense of entitlement as a compensation. Identification confers moral wealth, which becomes a renewable resource from the economic point of view of the psyche; although the process is circular and never resolved, masochist guilt and sadistic judgment are compensatory. Status, once achieved at the level of material prosperity, wealth, and property in its various examples, has been achieved at the moral level and because of what it confers on the self, multiplied when it is shared by a group identity. The theological-political imagination fosters a moral collectivity.

Theological-political movements are making significant incursion into the understanding and the efficacy of a private justice administered by those who have identified themselves as capable, as if elected, of passing judgments. The confluences of psychical operations are symmetrical and ideologically persuasive since the majority appear to be either persuaded by the projection of this reality or so manipulated as to be unable to respond in any way except acquiescence. It will be necessary, in an upcoming section, to add to the masochist-sadistic relation and to define the nature of our contemporary theological-political perversions; and though we have not been interested in applying our analysis to specifically sexual behaviour (which, given the sexual mores of the times, requires an extensive but separate analysis) we should at least mention the problem of perversion beyond the eccentricities of sexual acts. For just as the exhibitionist, for example, acts out fantasies of his desire and, aggressively so, without considering either the consciousness or the desire of his "audience," the political neurotic acts out an entire system of many-faceted perversions without considering how individuals in society may not reciprocate (express the same desire) and in fact find themselves not at all identifying either with their sense of self or aspiration. The ceaseless promotion of identities are, for many, an indifferent reality. For the vast majority of people, and citizens, morality is in fact not a day-to-day issues when it comes to the ideals of social justice; personal ethics are more immediate and require some care and attention. The public as a whole, however, has no status because of the ongoing mechanism of contemporary politics; and yet one can understand how, with so much advertisement, the susceptibility and contagion is an ongoing temptation. Becoming a member has its attractions and benefits. Submission is easier than opposition.

Freud continues to make quite remarkable observations; understood politically, they are pointed. "We shall not be surprised to hear that in certain circumstance the sadism, which has been directed outwards, projected, can be once more introjected, turned inwards, and in this way regress to its earlier situation" (19:164). Can we call this an infinite regress and one more piece of psychical knowledge added to the rest and since our beginning in the regression of group psychology? In an essay of 1924, Karl Abraham wrote: "The important instinct of sadism, as it exists in the infantile libido, also shows in two opposite pleasurable tendencies at work. One of these tendencies is to *destroy* the object (or the external world) the other is to control it."[49] *Destruction and control*: these two mutual impulses can continue to be part of our psychopolitical essay insofar as the moral control by the super-ego and the destruction by the death drive can now be understood within the context of a *circular* masochistic-sadistic bind involving inner and outer machinations. The circle is structurally closed and very difficult to impede in its movement or to break altogether. The defense of a closed system has to be perpetuated.

The "infantile libido," operating unconsciously in the politically motivated individual and various group, has been preserved as a remnant from an archaic source and from a particular set of pre-Oedipal experiences. The movements outlined from the beginning are each inter-related processes and determined by several factors. Can we now develop our earlier observations into a continuing unity, as Freud did, and with a phenomenon that we can more readily witness today? Will the theological-political nature of our liberal societies also reveal an undercurrent of masochism and sadism, each impulse, and its symptoms, recognizable in its effects? What could compel the individual (a group and, indeed, an entire culture) to so drive itself towards a sense of prevailing dissatisfaction and misery? What has compelled the fixated and obsessed individual and group to experience such negative emotions as rage and resentment? What internal pressures could act so decisively *against life* and lead the human individual (and, more seriously, entire societies) towards its own repeated anguish and self-destruction unless some enticing benefit could be identified, one that could be guaranteed to be a renewable, and infinite, source of perverse pleasure? More particularly, what are the reasons for an entire movement in today's liberal democracies towards the implementation of moral policies which, when more fully (that is, unconsciously) examined, shows traces of both sadism and masochism? Can we see a new kind of political gratification? Institutionalized incentives for the propaganda of shame and guilt are rampant. Shame and guilt is being imposed on society and with a universal *mea culpa*, with the demand of contrition as a permanent condition so as to weaken and deplete the ego even more.

To the questions above, Freud has a number of answers: connected to the nature of the introjected ego ideal, a certain relationship has become inviolable. Our familiar "ghosts" have indeed returned. "The super-ego retained essential features of the introjected persons – their strengths, their severity, their inclination to supervise and to punish" (19:167). All the previously mentioned theorists who invoked the reality of the "return of the religious" were, it seems, misled by a deceptive appearance – one strictly defined by the traditions of theology. The manifest appearance of religion was too closely observed; the concentration of perception, so apparent, severely narrowed the field of vision. The return has been, much more profoundly than a historical phenomenon – the theological or the political *on its own* – an antecedent psychological infantilism and primitivism that has been perversely collaborative in the splitting of the contemporary psyche. The super-ego and the death drive have been unconsciously able to unify two historical phenomena and instrumentally use them for their own ends. The more *only one* was perceived, the better it could conceal its necessary connection. The "introjected persons" have indeed been ghostly because they have been dead; their enforced resurrection has created one more element of the theological-political affect within individuals and their associations with groups. One significant change in the process of human development has been radically altered. An accomplishment has turned into the greatest danger. At one time, *prior* to the emergence of a theological-political epoch, "the course of childhood development leads to an ever-increasing detachment from parents, and their personal significance for the super-ego recedes into the background" (19:168). In the past, such a transition was an accomplishment reached by most individuals as a matter of course; today, however, it has led to the entire range of psychical processes we have outlined, with repetitions, up until now and from the starting point of a regression that is much more than a "detachment" from parents but their repudiation and substitution by the introjected dead ego-ideal. The movement from the identification with parents to the emergence of the super-ego has been deviated.

The connection between his social and political writings of the 1920s and the almost exclusive attention to the training of analysts was no coincidence. There was, for Freud, only one way to resist the drive of the perverted human: the training of analysts could at least make one real, if very private, difference in the life of individuals. *His* response to the inevitable increase in the neurotic afflictions of an entire society could only be offset with his full professional commitment: on the one hand, to present his diagnosis, on the other, to offer the only viable solution – the training of more analysts for the difficult and necessary therapeutic work to come. Freud saw himself, and psychoanalysis, as a system of thinking and life that, with enough commitment to its own ideals, could minimize and perhaps substantially transform the worsening symptoms. We should not be surprised in the least, and certainly not be cynical, when Freud soon begins to think and discuss the problem of human happiness; unless we recognize him for his deep commitment to the overall condition of humanity, psychoanalysis will be regarded incompletely and, according to its critics, with ongoing misperceptions.

When Freud uses three different descriptions to characterize the death drive – its destruction, instinct for mastery, or the will to power – we have moved, almost seamlessly, towards a much more direct awareness of the inter-related phenomena of politics and in the manipulation (or, to anticipate Freud's repeated word) *coercion* of individuals. Destruction, mastery, and power: each of them are part of a chronology and a fantasy for the future where culture and the human body will be newly created and from the unconscious exerting greater pressure on reality. His early consideration of the masochistic-sadistic bind has been on his mind, for social reasons, since "Instincts and their Vicissitudes." It was in a work on "*Triebschicksale*," on the *fate* or *destiny* of the strongest, most dangerous drives, that he remarked: "sadism consists in the exercise of violence or power upon some other person as object" (14:127). Once the violence and power could be deployed non-physically – without, that is, the heavy-handed tactics of typically totalitarian methods – it could then be much more effectively spread, through propaganda in the creation of moral liberal order. The super-morality can no longer proceed without accountability, not when Freud has so easily exposed its motives and methods. The biological understanding of the death drive has been replaced by a much more insidious political phenomenon; the biology was, after all, extremely accurate – but for different reasons that other psychoanalysts would have to reach (and, not surprisingly) when dealing with children, as did Klein. Far from the self-impulsive drive towards individual dissolution, the political death drive aims at the destruction of the old and the traditional and the historical in order to assert its mastery of a new foundation of reality. Reality will be created anew. Its aim is the annihilation of a consciousness of a culture and its substitute by debasement and a continuous self-recrimination, such that nothing positive or meaningful can be found in the efforts at making a world as it has been handed down. Civilizations are not made by the fainthearted nor by moral sensibility. As it happens, the everyday citizen who does not suffer from these neurotic afflictions (the guilt of territorial expansion and the movement of dominant civilization – that is, precisely how the world and empires have been made since time immemorial, *pace* post-colonialists) is made to endure the acrimony of the political neurotic who has found the most adequate field for the projection of a perpetual ambivalence, both a self-loathing and an aggressive and hostile hatred for anyone deemed to be culpable for a primordial crime: the creation of human civilization. The tradition of Oedipal "detachment" and acceptable resolution has been completely transformed by a new set of desire and fantasies. The once separate realms of the cultural and the natural, so irreducible, are now threatened by the attempt at a "revolutionary" break that is making the omnipotent attempt to transcend both simultaneously. Previous references to the death drive towards the biological, sexual, procreative body can be presented in an analysis by Melanie Klein and with a depth that requires to be understood from its individual expression to its effect on society. The nature of the "primal scene" as described by Klein can be interpreted from the foundations of our argument. She writes: "At its period of maximal strength, the child's sadism is centred around coitus between his parents. The death-wishes he feels against them during the primal scene or in his primal phantasies are associated with sadistic phantasies which are extraordinarily rich in content and which involve the sadistic destruction of parents both singly and together."[50] The "destruction of parents" can now be understood, in the context of the 21st-century fantasies of the human body, as the nihilistic repudiation of the parents in so far as they have been, individually, as a couple, a mother and a father, at the origin of the birth of the child and, more universally, the grounding examples of the continuity of civilization. Psychoanalysts are unmatched in their observations. "The potential for the perverse is not only borne from supplanting the genital father, from stripping him of significance or from destroying him, but also from a setting dominated by a non-genital father."[51]

Michael de M'Uzan, not without first asking, ironically, for permission, then followed by a pun, writes: "If I may so, the death instinct is alive and well."[52] Its "liveliness" has not made *us* very healthy. We return to responses only to be aware of how difficult the problem has been that Freud left us with. Other psychoanalysts have not hesitated to develop the ideas most necessary for our present consciousness. The hypothesis of the death drive has shown itself to be observable. "This is a hypothesis, a speculation, which would eventually impinge upon and modify the fundaments of Freudian metapsychology and create innumerous controversies."[53] The controversy has not been avoided. To mention only a few gives us more than an indication of how much onerous reaction can be expected.

The masochistic-sadistic bind will no longer be the extravagant indulgences of erotic individuals in the privacy of their acts – or their public spectacles of exhibitionism in the political realm. The whole of reality reflecting masochistic-sadistic principles of morality will be as severe as only Freud could have imagined it. Is this not the reason why he turned to his analysis of religion as a *screen* for politics and one of the reasons he had made several references to Kant's categorical imperative, of the super-ego, and recognized it for its compulsion to become a "dictatorial 'Thou shalt'" (19:55) and with the Soviets as his unique and repeated example? The dictatorship of morality is no longer hyperbole. The situation, especially now, is no cause for a dispirited resignation or the acceptance of an understandable pessimism. If, at this point, when the masochistic-sadistic bind has been identified as one of the many phenomena of the theological-political situation at hand, psychoanalysis must assume its responsibility with renewed and unfailing commitment. The analysand can once again take his place as an opponent of the political activist and on the principal virtues we began with: freedom and intelligence, love and creativity. Jonathan Sklar writes: "The examination of impediments to social freedom has parallels with the process of developing states of mental freedom… … Such complex matters include the need for the analysand to find new ways of expression."[54] While we have not always recognized the analysand for his ability to be independent from social movements (he should, after all, be capable of recognizing the mechanisms of self-deception and many other associated defenses) in this case we can be unwavering. The analysand has to declare his opposition to the theological-political initiatives of the times and most especially when they are guided by nihilistic values. An analysand, a scholar, a reader: he has an obligation to bring psychoanalysis into the heart of the matter and to defend the history of civilization as represented by the individuals who contributed to the continuity of culture and life.

The moral masochist-sadist is caught in a binding situation; and with one element now to be added to the rest. The experience of anxiety is consistent with the sense of self being unable to meet the expectations of the introjected ego-ideal. How could it? The ego-ideal is dead, and the process of mourning is perpetual and can never be resolved. The homage to the dead never suffices, not even when the supposedly sacred has become idolatrous. Mourning, anxiety, depression; the malaise of the political neurotic must be exceedingly painful; and the result is the particular enjoyment of the masochist and sadist who revolves in a private and recurring set of fantasies. Despite the complications of the masochistic pleasure of the political neurotic, the sadistic trend also finds its adequate expression. The introjected dead victim represents the symbolic justification for any persecution and destruction of others.

Parenthetically, and to raise a brief theological point, in the past notions of forgiveness (and mercy) were essential to the religious imagination. Today, in our secular condition, forgiveness has been eradicated from political consideration since it would interfere with the continuity of justified rage and reaction. There is one significant difference today than in the past. Freud believed that the super-ego "came into being through the introjection into the ego of the first objects of the id's libidinal impulses – namely, the two parents… … The super-ego retained essential features of the introjected persons – their strengths, their severity, their inclination to supervise and to punish" (19:167). One significant modern transformation has been presented; our changed historical circumstances in the 21st century requires added analyses. The introjection of the dead historical victim has, in many cases, displaced the parents in the psychical economy of the individual. The identification with the parents has, for many different reasons, undergone a radical shift and in many cases has been, if not completely severed, mutilated. The identification with any parent, father or mother, man or woman, has been severely compromised. The very tempered idea expressed by Thomas Ogden about parents who are "lovingly murdered"[55] is, today, much more than an oxymoron or irony. The political neurotic is at the present time in a situation of near psychical destitution – a stranger to himself, cut off from parental identification, and severely alienated from a despised society as a reflection of the earliest relationship with all objects outside the self. "The super-ego – the conscience at work in the ego – may then become harsh, cruel and inexorable against the ego which is in its charge." If the super-ego could be restricted to its relationship to the ego, then the difficulties would, perhaps, be less severe, for the individual and for everybody else. As the situation stands, the harsh cruelty of the individual's super-ego has turned against the external world and anyone in it who is deemed to be responsible for the dead victim – of history and of one's introjection. As the representative the three moral categories Freud outlined previously in his "Postscript" (justice, equality, and rights) the contemporary super-ego has managed to coalesce into the collective identity of many different kinds of groups; and though each of them may be rivals in their desire to be recognized, together they have created a social condition where any independence from group psychology has led to a more decisive separation than the one imagined by political thinkers in terms of *classes*. Despite not identifying with any group, the individual is under enormous pressure to agree and conform and live in accordance with the new directives being established as a matter of policy in private and public institutions. In many ways, because the changes are being accomplished in the name of the greater good, their dangers have not been completely revealed; they are simultaneously enforced and accepted – at least silently, with a pretended conformism but also not without increased suspicion and distrust. But if the cultural signs of liberal democracies are analyzed for their sadistic and destructive tendencies, then we can be certain that recent trends – which are more than a half-century in the making – are bringing us closer to the remarkable overhaul of Western culture, including the partial destruction of its libraries in the name of "de-canonization." Civilization has never been more loathed. It seems to be that only psychoanalysis offers both the most in-depth thinking of all the various symptoms of our times and the presentation of human ideals Freud has promoted and defended from the beginning. As we continue to move forward with the final section of *The Ego and the Id* and ahead to the two great works in the later half of the 1920s, we can anticipate a vigorous defense of the human despite the on-going cultural assault by those who believe they are creating a good, a better, a more perfect world.

Although Freud and psychoanalysis have been original in providing us with the interpretative concepts for our understanding, the contemporary situation allows us to be more specifically directed. The earlier and brief mention of sexual perversions, as such, are not relevant. The focus, for us, has to be strictly addressed to the perverse distortion of reality and how the three-part psychical condition of the group leads to a form of perversion – that is, perception that can only be absolute and that sadistically repudiates nothing less than what Stanley Ruszynski calls the "facts of life," the ones already defined as constitutive of terrestrial existence. The very worst of our human capacities are extended when theological-political sadism is unified in the misinterpretation of reality and the expression of domination, control, and the deprivation of human subjectivity. We continue to support the development of human intelligence while, with Freud, make ourselves aware of social manipulation. "What is deadly about the death instinct is the way in which meaning, and specifically difference, is attacked, resulting in the retardation of the development of the thinking psychological self."[56] We can no longer hesitate with a possible diagnosis of the extreme hatred for, precisely, "the facts of life" as they are ideologically driven today. The argument continues to be pressed, and in a work provocatively titled *The Triumphant Victim*. No resignation or pessimism can be accepted when psychoanalysts do not hesitate in exposing the danger of our times. "The issue of sadomasochism is central to a much deeper issue and which the quality of life – even the survival of civilisation – depends."[57] *The survival of civilisation*: the statement is grave. Can the apprehension be justified when the theological-political reality of our times has relied on one set of symptoms, the sadomasochistic, and in the associated neurosis of the gain from illness?

(h) The Social and Political Gain from Neurotic Illness

The opening of the last chapter of *The Ego and the Id* gives Freud the opportunity, as is so often the case, to alert the reader to the method of his exposition; although he has been aware of the individual expression to everything he has written, a turning-point can be witnessed that, by the time of

The Future of an Illusion, will be more fully active. His future writing will have greater expectations, for himself and for his readers. The "excuse," here, seems strategic. "The complexity of our subject-matter must be an excuse for the fact that none of the chapter-headings of this book correspond to their contents" (19:48). That will be especially true for V, "The Dependent Relationships of the Ego," and one feature in particular that requires extra attention: its psychical reality (for the present) can be analyzed as the cultural culmination of the three previous sections and as one more example, perhaps the most serious, of the masochistic-sadistic relation and everything he has been presenting, as a unity, once the shifts from one individual to the group were followed. First alerting us, in *On Narcissism*, to "all the dangers of a crippling dependence," he goes on to add that "the ego ideal opens up an important avenue for the understanding of group psychology" (14:101). *All the dangers of a crippling dependence*; the diagnosis is made with a certain amount of gravity, which is precisely the reason he had to return to the theme and explain its origins, mechanisms, and consequences. The preoccupations with the dangers of the group, as a political body, are still foremost in his mind; the narcissism was not solely individual. The convictions, as to the severity of the symptoms for groups, became more than guiding principles of his thinking. One senses a deeper commitments to psychoanalysis as a discipline, of understanding and therapy, uniquely capable of confronting the most deeply-rooted conflict in societies and most especially in the individual (his creative poet of myths) whose internal force and independence fostered the possibility of a lasting creativity. His mythic poet, who is creative and original because of his particular relationship to his time and society, can be highlighted as the complete opposite of the individuals in groups who have turned many illnesses into virtues. Has the drive of liberal societies inflicted all kinds of neurotic illnesses on as many people as possible, most especially the young, in order to profit from the gain of vulnerability, weakness, and hurt? The *gain from illness* is well-known as one more piece of psychoanalytic knowledge; can an individual disposition be developed, politically, for an entire society? Are we obligated to consider how a neurosis of a society may be both perversely pleasurable (and as perpetuated by a masochistic-sadistic bind) ideologically exploitable? Has the super-ego, among its other effects, produced a culture of traumatism? What could be more dangerous, for a doctor, than a patient – or a society as a whole – taking pleasure in an illness and actually exploiting it for its considerable benefits? Freud sought an answer to one more counter-intuitive condition. The traumas of war were one phenomenon. "And the same is true of neurotics in civil life. They complain of their illness but exploit it with all their strength."[58]

Returning to arguments already established in group psychology and then furthered because of the tripartite division in the psyche, Freud remained concentrated on the character of the super-ego; once he returned to the infant and the stasis of regression and tells us that the super-ego is formed through its identification "which took place while the ego was still feeble," the political consequences are inestimable for our present situation. The foundations are "feeble" – recalling one of the earlier theories of *Group Psychology* – because infantile and primitive. Freud always returns us (as the therapeutic technique of analysis demands) to the earlies experiences of childhood and how, more importantly, they are never overcome or forgotten as unconscious feelings and dispositions. The persistence of the psyche can, because infantile and primitive, overpower the rationality of a possible maturity. Processes leading to growth can be severely stunted. The circular process inherent in regression, previously defined as infinite, maintains a certain stability. Defenses endure and become more determined with the passing of time; the regression, once frenetic as it sought relief from internal and external pressures, settles and hardens. The feebleness of the infantile period of human life, so dependent, so fragile (and so aware of the fact) accounts for so much of the difficulties of the adult and, more comprehensively, social and political life for everyone. We have an infantile and primitive regression that, once embodied in the split super-ego, was fully organized to exploit all the power of a theological-political situation. How can we continue to develop all the interrelationships of a regressive psyche when it has also been determined by the morality of the death drive and the bind between masochism and sadism? The ideology of liberal democracy is unconsciously *salvific*; but whereas, in the past, human beings were defined according to "sin," they are now categorized, on the one hand, in line with various illnesses that have to be treated with social circumspection.

If we realize how the super-ego has re-directed the enfeebled ego to serve its ends, and to mete out punishment internally and externally, we can better understand one other psychoanalytic idea as a supplement to only a few of the most important ideas in *The Ego and the Id*: the gain from illness, a masochistic pain evenly (equally) distributed among everybody in society as a form of sadistic *equality*. Everyone will be made ill without prejudice or favour; equality will be become real and through all the losses Freud previously outlined. We can complement the idea of the pleasure in the gain from illness from its instrumental use. Illness has been produced; social neuroses have settled into their proper role. Today it serves a highly important function; and it prevents, most important of all, any real or lasting cure. The political neurotic has become a bureaucratic *administrator* of illness and guilt. Are we to put forward the argument that, perversely, the theological-political relationship of the liberal psyche has led to the acceptance of a widespread illness, forms of debilitation we have seen increase only in the last few decades – and with forms of withdrawal exhibiting classical form of psychic neurasthenia? The present condition of a controlling super-ego has led to the severity of the moral principles and the gradual and simultaneous control/destruction of the ego – that is, in conformity to the death-drive which is now a two-pronged operation: to render the ego as weak as possible and so incapable of resistance, or to consider its own re-affirmation, and to make the super-ego the single most powerful psychical agency. One relationship, which has been stated time and again but with my argument on the particular character of the analysand (as a reader, a thinker, and a writer), remains foundational in psychoanalysis. In a work called *Tragic Knots*, Roy Schafer has stated that "psychoanalysis achieves its greatest understanding through its close attention to, and interpretation of, the relationship between patient and analyst."[59] My belief in the possibility of psychanalysis initiating an infinite process is in part accomplished by the internalization of a *relationship* that is capable of resisting coercions from the world. The interminable process of the analysand is one long-lasting experience that can counter the infinity of the infantile and primitive psychical regression. Once the primary relationship, of analyst and analysand, comes to a formal end, however, the dialogue continues and can actually be developed in a relationship of reading. Finally, when the development is then made even more expansive by *reading Freud*, then it seems to be that there is the real possibility of advancing beyond any and all theoretical speculations. André Green was correct in emphasizing how any idea of drives can only be understood, first, in the analytic situation; but only outside, in the day to day life of an analysand, can the drives as they unconsciously permeate social and political life be effectively understood and remedied. The analysand is, for himself, a case history. The analytic process has allowed an analysand to perceive how the structures of liberal society reflect a self-imposed psychical destitution. More seriously today, the theological-political constitution of liberalism has turned illness into a virtue and traumas into a new ideological defense.

If social and political thinkers have been either unable or unwilling to recognize the depth-psychological problems of our contemporary reality, psychoanalysts have not hesitated to share uncomfortable truths. "Narcissistic traumas can act as a basis for ideology."[60] The transition from trauma to ideological rage is one significant symptom. One other concept informs us about the theological-politics of our present. Masud Khan's concept of "cumulative trauma"[61] is suggestive because of the way political neuroses can consciously construct how civilization has been developed unjustly, by territorial incursion, conquest, and primary cultural repetition (conceived exclusively as Western and European) as displacements for individual and infantile conflict. Thierry Bokanovski's concept of "traumatism"[62] can round off the brief comments when we can connect the ideology of trauma, in the present, to the psychical traumas suffered by the infant and when in the most difficult conflict with the primitive psyche and its fragmented objects. The expression of outrage by the political neurotic depends on the force of a still active primitive experience in infancy, with, eventually, all its deep-seated mechanisms of defense, and the simultaneous presence of the new introjected object from the historical past. The primitive super-ego and the dead introjected object are inter-relational and are a powerful combination in shaping the new moral world.

During his early collaboration with Josef Breuer, Freud reached one early conclusion – on the temporal and formal aspects of regression. A later essay summarized an initial finding. "We led the patient's attention directly to the traumatic scene in which the symptom had arisen, and we endeavoured to discover the mental conflict in that scene and to release the suppressed effect in it. In the course of this we discovered the mental processes, characteristic of the neuroses, which I later named 'regression.'"[63] Regression has been all-important for the analysis of the politicized group and its identity; as is the psychoanalytic understanding of a *trauma*, as an *ism*, a word whose currency has never been more valuable for political defenses, or, over-used as a personal experience. We are firmly in an epoch of the ubiquitous trauma; the concept has become politically expedient. The gain from what Vamik Volkan calls the "reactivation of a chosen trauma" is, today, being exploited as are other modern afflictions to become "entitlement ideologies."[64] The regression, as the psychical turning away from a present reality and the unconscious revival of a past experience (which, for the political neurotic, is both history *and* fantasy, each of them indecipherable on their own) will be understood as the repetition of an older, infantile conflict that the individual and the group attempt to remedy, with effects that today we can witness as intensifying. The description "the politics of affect" is a beginning, as is the sense of "affect and 'We' group identities and their concomitant attachments."[65] How does the attachment *in groups* and *to trauma* lead to a psychical response that has theological-political connections for social reality? "*Hysterical patients suffer from incompletely abreacted psychical traumas.*"[66] The classical formulation has become pertinent for politically-minded groups. The difference between Freud's observations of his first hysterical patients and the "traumas" of the political neurotic of the present time has been seen before, in the context of another aetiology – one, related to the *fantasy* of a trauma.

Freud's analysis from *Group Psychology* has been unsettling; the diagnostic, however, leaves room for the anticipation of a remedy, for individuals to begin with if not for our consensus society of public opinion. The derivation of a former identification "is a memorial of the former weakness and dependence of the ego, and the mature ego remains subject to its domination. As the child was once under the compulsion to obey its parents, so the ego submits to the categorical imperative of the super-ego." Once more, we should not simply pass by the repetition of *categorical imperative* nor, equally as important, the substitution of parents who, in addition to preserving the genealogy of the Oedipus complex, has also *regulated authority*. Once the super-ego was raised to the level of a supreme moral authority, all previous legitimacy (from the family, society, and conscience) was abolished and made the way for the attempt at a *new* social structure. The previous argument can be re-stated. Freud revisited the problem in the important year of 1924. The traditional viewpoint, for us, must be supplemented. Freud writes: "The object-cathexes are given up and replaced by identifications. The authority of the father or the parents is introjected into the ego, and there it forms the nucleus of the super-ego."[67] We have every reason to believe that this process, leading to the dissolution or at least the controlled modification of the Oedipus complex, is today in danger of being radically transformed. Freud left us with an intimation. We can interpret it for the argument at hand. "We may plausibly assume that we have here come upon the borderline – never a very sharply drawn on – between the normal and the pathological. If the ego has in fact not achieved much more than a *repression* of the complex, the latter persists in an unconscious state in the id and will later manifest its pathogenic effect" (19:177). My re-interpretation of the process when considering the contemporary situation leads me to the "dissolution" of the Oedipus complex but in a different way than envisioned here by Freud. The mechanism is the same; the psychical process requires to be viewed from a different perspective in order to recognize, to stress this again, how the introjected parents (mother and father, male and female) and society's moderate conscience are displaced by the hysterical introjection described before. The previous repression, which we can recognize for its largely beneficial effects as it made it possible for the individual to grow, develop, and mature, has turned to a fierce drive of super-ego rejection, unconsciously absolute and all the more powerful because of it. Freud had immersed himself in a harrowing reality. He often saw himself as an archaeologist of the depths. Approaching the middle of the decade, Freud has not been reluctant about leaving suggestive problems for later readers; which is the reason why, in a short piece, "The Loss of Reality in Neurosis and Psychosis," the earlier demarcation, of one side to the other, can be reconsidered and from what was earlier written not so much about "borderline" cases but perhaps a new phenomenon of the politically functional psychotic – and, again, with one necessary shift. "In both cases [neurosis and psychosis],"[68] Freud believes that they serve the power *of the id*. Our new conditions force us to reconsider which psychical agency is exerting the force necessary so that the self (caught between a despised reality and two antithetical drives in the super-ego) "will not allow itself to be dictated to by reality." The current situation does not allow us to single out the id as the active agency here. "Both neurosis and psychosis are the expression of a rebellion" from the psyche, with one difference: in neurosis, there are many ways to avoid or be independent for much of reality; the politically functional psychotic, however, accepts no compromise, cannot allow himself to admit to a historical or biological reality and so "disavows it and tries to replace it." The theological-political essay has been concerned, from first to last, with this highly motivated trend in liberal democracies and the unconscious force in attempting to "replace" (first by destroying) the reality of the world.

The first introductory statement of the last chapter of *The Ego and the Id* is the beginning of a tour de force of expository analysis, one that has the most direct relevance to our psycho-political present; because once the ego has been made to submit to the domination of the super-ego, it has been rendered (almost) incapable of resisting or, indeed, mounting a vigorous defense on its own behalf because it now had to deal with an irreconcilable ambivalence. The modern ego in liberal democracies has been so beaten into submission by the authoritarian demands of the super-ego that we can only wonder at the individuals – or the silent *majority* at large – that has made the decision to acquiesce with resignation (as is the case of some liberal democracies) or begin to respond, individually and with selected others, friends who can confirm a predicament. Thus far, dissent has been sparse and met with the most vigorous of denunciations. *Extreme* forms of opposition are simply the remnants of hysterical ideologies from the past. The super-ego has become so imperious and morally arrogant, to the point of believing in a telling self-possession (its infallibility), that moderate alternatives no longer seem possible. Any dialogue, for example, is today out of the question. The moderation and reason of a philosophical discussion have been repudiated by the certainty of a super-ego that only acknowledges itself. If Freud anticipated these circumstances, how does the conclusion to the work that explicitly introduced the super-ego and the death drive *lead us* towards a psychology of the ego strong enough to be indifferent to both the impositions of a hysterical guilt and human vulnerability and therefore create the conditions for the ego to regain *its strength*? Any gain from illness is to be renounced as a condition of intelligence and freedom. We can no longer give ourselves the assurance that, as may have been the case earlier, that only in severe pathological states does the super-ego turn against itself and others. Although the super-ego can turn against itself and, in the extreme cases of melancholia lead to self-destruction – slow, drawn-out, or with the finality of an act – our concern is how the super-ego can turn against the *reality* of existence with intensity and obsessive dedication; reality as a whole and the people who are there to perpetuate one version of it. Self-destruction is one problem; a social death drive is much more inclusive. A reminder is in order. "The death instinct would thus seem to express itself – though probably only in part – as an instinct of destruction directed against the external world and other organisms" (19:41). The "external world" is civilization. As for *other organisms*, these are living, sentient beings. The often-repeated word, "destruction," stands out; but if we recall Abraham's two descriptions (of both control and destruction), we can better appreciate the acting-out of the super-ego in its modern forms. Other organisms. Other life. The bureaucratic organization of the super-ego within society, more than the state, has been one more method of disavowing the reality at hand and forcing the individual to conform to the vision of a new one. One of the most telling has been the production of social illness.

Freud's own "two sides" can be reconstructed further. "We shall best appreciate these relations by turning to certain clinical facts, which have long since lost their novelty but which still await theoretical discussion" (19:49). Before turning to Freud's observation of his patients, the "clinical facts," we should be aware that at the same time as he presents the accumulated knowledge of his therapeutic findings, he has another and equally if not more important set of arguments: *his patients* are exemplary. A historical example is not irrelevant. We know from Freud's writings that once the super-ego became more a focus of concern for individual patients and how it coincided with his ever-widening interests in the external world and civilization as a whole, his professional duties shifted. "From about 1920 onwards it became his custom to take patients only people who intended to become analysists."[69] As Freud took greater notice of the power of the super-ego to make individual lives difficult and so transform the nature of society and the temptation to rule it with authority, his professional duty towards the training of analysts can be understood within the framework of his discoveries. The point must be emphasized: once he came to the conclusion that the modern ego was on the way to being severely restricted in its freedom and intelligence and creativity due to the super-ego, his writings would have to be complemented by a renewed dedication to the supervision of the training of the next generation of analysts who would be made aware of their individual responsibilities. His legacy has not been altered. Any devoted reading of the psychoanalytic literature confirms the tradition of an *ethos* – a therapeutic one dedicated to the alleviation of suffering and the overcoming of forms of illness most especially when (as in the case of chronic defenses) they are perpetuated at all costs and with the delusion of their benefit.

The added constraints of society would have to be addressed in the clinical situation and for the purposes of the patient's well-being. Only the future analysts who were themselves fully aware of the impact of the super-ego on their patients would be in the position to minimize, if not completely eliminate, the most destructive aspects of the super-ego. Some have not realized what the shift actually meant for Freud. "In 1925," Martin Bergmann writes, "something happened that no one had expected: Freud lost much of his interest in psychoanalysis as a method of curing mental illness and turned to a broader interest in the future of civilization."[70] This is misleading. Freud never "lost interest in curing mental illness." He did, however, come to the realization that the concentration on individual neurosis was not enough if the pathologies of societies were going to continue and become worse. The processes had to be both clearly explained, in writing, and through the training of analysts who would become aware of the power of the unconscious psyche to determine the nature of reality and the social and political life of humanity. Although the example, here, is specifically about "word-presentations" (and we can therefore recall the message of propaganda) Freud's psychical understanding has endured, and for good reason. The most important of psychoanalytic ideas are repeated.

> The part played by word-presentations now become perfectly clear. By their interposition internal thought-processes are made into perceptions. It is like a demonstration of the theorem that all knowledge has its origins in external perception. When a hypercathexis of the process of thinking takes place, thoughts are actually perceived – as if they came from without – and are consequently held to be true.
>
> (19:23)

The psychical knowledge of this phenomenon, even if well-known, when it was declared with such precision, gave the reader not only the opportunity to understand it as the immediate declaration of a concept; the insight clarified several processes at once.

One can better appreciate what Freud calls "the clinical facts" and the example of an analysand who has developed a "negative therapeutic reaction" by abstracting from the analytic situation to the everyday life of the political neurotic. The correlation will be revealing insofar as Freud presents us with a general case history of any individual to the political analogy. "There is something in these people that sets itself against their recovery" (19: 49). We have arrived at another of Freud's cumulative ideas when we move from the individual *in analysis* to political groups, and a segment of an entire population of a society, that whatever social improvements are actually and objectively made, will respond with a *chronic* dissatisfaction. The negative therapeutic reaction noticed in a clinical setting, then, has implications for society as a whole; despite all the best conscious intentions and the real progress made in questions of justice, for example, the complications of concealed motives makes the attainment of social ideals impossible – because for them to become realized, as accomplishments, would render the affective pleasure of dissatisfaction moot. If society did become just and equitable, they would have to forego the elaborate psychological edifice of the defenses that were strengthened during the process of regression. Being infantile and primitive is an enormous advantage. To admit to the possibility of a gradual improvement in *their* condition would force them to modify their internal grievance and acknowledge the changes in social and political reality. The "gain from illness" Freud diagnosed for a patient is only an illustration of a far more widespread phenomenon; the chronic dissatisfaction with the social and political conditions is essential to the absoluteness of the mechanisms fully operative in the super-ego. The matter can become graver still and in terms of "deterioration." Our society has so ordered its reality that "expectation of secondary gain can increase feelings of illness and, thereby, stimulate *deterioration* in a psychiatric and somatic sense."[71] The somatic is no less important in some cases since the illness is rationalized by medical diagnosis and given support by institutions (educational, for one). This is when the introjected ego-ideal, because dead and a victim of history, can never, under any condition, be satisfied. The idea of "reconciliation," for all its promise, is effectively impossible by the very structure of the psyche as it perpetuates a certain state of reality in order to maintain its advantage over everyone else.

One preliminary conclusion can be modified given the conditions of the present. The morality of a theological-political society are exacting as they proliferate to create, as much as possible, a totality. Freud writes: "In the end, we come to see that we are dealing with what may be called a 'moral' factor, a sense of guilt, which is finding its satisfaction in the illness and refuses to give up punishment or suffering" (19:49). Our previous discussion of the masochistic-sadistic bind can be emphasized in the discussion of the gain from illness since the "moral factor" Freud noticed with such clarity is intimately tied to guilt – a condition now promoted and inflicted on others so as to force everyone to bear responsibility for the process of civilization in Western history. The need for the punishment and suffering – that is, for the masochistic-sadistic relation to *endure*, it must be perpetually activated; and that is also the reason that, in the end, the control of self and others is inseparable from the death drive. As long as the bind can be dynamically renewed, from the masochism of guilt to the sadism of retribution, the psychical circularity will never be altered. The infinitely renewable pleasure cannot be relinquished.

As a brief conclusion to the problem of masochism as Freud began to outline it in 1924 (as a supplement to his political argument), we can turn to Sergio Benvenuto and his study of perversion. In the Appendix, "Freud and Masochism," he writes: "The moral masochist is not someone who seeks pleasure through unpleasure, but one who arranges things so as to be forever unsatisfied and unhappy."[72] The "discontent" Freud wrote about, which for him required an analysis of the causes for a general dissatisfaction with social life, has been transformed today into an affective state, one that serves definite ends. To be chronically dissatisfied with the conditions of social life means one will experience, perpetually, a personal malaise no outward, "objective" change will in effect be able to alter. To justify the re-ordering of society along the most stringent of ideas and methods, the inherent problems (as perceived) can *never* be satisfactorily overcome. Propaganda ensures its own perpetual life span by continually making the same claims. This has been one of the enduring problems of academic "critical theory."

We will see how Freud's manifest critique of religion in the two outstanding works of the late 1920s sum up the reality of our day. Religion, rightly or wrongly, was once thought to be a form of thinking inimical to life and (because it so devalued existence) it betrayed itself by positing the idea of a metaphysical afterlife where the soul, at least, would be redeemed – unless, of course, it was condemned to eternal suffering and reflective of the perversity of a medieval imagination. Damnation, however, is no longer a metaphysical problem. Once we accept the premise and transfer these ideas to the political realm, then we can begin to provide a better understanding of a new phenomenon in the *welfare* conditions of a liberal society. The commentary on *The Ego and the Id* will be the opportunity for us doing so. To be "forever" and infinitely unhappy will have been relatively easy to achieve for the melancholy post-colonialist historian, the individual and the many groups whose psychology, identification, introjection, and projection, depend on a double operation: the ceaseless critique of history for its traumas (some of which, of course, are *real*) and then its time filled up with as many phantasies as can be created. While we can once again, cautiously, state a truism that "the superego system of the individual is clearly associated with the predominant morality of the society in which the person lives,"[73] any notion of our "morality" can no longer be evaluated without also considering all subsequent developments in our specifically liberal societies and during an epoch that has established human debility and guilt as associated conditions of being. At the level of what has been stressed all the way through, the prevalence of a political unconscious in liberal democracies, we continue to make one comprehensive argument – and, here, with one more addition: the viral drive of super-ego psychology that seeks to make everyone ill while at the same time supervising them with a systematic solicitude.

The diagnosis of the power of the super-ego is having (will continue to have) a number of adverse effects. Originally aware of the individual's propensity to think and act alone, as an individual, and consciously refusing to follow the contagion of groups, Cornelius Castoriadis believes "society replies by attempting to bring about the full impotence of their thought, and ultimately *tout court*, as the only means to limit the acts. Forbidding to think has thus appeared as the only way to forbid the acting. This goes *much further* than the "severe and cruel superego" of Freud; history shows that it has actually entailed a mutilation of the radical imagination."[74] The "mutilation" has gone much further than the imagination. The morality of the super-ego and the death drive have reduced human beings to vulnerable and weak beings who need the support of society (morally and institutionally) and who must, at the same time, fully accept the guilt imposed on them by the fantasy-history of its civilization. It seems that the psychoanalytic response to the continued and worsening mutilation of thought as such will demand a response, first of all from individuals, who will minimize and in the best possible cases eliminate completely what the mutilation is *serving*. When the sadistic is understood to be psychical manipulation, then the response will have to be devoted to the interior work of freedom. Our two initial themes have not changed; if anything, because they have been omnipresent as our psychoanalytic ideals, intelligence and freedom will be the only ideals defended with as much commitment as possible. How Freud continues to argue for the necessity of human freedom and intelligence against all the many social factors for its control and abolition will soon turn to a writing that has been interpreted far too one-dimensionally. One *illusion* will lead to others.

The moral sense of guilt and the need to perpetuate the illness *for good* – always and for the sake of morality – will not be simply felt, unconsciously, in the perversion of a sado-masochistic self-relation. It has become more than evident that the neurotic political activist has been able to exploit himself at the same time as justifying the punishment and suffering *of others*, everyone who is held to the highest of moral standards and who will inevitably fail to live up to idealist expectations. We should not underestimate the real-life consequences of a political acting out in terms of inflicting the most aggressive kind of punishment on anyone who is perceived to be culpable for the moral wrongs of the world. At the same time as the introjected dead victim is causing all kinds of internal malaise, there is at the same time the desperate need for a complete projection and an evacuation of the decomposing subject of history. The process is, however, always and necessarily at an impasse. The circulation between the introjection of the dead subject and the projection into a world that will always be judged to be inadequate and morally woeful ensures that the psychical drama will continue without interruption no matter what happens in the world of objective reality; and no different than the ethical bureaucrats in and out of institutions who are now the guardians of equality and justice and rights that, in principle, will never be achieved and precisely due to their overbearing tactics in the guise of "education."

Freud's conclusion leaves us, for the moment, with a pause: "We shall be right in regarding this disheartening explanation as final" (19: 49). Is he, then, as "pessimistic" as many people claim? What progress can then be made? For the analysand, as long there is no abandonment of the daily obligation, there will always be the opportunity for a modification of a position – with the assistance of the analyst and when the positive transference can make a real difference, eventually, in daily life even long after termination. The political neurotic, however, has no such hope since his transferences occur mostly in and through his libidinal ties with people of his own persuasion (one or more characteristics and identities) and depend on the perpetual experience of a masochist-sadistic bind. "It is also particularly difficult to convince the patient that this motive lies behind his continuing to be ill" (19:50). The analytic analogy, once it serves our psychopolitical analysis, proves to be highly effective as an explanation for the current intensity of political sensibilities in society. There is no desire to be either callous or cynical. Human suffering is all too real; but there seems to be a general infatuation with trauma today, as if the experience of any suffering from the past will be regarded with utmost care and ensure that the individual will be treated well and assuage any feeling of neglect. The Greek term *trauma* (or wound) can be medically attended to; or it can be used, infinitely, for many different social and political reasons. There are a few indications that we are more content to create a society of traumatized individuals who (in a perpetual state of debility) can count on the attention of those whose bureaucratic positions further their causes. The bureaucrats of care require individuals who come to them for assistance. There are, now, departments organized for such tasks. At this point, when each of our arguments have been presented along the way and, in the final section, have exhibited the most serious consequences, we have a decision to make – or, better yet, in what way do we continue to access Freud's writings in the 1920s as both a social diagnostic and, finally, the proposal for a remedy? The "Postscript" to *Group Psychology* has, hopefully, been retained. The force of human creativity can be suppressed; but it cannot be abolished since Eros is the one constitutive essence of being that will not capitulate to Thanatos. How does Freud's work on illusion continue the still unfinished analysis of civilization and its discontents?

Notes

1 Reiner, Anni. *The Quest for Conscience and the Birth of the Mind.* London: Karnac, 2009. Reiner's study can also be emphasized for introducing the concept of the "spirit" in a ways that does not accept the traditional dichotomy of religious and secular. She makes an important argument when the idea of the spirit is thought about as an aspect of a "mental development" not restricted by traditional prejudices and definitions. Keeping in mind the distinction between mature development and regression is one way to differentiate a healthy conscience from the pathologies of the super-ego. Her added investigation of the root conscience – as the Latin *conscientia* – gives us its double sense of knowledge and consciousness. The regression of our primitive present is minimizing our epistemological and perceptual capacities.
2 Carveth, Donald L. *The Still Small Voice: Psychoanalytic Reflections on Guilt and Conscience.* London: Karnac, 2013, 20. In his Introduction, Carveth writes that "it is time we began rethinking the psychoanalytic theory of morality."
3 Jurist, Elliot L. "Whatever Happened to the Superego? Loewald and the Future of Psychoanalysis," 489–501 in *Psychoanalytic Psychology*, Vol. 31, No. 4, 2014, 498. Jurist adds that "the superego seems so antiquated," 494. Primitive is, for me, closer to the truth.
4 The quote comes from the short introductory notes made by R.D. Hinshelwood to the essays collected in *Influential Papers of the 1920s*. Ed. R.D. Hinshelwood. London: Karnac, 2014, 2014, 218.
5 Merkur, Dan. *Unconscious Wisdom: A Superego Function in Dreams, Conscience, and Inspiration.* Albany: SUNY, 2001, 56.

6 Donnet, Jean-Luc. *The Analyzing Situation*. Tr. Andrew Weller. London: Karnac, 2009, 173.
7 Frank, George. "Freud's Concept of the Super-ego: Review and Assessment," 448–463 in *Psychoanalytic Psychology*, Vol. 16, No. 3, 1999, 455.
8 Lapsley, D.K. and Stey, P.C. "Id, Ego, and Superego." 393–399 *Encyclopedia of Human Behavior*. Second Edition, 2012, 397.
9 See, for example, Paul Terry's work with one such patient in "Working with Psychosis: Part 2 – encounters with an omnipotent super-ego," 45–59 *Psychodynamic Practice*, 10(1), 2004.
10 Horney, Karen. *New Ways in Psychoanalysis*. Oxford: Routledge, 1939, 211.
11 Carverth, Donald L. "Why we should stop conflating the superego with the conscience," 15–32 *Psychoanalysis, Culture & Society*, Vol. 22, No. 1, 2017. John F. Crosby has made the same argument in Chapter 4, "Conscience and the Superego" in his *Personalist Papers*. Washington: The Catholic University of America Press, 2004. Not surprisingly, analysts and others who are nuanced about religion can make the distinction better than most. Has one of the effects of the superego resulted in the suppression of a moderate conscience since only a balanced view of good and evil allows for a rational discernment of the facts? Has the death of God also resulted in the suppression of conscience and the unbridled domination of a new kind of morality? The *Future of an Illusion* will not avoid these and other neglected questions.
12 As one other description added to many others, see Les Fleischer's "The Corruptibility of the Superego Revisited," 86–106 in the *Canadian Journal of Psychoanalysis*, Vol. 28, Issue 1, 2020. One of his more memorable statements is on "the venality of the superego."
13 Askay, Richard and Farquhar, Jensen. "On the Nature of the Human: Sigmund Freud," 73–88 *Contemporary Psychoanalytic Studies*, Vol. 12 (2011), 76–77.
14 Jones, Ernest. "The origins and status of the super-ego," *Influential Papers from the 1920s*. Ed. H.R. Hinshelwood. London: Karnac, 2014, 222.
15 Green, André. *Illusions and Disillusions in Psychoanalytic Work*. Tr. Andrew Weller. London: Karnac, 2011, 60.
16 Holmes, Jeremy. "Superego: An attachment perspective," 1221–1240 *International Journal of Psychoanalysis*, Vo. 92, No. 5 (Oct 2011), 1230, 1230.
17 Weiss, Heinz. "A brief history of the super-ego with an introduction to three papers," 724–734 *International Journal of Psychoanalysis*, Vol. 101, No. 4, 2020.
18 Grotstein, James S. "Notes on the Superego," 257–270 *Psychoanalytic Inquiry*, Vol. 24, Issue 2, 2008, 267.
19 Sedlak, Vic. "The psychoanalyst's normal and pathological superegos," 1499–1520 *International Journal of Psychoanalysis,* Vol. 97, No. 6 (2016), 1506.
20 Lacan, Jacques. "Discourse to Catholics," in *The Triumph of Religion*. Tr. Bruce Fink. Cambridge, UK: Polity Press, 2013, 16.
21 Britton, Ronald. *Sex, Death, and the Superego: Experiences in Psychoanalysis*. London: Karnac, 2003, 104.
22 Schmidt-Hellerau, Cordelia. "How Demagogy Works: Reflections on Aggression in Politically Fraught Times," 234–242 *Psychoanalytic Inquiry*, Vol. 40, No. 4, 2020.
23 De Masi, Franco. *Working with Difficult Patients: From Neurosis to Psychosis*. London: Karnac, 2015, 91–92.
24 Nobus, Dany. "Freud's Infernal Trinity: On the Vicissitudes of the 'Tripartite Model'." *Drawing the Soul: Schemas and Models in Psychoanalysis*. Ed. Bernard Burgoyne. London: Karnac, 2000.
25 Freud, Sigmund. "Analysis Terminable and Interminable." SE 23:244.

26 Virsida, Anthony R. "The Death Drive: psychic construction or destruction," 511–523 *Psychoanalytic Review*, Vol. 88. No. 4, Aug. 2001. I need not belabour the point made from the beginning. "Killing" something, God or a concept, does not at all means it has been "laid to rest."

27 Schaffner, Anna Katherina. *Exhaustion: A History*. New York: Columbia University Press, 2016, 158.

28 Black, David M. "Mapping a Detour: Why did Freud Speak of a Death Drive?" 185–198 *British Journal of Psychotherapy*, Vol. 18, No. 2, 2011, 195. The conclusion to his essay did not prevent him from outlining several important points that merited further consideration.

29 Razinsky, Liran. "Driving Death Away: Death and Freud, Theory of the Death Drive," 393–424 *Psychoanalytic Review*, Vol. 97, No. 3 (Jun. 2010), 394, my emphasis.

30 Laplanche, Jean. *Essays on Otherness*. Ed. John Fletcher. London: Routledge, 1999, 122.

31 Frank, Claudia. "On the reception of the concept of the death drive in Germany: expressing and resisting an 'evil principle'," 425–444 *International Journal of Psychoanalysis*, Vol. 96, No. 2 (2015), 427.

32 Novick, Jack and Novick, Kerry Kelly. "The Superego and the Two-System Model," 232–256 in *Psychoanalytic Inquiry*, Vol. 24, Issue 2, 2008. Far from considering it irrelevant, one of the important aspects of their paper is the idea of an "omnipotent sadomasochism," one that will be analyzed further.

33 Girard, René. *When These Things Begin: Conversations with Michel Treguer*. Tr. Trevor Cribben Merrill. East Lansing: Michigan State University Press, 2014, 106–107.

34 Žižek, Slavoj. *The Sublime Object of Ideology*. London: Verso, 1989, 4–5.

35 Dare, Christopher, Anna Ursula Dreher, Alex Holder, & Joseph Sandler. *Freud's Models of the Mind: An Introduction*. Routledge, 1997, 174.

36 Montgomery, Scott L. "A Case of (mis) taken Identity? II: Freudian Language in the Ego and the Id," 51–81 *Psychoanalytic Review*, Vol. 88, No. 1 (Feb. 2001), 52.

37 Chabert, Catherine. "Can we do without the death drive?" *International Journal of Psychoanalysis*, Vol. 100, No. 6, 2019.

38 Zilbersheid, Uri. "The Historical Character of Human Nature in Freud's Theory," 184–204 *American Journal of Psychoanalysis*, Vol. 93, No. 2 (Jun 2013), 192.

39 Klein, Melanie. *Envy and Gratitude and Other Works*. London: Virago Press, 1957, 72.

40 Kernberg, Otto. "The concept of the death drive: a clinical perspective," 173–190 *On Freud's Beyond the Pleasure Principle*. Ed. Salman Akhtar and Mary Kay O'Neil. London: Karnac, 2011, 176.

41 Lear, Jonathan. *Happiness, Death and the Remainder of Life*. Cambridge, Massachusetts: Harvard University Press, 2000, 87. Theory is my emphasis.

42 Levine, Howard B. "Aggression and Psychoanalysis: Reflections," 43–59 *Canadian Journal of Psychoanalysis*, Vol. 25, No. 2, July 1, 2017, 48.

43 Ansermet, François. "Freud's Death Drive: the paradox of destructiveness," 71–77 *Freud and War*. Ed. Marlène Belilos. London: Karnac, 2016, 75.

44 Steinbach, Oscar. "Aggression, the Death Drive and the Problem of Sado-Masochism: A Re-Interpretation," 857–881 *Psychoanalytic Review*, Vol. 93, No. 6 (Dec. 2006).

45 The title of the last chapter in Jeffrey Rubin's *The Good Life: Psychoanalytic Reflections on Love, Ethics, Creativity and Spirituality*. Albany: SUNY, 2004.

46 Mills, Jon. "Reflections on the Death Drive," 373–382 *Psychoanalytic Psychology*, Vol. 23, No. 2, 2006, 374.

47 Hageback, Niklas. *The Death Drive: Why Societies Self-Destruct*. Las Vegas: Gaudium, 2020.
48 Rothstein, Arnold. *Making Freud more Freudian*. London: Karnac, 2010, 42.
49 Abraham, Karl. "Melancholia and Obsessional Neurosis: Two Stages of the Sadistic-Anal Phases of the Libido." (1924), in *Selected Papers on Psychoanalysis*. London: Karnac, 1988, 428.
50 Klein, Melanie. "Early Stages of the Oedipus Conflict and the Super-ego Formation," in *The Psycho-analysis of Children*. Tr. Alix Strachey. London: Virago Press, 1989, 32.
51 Manninen, Vesa. "The face of fear: castration and perversion," 193–215 *The Scandinavian Psychoanalytic Review*, 23:2, 2000, 196.
52 De M'Uzan, Michael. *Death and Identity: Being and Psycho-Sexual Drama*. Tr. Andrew Weller. London: Karnac, 2013, 4.
53 Falcão, Luciane. "Death drive, destructive drive and desobjectalizing functions in the analytic process," 459–476 *International Journal of Psychoanalysis*, Vol. 96, No. 2, 2015, 463. She adds. "As many psychoanalysts today believe, death and life drives may be Freudian myths, but myths are also our frames of reference," 473.
54 Sklar, Jonathan. *Dark Times: Psychoanalytic Perspectives on Politics, History and Mourning*. Oxfordshire: Phoenix Publishing House, 2019, 2.
55 Ogden, Thomas H. "Reading Loewald: Oedipus Reconceived." 651–666 *International Journal of Psychoanalysis*, Vol. 87, No. 3, June 2006.
56 Ruszynski, Stanley. "The problem of certain psychic realities: Aggression and Violence as perverse solutions," 23–42 *Lectures on Violence Perversion and Delinquency*. Ed. David Morgan and Stanley Ruszynski. London: Karnac, 2007, 41.
57 Miller, J.F. *The Triumphant Victim: A Psychoanalytical Perspective on Sadomasochism and Perverse Thinking*. London: Karnac, 2013, 214.
58 Freud, Sigmund. "The Question of Lay Analysis." SE 20:222.
59 Schafer, Roy. *Tragic Knots in Psychoanalysis*. New Papers on Psychoanalysis. London: Karnac, 2009, xiv.
60 Laine, Aira. "On the edge: the psychoanalyst's transference," 1171–1183 *International Journal of Psychoanalysis*, Vol. 88 (Oct. 2007), 1172.
61 As presented in *The Privacy of the Self*. London: Karnac, 1996.
62 In "Variations on the concept of traumatism: traumatism, traumatic, trauma," 251–265 *International Journal of Psychoanalysis* 86, 2008.
63 Freud, Sigmund. "On the History of the Psycho-Analytic Movement," SE 14:10.
64 Volkan, Vamik D. *Psychoanalysis, International Relations, and Diplomacy: A Source-book on Large-Group Psychology*. London: Karnac, 2014. Howard B. Levine wrote the Foreword, "Psychoanalysis and Political Conflict: Is Psychoanalysis relevant?" and introduced one of the most significant concepts for us in terms of how a "chosen trauma" can "cause individual and large-group regression," xiv.
65 Sarra, Nicholas. "Attachment and Trauma in Groups and Organizations," 263–272 in *British Journal of Psychotherapy*, Vol. 35, No. 2, 2019, 266.
66 Freud, Sigmund. "On the Psychical Mechanism of Hysterical Phenomena: A Lecture." SE 3:38.
67 Freud, Sigmund. "The Dissolution of the Oedipus Complex." SE 19:176.
68 Freud, Sigmund. "The Loss of Reality in Neurosis and Psychosis." SE 19:185.
69 Nissim Momigliano, Luciana. *Continuity and Change in Psychoanalysis: Letters from Milan*. London: Karnac, 1992, 8.
70 Bergmann, Martin S. "The Dual Impact of Freud's Death and Freud's Death Instinct Theory on the History of Psychoanalysis," 664–686 *Psychoanalytic Review*, Vol. 98, No. 5 (Oct. 2011), 672.

71 Van Egmond, J.J. "Beyond Secondary Gain," 167–177 *The American Journal of Psychoanalysis*, Vol. 65, No. 2, June 2005, 169.
72 Benvenuto, Sergio. *What are Perversions? Sexuality, Ethics, Psychoanalysis*. London: Karnac, 2016, 148.
73 Barrett, Bernard. *You Ought to! A Psychoanalytic Study of the Superego and Conscience*. London: Karnac, 2007, 150.
74 Castoriadis, Cornelius. "Psychoanalysis and Politics," 1–12 *Speculations after Freud: Psychoanalysis, Philosophy and Culture*. Ed. Michael Munchow and Sonu Shamdasani. London: Routledge, 1994, 8.

3

THE PRESENT OF OUR ILLUSIONS

> If you want to expel religion from our European civilization, you can only do it by means of another system of doctrines; and such a system would from the outset take over all the psychological characteristics of religion – the same sanctity, rigidity, intolerance, the same prohibition of thought – for its own defence.
>
> *The Future of an Illusion*

(i) The Extra-Religious Dimension of Freud's Analysis

The development of Freud's thought as he became increasingly preoccupied with social and political problems reaches one more important juncture when the super-ego and the death drive relation are brought into prominence in a work that has been often too-narrowly interpreted as a critique of religion and, moreover, as the personal testimony of atheism. A proposal will be made from the outset: to abandon a commonplace agreement on Freud's view of "religion" and examine, instead, the psychoanalysis of the unacknowledged transference between one system of doctrines and another one (from the theological to the political) and its internalization to create a new social reality in the 21st century. Anyone who gives themselves the illusion of the authoritarianism of religion as unique and somehow self-contained are, according to what follows in Freud's argument, too focused on the particularities of one human institution instead of following his *expository method* – which requires attention, above all, to the multi-leveled structure of *The Future of an Illusion* and its thematic chronology as it both recollects the regression to infantile and primitive defenses and their sanctimonious, rigid,

DOI: 10.4324/9781003410911-4

and intolerant characteristics. The reception of the work can, today, be re-assessed and its extra-religious dimension be presented.

One view has been traditional, consistent, and often repeated. *The Future of an Illusion* has been characterized as "Freud's most sustained analysis of religious belief" and "a powerful undermining of Christianity."[1] This kind of statement could be multiplied and added to many others, sometimes of a more emotional tone, to become a virtual compilation – such as the belief in "his abhorrence of religion."[2] One other can leave us with traditional impressions. "Convinced of the falsity of belief in the existence of God, Freud explain the origin of the religious world-view in these words."[3] The precise words will be spared; they are not as evident as has been assumed, in one place and in others. As for the existence of God, that *one* metaphysical belief was not ultimately Freud's concern; rather, the psychical origin and condition of *any* decisive belief was one of the goals of his analysis of the nature of illusions, as such. Before a few more typical assessment are mentioned, my argument can be stated and without in any way choosing the option of being *against or for* religion, the inadequate logic of an either/or. An analysand, in any case, should not be satisfied with one or two choices – not once the experience of a dilemma was understood from the perspective of psychical processes; overdetermination is, always, to be taken into consideration. This or that interaction is never enough; and surely Freud was motivated by something far more intricate in the religious imagination (and, at times, delusion) than denying the belief in the existence of God. Infantilism is not a theological condition *per se*. Therefore, the possibility of another reading and interpretation will be offered and one based on the ability to translate, as Freud does, the dynamic of the psyche into writing; levels are multiple and varied, their meanings consciously over-determined and systematically presented to offer much more than a simple critique of religion. The unconscious transference from the religious to the political illusion (and its theological-political reality) has not been examined with the attention the theme deserves and in the individual way Freud approached it with all the force of his analysis in *The Future of an Illusion*. The 1927 work is, to use an inadequate because spatial word, layered; the layers are *temporal* and thematic insofar as one statement cannot stand alone or be exclusive. Cross-references, in terms of reading, are essential if Freud's meanings are to be fully appreciated during a period of highly perceptive acumen. His opening statement should make us conscious of how easily *one system of thought* can be transferred to another. The theological-political argument can be given more support once *The Future of an Illusion* is *psychoanalytically* read as a treatise on the shifts from one illusion to another; splitting (a concept alluded to and to be further examined) facilitates their back and forth. Orthodoxy – "right" ideas – are not exclusive to one world-view; the reliance on dogma was neither invented nor perfected by religion. Other institutions are no less capable of being imperious.

Many traditional readings of Freud's 1927 work are, today, outdated and incomplete; they seem far less a reflection of Freud's analysis than the self-congratulatory attitude of agnostics, atheists, or cynics who are satisfied with a dogmatic finality and therefore emulate, by being diametrically opposed to, their equally self-possessed theological rivals. Reactions against religion does not abolish its persistence. His conscious transference, to a reader and an analysand, has a purpose that has not been discussed. The readiness to follow customary attitudes has been too strong to avoid; if for no other reason, Freud would make us aware of the meaning of consensus and opinion and how it can distort our individual perception in the act of reading, interpretation, and reflection. Self-righteousness, to mention but one attitude, might be an appealing privilege to some; to others, it represents a danger to independence of mind as both the intelligence and freedom at the root of Freud's psychoanalytic ideals. The resolve of an analysand must be sustained for a considerable period of time and without rushing to facile conclusions.

One original thinker can prepare us for the interpretation ahead; intimations have been mentioned in the Introduction. In a short piece, "Materialism," Georges Bataille writes: "Most materialists, even though they have wanted to do away with all spiritual entities, ended up by positing an order of things whose hierarchical relations mark it as specifically idealist." How did he reach this philosophical position? "It is from Freud," Bataille continues, "that a representation of matter must be taken. It is of little importance that the fear of psychological complications (a fear that only bears witness to intellectual weakness) causes timid souls to see in this attitude an aversion or a return to spiritual values."[4] *Aversion or return.* The theme of the "return of the religious" can be made explicit once more. Our present is no time for either "timid souls" who would avoid the complications of reading Freud psychoanalytically or revert to the widely accepted either/or, which requires neither courage nor originality. Still, more or less accepted readings can be cited. Alternatives will not be withheld; the argument overall depends on recognizing Freud for the thinker he is and for the individual who transformed the act of *writing psychoanalytically* and so not readily accessible without interpretative commitment.

"Freud's antipathy and preoccupation with religion are well known."[5] The two are quite different. Preoccupations are not at all like antipathies: one is *interested* (as in *inter-esse*, being between and inside, committed and involved) the other is an emotional reaction. Anyone who has no sympathy to religion must also ignore – first of all, its foundational writing – and then the responsibility of a personal obligation of acts of interpretation without relying on pre-established approaches, ecclesial or academic. One other comment sums up in many ways what has been one kind of reading; to call it, simply, *manifest*, is a beginning to Freud's individual composition. How does anyone respond to this kind of statement? "Freud defined religion as the folk beliefs of European Jews and Christians."[6] To reduce Judaism and Christianity to "folk beliefs" is, unfortunately, simply dismissive. Such a statement does not do any justice to Freud's thinking much less to the profound metaphysics of biblical thought and writing as he analyzed it. Any presumption of supplanting one of the essential elements of a civilization had better be prepared for the inevitable – what Freud called *another system of doctrines*; they have indeed taken the place of a manifest religion, a phenomenon that has been, for the most part, ignored by the commentators who were satisfied with the superficiality of atheism since that view served the illusion of our secularism. If we are going to be responsible to our own interpretations, the least we could do (as Freud reminded his readers) is to be aware of our prejudgments and prejudices, which are so often unconscious, and be attentive to "the psychic function of ideology."[7]

That word (ideology) can be mentioned for this one reason even though propaganda is today more accurate and representative of our times: since the 19th century, when the concept became philosophically prominent in the context of revolutionary politics, ideology was a phenomenon indicative of wealth, power and, above all, class. No one since that time, however, has had the psychological courage or audacity to turn it back on themselves to see how *they* were ideological. The political responsibility was always adopted *theoretically* but rarely as an individual obligation. Critical theory has always been projective; *others* were ideological. The social critic was exempt. Are we, today, in exactly the same position when it comes to certain readers of Freud who notice the manifest level of an anti-religion discourse and nothing else? Beginning with the title of *The Future of an Illusion* itself, and its far-from obvious meaning (for one, because of the specific emphasis on the *future* – that is to say, our present and our illusions) will prepare, as a foundation, the interpretation to come on Freud's work. Much more than any straightforward critique of religion, he anticipated the possibility of dangerous effects – the very same ones that, exhibited by group psychology, undermined freedom, intelligence, creativity, and love. All the previous analyses of group psychology, the super-ego, the death drive, the masochist-sadistic bind, perversions, and the gain from traumas and illness are to be brought forward into the illusions of secularism. The now almost complete confidence of our liberal democratic secularity, once examined first from the perspective of an analysis of certain characteristics (Freud's ideas on the "sanctity, rigidity, intolerance, the same prohibition of thought" of what replaced religion) reveal features that have been rationalized due to their moral necessity. The social ideals of groups had to be attained. Equality, justice, rights had to be served, at all costs; and only Freud, remembering the "Postscript" to *Group Psychology*, presented its origins and its unconscious fixations. Notes from the introduction on the nature of our theological politics can mentioned again with a comment that needs to be revised, once again, for emphasis. Victoria Kahn writes: "Freud is one of the great political theologians of the early twentieth century."[8] While the beginning of the statement is correct, my emphasis has been, and will continue to be, how Freud's singular psychoanalytic interpretations allowed him to recognize how 20th-century politics was going to become, unconsciously, theological and be driven by a "super-morality." Have we mis-read *The Future of an Illusion* as a critique of religion when a more intricate and layered thought process was being presented by Freud on the psychoanalysis of the theological-political status of liberal democracy? "Atheism" and secularity have become more moralistic and dogmatic than when the church was, by necessity, limited by society and the state. The orthodoxy of our times is not a mystery and is not at all hidden. Religion may have been usurped, but only in appearance, as a mere *decision* about history, as if the power of the will alone could accomplish the impossible; the confidence of a secular modernity gave itself the unparalleled drive towards reconceiving life and society and without recognizing how its regression and resulting obsession – in perfecting, impossibly, the very human past of creating and building a civilization – was bound to lead to uncontrollable *desires*.

My interpretation continues to advance one argument on the nature of a writing that has been neglected: if Freud's particular kind of thinking and writing in *The Future of an Illusion* is given more attention than usual, then an added element can also be traced. He alerts us, first of all, to the manner of his exposition; the language should be well-known. Analysands with good memories should not be surprised. How Freud writes – organized by intentional screens and displacements (as an emulation of a *conscious* free association) will lead us toward a certain kind of interpretative responsibility, one that starts out from multiple possibilities and where nothing is editorialized for expediency. The act of reading should not be altogether different, in principle, from the cooperative work between an analysand and his analyst; exchanges are multiplied until affects act as confirmations and internal conflicts minimized or overcome. One initial comment from the work can make us aware of how organized Freud has been – throughout the whole course of psychoanalysis since its inception. "If I am now trying to add the other, less deeply concealed part, you should not accuse me of contradicting myself… … It is, of course, my duty to point out the connecting links between what I said earlier and what I put forward now, between the deeper and the manifest motives" (21:23). If this one statement makes us aware of a certain quality of his writing (and so for our reading) then the "deeper motives" of *The Future of an Illusion* may not be about a critique of religion – which, after all, is commonplace and hardly original and, ultimately, *not interesting* because over-saturated – but leading us toward a much more complex analysis. His conscious displacements are to be interpreted no differently than the manifest content of a dream. A manifest reading is no longer sufficient; his many-layered latent exposition deserves a certain attentiveness. Fortunately, a few readers with nuance have avoided making hasty judgments; prudence and care, for and with meaning, are not incidental. Marsha Hewitt writes: "If one is to do proper justice to *The Future of an Illusion*, one ought not to read it as an atheist manifesto nor as exclusively representative of Freud's thinking about religion."[9] And we therefore come to one of the pivotal moments of our psychopolitical essay and add another argument to the whole; and doing so by recollecting, as we can often do, Freud's individual, and original, perception. For example, in "The Future Prospects of Psycho-Analytic Therapy," he writes: "It is clear that every advance in our knowledge means an increase in our therapeutic power."[10] Too aware, by now, of our psychological tendencies to neglect knowledge if it was inconvenient or simply too threatening, he made sure to talk, in this particular case, directly to his fellow analysts and to make them once again conscious of their personal duties. Therapeutic power also required a constant self-reflection. "We have noticed that no psycho-analyst goes further than his own complexes and internal resistances permit" (SE 11:145). The statement is equally true for a reader; the analysand has confronted *himself* on the matter many times. Although the lecture was directed at practicing psychoanalysts, the overall intentions are not to be limited to the therapeutic situation. Readers may want to be equally aware of their motivations; the concept of *resistant reading* can be put forward without controversy. Surely it should not surprise anyone that certain interpretations of Freud have been suppressed. The repression of psychoanalysis has been concealed by no one.

We can sense how, only a couple of years before the publication of *Totem and Taboo*, preoccupations which would last a lifetime were already central for him as a thinker and writer. One can here notice so much of what has already been discussed and what will become even more prominent. The 1911 lecture was delivered in the same year as the foundation of the International Psychoanalytic Association. The reference to the "impoverishment of the ego," one of our main preoccupations, is not redundant in a discussion on our illusions.

> Only very few civilized people are capable of existing without reliance on others or are even capable of coming to an independent opinion. You cannot exaggerate the intensity of people's inner lack of resolution and craving for authority. *The extraordinary increase in neuroses since the power of religions has waned* may give you a measure of it. The impoverishment of the ego due to the large expenditure of energy on repression demanded of every individual by civilization may be one of the causes in this state of things.
>
> (SE 11:146)

One has to at least italicize a part of Freud's extraordinary statement. What can we learn from this passage that, for anyone much too confident in secularity – or in a mere intellectual critique of religion – is required to give the matter some thought? Once Freud presents one fact – *neurotic afflictions have increased due to the waning of religion* – then our interest is all the more inspired to find out how, today, the individual is under enormous pressure to *conform* to a specifically moral authority while at the same maintaining the most strict separation from any kind of religious thought. Irreligion, the more self-assured the better, gives secularity the illusion of its own independence. The consequences have, however, been dire for individual freedom and intelligence, as well as two other of Freud's most pronounced ideals: *courage and originality*. The individual, far from being free from orthodox dogmas, is under more pressure than ever and is *systematically* made to be "impoverished." Has the ego ever suffered as much? Hasn't Freud been telling us precisely how the ego has been thwarted from its own proper (and human) self-development because internal debility has been exploited for political reasons? Equally important, neuroses have not only increased; there are now more pathologies and they are being created, some unconsciously, some not, as a new kind of social engineering in the guise of moral education. If my main argument is going to be furthered, then Freud's work should be regarded with particular attention, with two first interpretative responsibilities: on ourselves, as readers, and in accompanying Freud in one of his most important texts on the relationship between the proliferation of neuroses and in the *conscious decline* of religion. We cannot allow the affirmation to be lost: Freud believes the loss of religion has led to the increase in neurosis. *How* has been, in part, the subject of this psychopolitical essay – *not to return to religious values*, as if they could remedy the situation, but to indicate how complex, and precarious, our situation has become because our psychical reality has made us less capable of thought. Our self-congratulatory interpretations have made us unable to understand the betrayal of our contemporary theories.

Could Freud, at this particular time in his life, waste his energy on the kind of critique of religion that was commonplace? Jonathan Lear may be focusing on the wrong issue of the illusion. "If we are to reassure ourselves that we are free of its [religion's] lingering residue, it is imperative to return to Freud's argument and determine just how good an argument it is."[11] Lear seems to want to undertake a critical appraisal of Freud's "argument." But this must presuppose that the argument has been rightly identified – which I believe is not as transparent as most people believe. As for Lear's fear of what he calls a "lingering residue," the situation presented thus far makes his examination of Freud's argument, ultimately, irrelevant because too superficial. *The Future of an Illusion* is *not* a critique of religion; and its arguments, as long as they are mis-interpreted, will not reveal Freud's ultimate intent. The 1927 writing is part of an inter-related and systematic psychoanalysis of how the theological-political consequences of secularism would eventually lead to a full-fledged theocratic imperative and with the simultaneous drive of the super-ego and Thanatos. As long as the argument is believed to be, simply, an either/or between religion and secularity, or faith and atheism, then we have reduced Freud's psychoanalytic vision and failed to recognize the implications of his thinking. We can continue to make accepted assertions such as "Freud visualized the relationship between psychoanalysis and religion as one of permanent animosity,"[12] and so remain only at one deceptive level of Freud's psychoanalysis of a future illusion – today, our own. His multiple perception has been severely restricted by our myopia, by our deceptive desires and the need to include him as one critic among others. We can refer to the section of a work called "the problem of religion" (that *title* is perfectly justified) and the statement: "finally, this brings us to the question of religion, i.e., the God question."[13] This one declaration sums up the difficulty: the problem of religion, as Freud presents it psychoanalytically, is only related to the "God question" insofar as it introduces all kinds of other issues. The *human questions* are the most serious one. Terry Eagleton, self-consciously perplexed, asks: "why are the most unlikely people, including myself, suddenly talking about God?... ... Why, just as we were confidently moving into a posttheological, postmetaphysical, even posthistorical era, has the God question suddenly broken out anew?"[14] Is it not because any confidence or anticipation of the *post* was, simply, not true, more a function of fantasy and desire than a set of identifiable circumstances? The post has been the illusion of a partial or complete supersession. What has "broken out" is a sign of our deep misgivings; thankfully, a few (like Eagleton) are honest enough to pause and reconsider that *status quo*. Others are intent on doing more than making observations about a set of phenomena; they have, because of Freud or their own unique thinking, identified one of the fundamental problems of our age. There is, indeed, the return of the religious in a decidedly unconscious form within politics; from all appearances, it has been duly noted, by a few individuals, and yet almost completely ignored as a social reality and as suppression and amnesia becomes more regulated.

A reminder of Freud's "Preface" to *Totem and Taboo* is not without relevance for us now. The four essays of the collection "represent a first attempt on my part at applying the point of view and the findings of psycho-analysis to some unsolved problems of social psychology [*Völkerpsychologie*]" (SE 13:xiii). Since *Group Psychology*, the interests have been on the dynamic of group ties and what they can lead to – independently of the state. If my interpretation can be sustained, then what Freud accomplished in *The Future of an Illusion* is one more element to an in-depth vision of political life, for his time and ours. Has it been confirmed today? This is the responsibility of the work as it continues to unfold and as it reaches its culmination with the work on the malaise of our culture. Adrian Johnston writes of "Freud's 1927 anticipation and endorsement of scientifically-driven secularization."[15] The idea of an anticipation is correct; an "endorsement" is an entirely other matter and may be more of an indication of a desire, to align Freud to strict definition of science, than a theoretical fact.

Once we examine *The Future of an Illusion* within the context of Freud's writings of the 1920s, another portrait comes into view – one, however, that is not self-evident; the hard work of interpretation is indispensable. Cristopher Bollas makes a provocative comment for anyone who approaches some of the more challenging aspects of psychoanalysis: "the history of psychoanalysis can be read in terms of writers who focus on what they can tolerate, leaving it up to colleagues to write up the rest."[16] For our purposes, it might be accurate to lay the responsibility on us as readers of Freud and what we, perhaps, cannot tolerate because the assumption of a facile atheism, or the nexus of science and secularism, is easier to accept than to acknowledge the religious nature of the super-ego and how its many effects have permeated contemporary life.

From the entire history of Freud's creation of psychoanalysis, one interconnected focus can only be fully appreciated for its reality today. The psychoanalytic writings in the 1920s reveal the same method of complex presentations; but, in our case, the sheer number of conceptual relations could only be confirmed at the appropriate time and which had little to do with either personal or historical events. Were his writings, at the *manifest* level, on religion, while at the same time operating on a completely different level and working towards showing how suppressions and displacements could be more effective since they were concealed by a complex number of screens? The opening of *The Future of an Illusion* does not mention religion at all. The introduction is both a recapitulation of the theory of the super-ego and the death drive, and for very specific ends. Freud is writing with particular care and for readers who would not be convinced by superficial appearances. The impressions are as noticeable as they are divided. "One has to consult the book anew, and compare it to Freud's other words stylistically, to appreciate how bald an attack it is, how lacking in the usual graces of Freud's prose, how fiercely intent it is on hammering home its point."[17] A few more moments in consideration of the reception of this work is not without its rewards. Could Freud really be so concerned about "hammering home" his godlessness? Or were there not other, much more concealed, much more nuanced arguments being raised that (as I believe) are more relevant for today, Freud's future, than they were in his own lifetime? Parenthetically, we as readers are often at our worst when we give ourselves very generous latitude. Turning the issue back on Freud to talk about *his* illusion is, perhaps, daring; but wise it is not.[18] Once we pursue the re-introduction of *The Future of an Illusion* and the effect of the super-ego and the death drive on the religious unconscious of today's politics, then our task becomes both more clear and more challenging.

Once the traditional power of religion to unify a people into the collectivity of the church had been (for some) abandoned, the ensuing fragmentation gave everyone the few-found "freedom" to *represent* themselves. Liberal democracy has achieved its present-day status by renouncing any conscious reliance on the existence of God, king, leader, father. The prior attention to the social transformation from the individual leader to the introjected ego-ideal continues to be a permanent issue. Others have their own interpretation of the lacunae. First posing the question ("where have all the leaders gone?"), Michael Hardt and Antonio Negri answer: "To confront the leadership problem we need to recognize, first, that the lack of leaders in the movement today is neither accidental nor isolated: hierarchical structures have been overturned and dismantled within the movements as a function of both the crisis of representation and a deep aspiration to democracy."[19] I'm afraid that their conclusions are, for me, far from representing the real nature of the facts, which threaten to completely undermine their arguments. Their *political* analysis remains mired in traditional assumptions; their perceptions are far more about ideals that about the real matters at hand. The striking contrast between their deceptive idealism ("hierarchical structures have been overturned and dismantled") and the theological-political analysis offered by Freud on how all kinds of power and domination is deployed as substitutions for a leader is, again, re-affirmed. The logic of critical theory can no longer be sustained because its foundations have never altered and only one "enemy" has been identified – the outward one. Hardt and Negri believe that the absence of a leader somehow represents "a deep aspiration to democracy." My analysis shows something quite different, and antithetical to, any serviceable idea of democracy *for the people* and one, instead, ordered almost exclusively *by groups*.

Freud's writing on the future of our illusion has been interpreted, for the most part, with the carelessness of projected desire and without the awareness of our psychological dispositions as readers, which can be determined by internal and unconscious inclinations as any other human experience. Before the act of reading, making ourselves conscious of our own assumptions. Would seem to be a first requirement. One of the most attentive of Freud's readers has given us pause; individuals always stand out. "We too become overly reductive if we take them [his arguments] as a sign of Freud's actual view of religion."[20] *We become reductive*; we reduce ourselves – as if the regressive and the projective ended up emptying the human of its resources, intellectual and otherwise. Understood psychoanalytically, the outcome of a superficial reading means we are undermining ourselves (we impoverish ourselves) to one simplistic perspective – in other words, we as readers exemplify the characteristics of the infantile and the primitive and remain determined by archaic conflicts that never become conscious, are never resolved, and are perpetuated as defenses. Once Freud began to notice the increasing power of the super-ego to unsettle the life of his patients and both its origin and its consequences, he saw its destructive potential in all of social life. Psychoanalysis added one more responsibility to its therapeutic endeavors: its clinical work would have to devote itself more and more to assisting the analysand in working through the manipulations of the superego and to become strong enough, independent enough, autonomous enough, to resist the coercions of moral imperatives and to avoid falling into a compliance that, today, has become such a characteristic of the life within liberal democracies. Coercion, compliance, consensus; they operate as relational and with one goal in mind: to force the individual to submit to the ideals of a group who, by the power of their will, has driven itself to one supreme influence. Freud's analysis of the future of an illusion can be diverted from the assumption of its principal task; commentaries are brought forward to show how one perspective has been dominant. Many examples of the kind "he [Freud] writes with contempt about spirituality"[21] are all too common. Others are moderate in their views and are willing to consider other factors. *The Future of an Illusion* "is not a triumphant, anti-religious pamphlet but a study of the future or religion and culture as Freud sees it."[22] Religion and culture; or, for us to be more precise, the complicity between an unconscious theological-political matrix and its many consequences of all areas of social life is now the sole responsibility of the psychopolitical essay moving forward.

One interpretation of Freud's "pamphlet" shows him to be, understandably, at the height of his analytical powers and with an intricacy of thought that can only be appreciated by highlighting, as we will do here, the recurrent themes – beginning with his preoccupation with social and political *coercion.* That word is often repeated. Freud advances one antidote: independence and originality of thought. His defense of human freedom and intelligence will not be neglected, nor will the sense of individual originality. Once the exercise of social and political power is traced to the mechanisms of the super-ego, with some of its most analytically processes identified, then Freud's work and his analysis of an illusion can be placed in a much wider contest of the achievements of psychoanalysis as a thought and practice and its singular dedication to the therapeutic health of the individual. There are specific reasons for Freud opening *The Future of an Illusion* with re-affirmations made earlier and on the super-ego/death drive relationship. Before turning to the rhetorical complexity of Freud's presentation, a few reminders of previous ideas are necessary so that the whole is not forgotten. What does he tell us in the first two sections, that is, before religion is even mentioned, as the foundation of the argument to come? His axiomatic conviction in the super-ego and the death drive remains unwavering and presents him with problems still to be addressed. His assessments of what he calls culture or civilization includes an observation that, going forward, will be central to our psychopolitical concerns; because once Freud comes to the conclusion that "civilization is something which was imposed on a resisting majority by a minority which understood how to obtain possession of the means of power and coercion" (21:6), the developments within culture today are exhibiting precisely the same features, except for the fact that, in liberal democracies (unlike *traditional* totalitarian states) the majority has not been able to respond. The power and coercion of a minority is being continually exercised, but with refined methods. While it may be true that "every civilization must be built up on coercion and renunciation of instinct" (21:7), today the drives of the minority are *total*: they are simultaneously coercive with *selective* moral issues and *permissive* on others – as long the foundations of tradition are undermined. Radical permissiveness and taboo restrictions are fatally intertwined. Traditional instincts are disparaged; *new* ones are given propaganda support, promoted by groups and their various media and institutional allies. In the meantime, Freud solidifies his earlier theory of the death drive and tells us that "one has, I think, to reckon with the fact that there are present in all men destructive, and therefore anti-social and anti-cultural, trends and that in a great number of people these are strong enough to determine their behaviour in society" (21:7). When the thinking and acting ends up being antithetical to intentions, psychoanalysis has found its focus.

At the time of writing, Freud's social analysis led him to the double-imperative of society: the necessity of work and the renunciation of instinct. Both the nature of work and desire have been transformed in our time, leaving us with the repeated emphasis of "the rebelliousness and destructive mania of the participants in civilization" (21:10) as well as his awareness of the manner in which "external coercion gradually becomes internalized." The necessity of a normal, non-pathological conscience has in the meantime suffered from distortion. The *privacy* of conscience has been undermined by a collective re-organization of our sensibilities. The analytic idea of a "destructive mania" should not be minimized. But this is where conditions in liberal democracies have altered the previous force towards a more or less steady balance. The moral and the nihilistic were both essential to the historical movement of civilization; they were antithetical. Today, however, we can witness a most unusual set of circumstances: while the moral imperatives of the super-ego have been heightened to a particular strong degree, the nihilistic has been (and is) equally forceful. Both are expressed from the same split drive. In the past, unconscious impulses had to confront super-ego restrictions, a dynamic inter-relation evident, for example, in the nature of the dream-work. It is no longer the case that a suppressed people (i.e., the proletariat) are resisting the order created by what used to be called the owners of the means of production. *That* conflict is barely acknowledged today; can one even invoke the idea of class without being outdated? We are not living in a time when classes of the traditional sort can give us a sense of our social existence. In the past, and with the awareness of the unfolding of the Russian

Revolution and the formation of Soviet society, Freud could confidently say that a certain number of people in a given population were "not prepared to acknowledge the prohibitions," for understandably "they are intent on destroying the culture itself, and possibly even on doing away with the postulates on which it is based" (21:12). The previous conflict of classes, though it can still be readily seen in the perpetual historical difference of wealth and poverty, for families and nations, has been replaced by a different force and with characteristics that makes it historically unique. *The Future of an Illusion* opens with the death drive and super-ego for very specific purposes and before even mentioning anything about religion. While many have focused on the obvious, manifest, argument, some time spent analyzing and understanding his unique composition will make reading him more revealing. The concept of overdetermination can be kept in mind as one more Freudian originality on interpretation. The passage to follow includes, on top of the manifest content, a hint at the *censorship of a reader*.

> I must now turn to consider a further complication to which I would certainly give no space if I were a man of letters engaged upon the creation of a mental state like this for a short story, instead of being a medical man engaged upon its dissection. The element to which I must now allude can only serve to obscure and efface the outlines of the fine poetic conflict… … This element would rightly fall a sacrifice to the censorship of a writer, for he, after all, simplifies and abstracts when he appears in the character of a psychologist. But in the world of reality, which I am trying to depict here, a complication of motives, and accumulation and conjunction of mental activities – in a word, overdetermination – is the rule.[23]

Can we regard Freud's "complication of motives" with renewed attention to his writing and to the reality of a new knowledge of a particular kind of transference? One comment can prepare for the section to come. "As well as being famous for their literary quality, Freud's writings have the merit of corresponding, usually, with the patient's own words."[24]

(j) Transferential Free-Association

The attention to *The Future of an Illusion* has been on its extra-religious dimensions and how Freud organized a specific form of communication, in writing, to convey a message that was multiple and over-determined; for the purpose of analyzing his conscious transference, one issue can be set aside. His cultural knowledge of the word, and his extensive erudition, does not matter as much the intent of his writing and specific nature of his composition. Is there anything unique in the form of his writing and has it been underappreciated? Did his transmission include both *ancient* kinds of expression (first presented in the writing of myth – as Plato tells us) as well as the newfound interpretation of meaning as revealed by the *work* of dreams? Many have added considerable areas of interest on "Freud's work in the context of various literary traditions"[25] and so necessarily examined his writing and its antecedent inspiration. Still, our main and guiding focus continues to be on his theological-political analysis and how, through various ways of expressing himself – in a writing that cannot examined strictly in terms of rhetoric or style because it requires a different sensibility to the act of reading – he manages to convey (to *transfer*, extra-linguistically) other meanings than the most apparent one. Michael Jacobs has an immediate statement on one of the problems that has been recurrent. There is, indeed, a "popular view" of Freud. Today, it is almost wholly negative except, of course, where he remains pre-eminent; both him as an individual and psychoanalysis have suffered from all-too-common impressions. In general, the assessments from a public and by others tends towards the dismissive and not a little hostility.

> One of the Freud's major problems (or would if he were alive to witness it) is that many of those who quote him have failed to read anything he wrote. Instead they speak from passing knowledge, from reviews and critiques of his work, and from the popular view that pervades our culture. But Freud cries out to be read.[26]

We should give some critical *readers* the benefit of the doubt. They have been, one presumes, diligent when doing their homework. How is, of course, always another question. Detractors rarely hide their feelings; the origins of their personal sentiments, and their animosity to Freud personally and to psychoanalysis, are theirs to trace, or not, depending on their attitudes and motivations. An analysand has his own obligations. Reading *The Future of an Illusion* otherwise than is common can be a start for us. In a section called "the dimensions of Freud's writing," Giovanni Foresti remarks. "Let us try to free ourselves from traditional methods of reading and use a method often claimed as necessary: the *close reading* of the Freudian texts."[27] The sensibility of a *close reading*, which has a long and pronounced history (one extending to the Greek sensibility of *exegesis* and the Jewish rabbinical *midrash*) gives us one possibility. The close reading has to be more precisely defined.

Freud's writing cannot be fully understood, across its range, without at the same time a dual process of reading and listening that approximates the analytic experience. The attention of an analysand is more than ever necessary, for himself, first and foremost, and on the objects of his interest. The depth of language, as a form of human communication, has been only one of the perceptions of note during the analytic experience. The idea of the extra-linguistic can be repeated. While remaining focused on the problem at hand

and the uniqueness of *The Future of an Illusion*, we can again turn to the responses from theorists and analysts. Once the preliminaries have been made explicit (on the super-ego, the death drive, and the question of the nature of the theological-political as a psychical phenomenon – as a unity) Freud moves on to the scope of the work with one more decisive element. Although the specific nature of the writing is not new, he makes sure to alert the reader to a particular dynamic he has inherited from the most affective of world writers – first of all, from myth – as well as from discoveries he made during the period leading up to the completion of his monumental work on dreams – "the royal road to the unconscious." Freud's particular kind of thinking can be observed in the different levels of writing of this one document and how he presents a mode of expression that reflects the complexity of a psychical system as a whole. How can writing devote itself to adequately representing the workings of the psyche when, since the tripartite structure, the complexities have increased? His writing is certainly *energetic*, in the Greek sense of *energeia* and *ergon* (work), which is disciplined and multiple, emulating both the inter-action of systems, in concordance or conflict, and in the attempt to unify them for our understanding and interpretation. How he does so, and to what end, will be presented in the forthcoming arguments on the neglected aspects of Freud's *consciousness*, in the act of writing, as he presents an antidote to infantile defenses and the phenomenon of splitting. Any sense of Freud's literary *style* is going to be partial.

At the beginning of *Freud as a Writer*, Patrick Mahony writes: "I use the term *style* in a comprehensive sense, referring not merely to the deployment of various figures of speech, but also including the other parts of classical rhetoric, such as manner of delivery, logical structure and organization."[28] One "dimension" of Freud's writing will have to be acknowledged above the others mentioned by Mahony. Relying on rhetorical figures no doubt has its benefits in the interpretation of the work and in order to reach certain kinds of conclusion. Freud, however, is not overly preoccupied with tropes or any figures of speech; the following observation, however, can be noted. "Metaphors shape concepts and expressions that instil additional sense to the text and may at times undermine the titular argument made by sliding (latent) meanings in an unexpected direction."[29] A reading of Freud's writing, with the sensibility of an analysand, does not reveal so much any outstanding metaphors as, on the whole, a kind of communication evident in the transference of a clinical situation, both in terms of what is said and what is, also, conveyed. Freud writes as if making interventions for an analysand to hear – acutely because with multiple meanings. He adopts techniques that are well-known to him – he did, after all, invent its form in its finer details after Breuer's beginnings; they require, from the reader, a special kind of perception if, also, a psychoanalytically traditional one. Neither the technique nor the example is new. Did Freud surreptitiously use his own discovery in the interpretation of dreams to create a specific way of writing when a special occasion called for it? One distinction can serve as the first element of his writing. "What is clearly the essence of the dream-thoughts need not be represented in the dream at all. The dream is, as it were, differently centred from the dream-thoughts – its content has different elements as its central point."[30] Can we call the coming exposition, on Freud's message, the difference between the manifest writing and *Freud-thoughts*? Does he not, at the same time (in 1899) also write "Screen Memories" as one more indication of how his thinking and his writing are not as apparent as the reasoned-out thesis, with all its examples and arguments? In the first of other markers in the composition of *The Future of an Illusion*, he writes:

> An enquiry which proceeds like a monologue, without interruption, is not altogether free from danger. One is too easily tempted into pushing aside thoughts which threaten to break into it, and in exchange one is left with a feeling of uncertainty which in the end one tries to keep down by over-decisiveness. I shall therefore imagine that I have an opponent who follows my argument with mistrust, and here and there I shall allow him to interject some remarks.
>
> (21:21)

One could easily ignore Freud's self-reflection here and one of the imperatives of psychoanalytic free-association: the temptation to "push aside" thoughts emerging at the same time as the speech at the particular moment. Censorship can be present in many different situations; the act of reading may also be repressive.

The characterization of an "opponent" is not, exactly, a ruse. Freud does, however, establish a certain co-operative relation from the beginning – one that is inseparable from the early stages of an analysis in its clinical setting and how an analysand can be expected to talk – and to respond to interjections, including to the heaviness of silence, which is an initial burden to withstand. The whole of *The Future of an Illusion* to come from Section IV on will demand a certain perception. The work of Paul Ricoeur on the "hermeneutics of suspicion" and on the dedication to "How to Read Freud"[31] is not a superfluous reminder; except in our case, our reading will be directed towards a unique kind of attentiveness more than any sense of hermeneutic suspicion. We have, as one more preliminary responsibility, the exigency of an overdetermined reading – which is to say, quite the opposite of the majority who have consensus opinions. The concept of overdetermination seems to be one of the most appropriate antidotes to dogmatic orthodoxy, which establishes itself within certain well-defined limits. The production of meaning can be expedient; the act of reading as Freud conceives of it has unique kinds of demands. An analysand can make for one ideal reader because drawing on the experience of listening, interpretation, and understanding.

Not one among others of our commentators, in this case from Julia Kristeva, a philosopher and psychoanalyst, has one initial comment: "A superficial reading of The Future of an Illusion (1927) allows us to think that Freud reduced belief to an illusion."[32] Although the religious argument has been made time and again, the psychopolitical one is the more necessary one since it allows us to witness Freud not as a simple critic of religion (after all, that's commonplace) but as the consummate psychoanalyst who, at this point in his life as a thinker, could rely on the entire range of his concepts to analyze an unconscious phenomenon in culture. Kristeva's warning of a "superficial" reading is also the anticipation of our possible *oversight* – a word suggestive for us because of its divided meaning, as both watchful and, potentially, an omission. We can, with the dedicated work of Ilse Grubrich-Simitis, go "back to Freud's texts,"[33] and though her exacting call for a review of the translations, editions, and various forms of manuscripts of Freud's work to be part of the ongoing work of scholars of psychoanalysis, the equally important dedication to the interpretation of Freud's writing is, for me, essential in *The Future of an Illusion* in particular. Once we begin to read Freud's 1927 work, in part unconsciously, freely, and without the prejudice of anticipation, then we can recognize an entirely different thesis than the one superficially, and incompletely, noticed by those who are satisfied with the version of its anti-religious presentation. The illusion is not, strictly speaking, religious; the illusion (which will soon transform itself into a political one) is the belief that secularity could be free of the religious once and for all and fail to recognize how a theological-political transformation in society had come about. Remarkably, one of the most obvious of psychoanalytic ideas could be so easily ignored, which proves the power of desire, and the need for illusion, to perpetuate a narcissistic view of ourselves. That illusion was one of most concern for Freud; and its truth is more relevant now than it was a century ago.

In his "Introduction," Salman Akhtar believes that Freud's interlocutor, otherwise described as an opponent, is someone who believes in God and is religious.[34] The assessment is too one-sided, presenting an either/or relation, between Freud the atheist and the presence of someone who, time and again, is given the opportunity to respond as a defendant of religion. Freud has not constructed *an argument*, as such, with each side presenting their beliefs in the manner of a rational and worked-out exposition; that would be much too standard as an exercise and lacking all the complications of an analytic speech situation. An analysand who *argues* is doing something other than analysis; as does the analysand who talks about Freud or psychoanalysis (theoretically) instead of himself. Resistance in analysis takes many forms. We cannot simply proceed with the assumption that Freud is the atheist and, in Peter Gay's words, the "godless Jew,"[35] while Freud's opponent represents, perhaps, a Viennese Catholic. Is it likely that "Freud structured *The Future of an Illusion* as if were addressed to a hypothetical adversary who argues against his assertions?"[36] There is, as such, no argument against an opponent being conducted in the work. Freud is expository – and for reasons that are directly related to his *future* reader who will experience a transference (in perception) in the act of reading. The either/or thesis has been rejected from the beginning as inadequate because it conforms to a rational logic and, in itself, cannot account for the layers of the psyche. Freud is acutely aware of the irrelevance of rational arguments when drives are overactive and perceptions are determined from unconscious sources. His resources are psychical, at once informed by the dreamwork and by the nature of screens.

Are we now in a position of understanding Freud's writing as many layered, conveying different simultaneous impressions, that both reveals and conceals, consciously, and so doing to activate the interpretation of the reader, as a kind of provocation for those willing to extend themselves beyond the manifest content of a screen? In his address when receiving the Goethe prize, he concludes his speech with a typical "inside" comment. "Goethe was not only, as a poet, a great self-revealer, but also, in spite of the abundance of autobiographical records, a careful concealer."[37] The concluding quote, from Goethe's *Faust*, "the best of what you may know may not, after all, be told to boys," makes a reader all the more aware of how wily Freud could be. He was no stranger to a specific kind of indirect communication; the subject of religion proved to be his most daring exercise in analytic thinking and exposé. There is no intent on his part to conceal what he wants to convey to the reader; he will, however, not make it so transparent and accessible that it will be read by *anyone*. The over eager predisposed by convictions, of an anti-religious type, would miss the mark. If the revealing/concealing distinction can be maintained, Freud makes the work of reading and interpretation more than simply an exercise in receiving information, as if the author was merely preoccupied with telling the reader his views about religion and allowing an interlocutor to make comments on the side, agreeing or not. Can we adopt one of Leo Strauss' arguments, in this case for Freud – and making the writing more pronounced since, leading up to his declaration, there has been the attempt to provide a number of inter-related processes of readings which have been outlined in terms of screens? According to Strauss and his distinction between esoteric and exoteric writing, certain authors will

> employ a peculiar manner of writing which would enable them to reveal what they regard as the truth to the few, without endangering the unqualified commitment of the many to the opinions on which society rests. They will distinguish between the true teaching as the esoteric writing and the socially useful teaching as the exoteric writing; whereas the exoteric writing is meant to be easily accessible to every reader, the

> esoteric teaching discloses itself only to very careful and well-trained readers after long and concentrated study.[38]

There is no doubt that Freud was writing both for a lay reader, his fellow psychoanalysts, and analysands. The back-and-forth gave the reader the opportunity to examine both sides *and more*. At one level – a conscious one – Freud and his "opponent" are discussing the problems and merits of religion in culture. Many have chosen to remain at this one level instead of making the psychoanalytically necessary effort to interpret the work according to several of Freud's concepts – of which only three inter-related ones, among the many others possible, will be mentioned and all from the creative period during the writing of *The Interpretation of Dreams*: the manifest/latent distinction, the work of displacement and condensation, and the screen which has its first historical example in the writing of ancient myths. What, then, is behind the *screen* of *The Future of an Illusion*?

A few selected passages from "Screen Memories" will orient our reading of Freud's work on religion and its meaning for social and political life. The most significant issue is not the recollection of a memory – or its omission. The screen operates psychically in more ways than in remembering and forgetting. "We must first enquire why it should be that precisely what is important is suppressed and what is indifferent retained."[39] If we abstract from Freud's explicit argument on the nature of remembering and forgetting and we use our examples, is it possible to consider a political retention and a religious amnesia? Does the political imperative exist only by virtue of a noticeable amnesia and perpetual suppression of the religious? Are we going to notice how the specific word illusion, as it makes its appearance here, will return at a later time and in the context of politics and so show the transference between one and the other? Can we continue to advance our overall argument by stressing how the illusion of religion is introjected into the politics of liberalism to sustain it as a moral project? The important distinction between a conscious suppression makes all the difference in this case. Due to the apparent elimination of religion from consciousness and from social life (or rather, the attempt to make it so) the political can take its place without any apparent interference. Its jurisdiction is unhampered and complete. The political gives itself the illusion that it no longer has any rivals; and yet, the more one examines its contemporary characteristics, it seems more theological than ever, with "the same sanctity, rigidity, intolerance, the same prohibition of thought," the analysis Freud gives us in *The Future of an Illusion*. The freedom of the political from the religious gives it the illusion of secularity. The political would be the confidence of a supersession of the religious; the illusion has been how secularity, divested of God and faith and all the other attachments of a certain prejudice, can now emerge in itself and so be free. Without religion, then, the modern subject, and society as a whole, can give itself the illusory comfort of being entirely secular and proceeding along purely rational and "scientific" principles, though always keeping in mind that, early on, Freud recognized a peculiar and, perhaps too, a historically novel problem to be analyzed: "obsessional neuroses as a pathological counterpart to religion" (9:126). When the latter is given up, the former can take its place without so much as an inkling of the process. *Why* this has occurred has been a constant preoccupation in Freud's thought. One writer has been forthright, even as he mounts an extreme critique of Freud. "Sigmund Freud believed that the modern susceptibility to neurosis and paranoia could be explained as a side-effect of the process of secularization."[40] "Side effect" is a mild way of describing the situation.

Freud's reminder of the relationship between remembering and forgetting is all the more relevant for our specific topic. There are, for Freud, "two psychical forces" at work. "One of these forces takes the importance of the experience as a motive for seeing to remember it, while the other – a resistance – tries to prevent any such reference from being shown" (3:307). The psychical mechanism discussed by Freud in "Screen Memories," in part as one more outcome of his knowledge of dreams, becomes one explanation for the modern phenomenon of psychopolitics. The religious has been resisted and suppressed in order for the political to give itself absolute independence and so carry out any and all programs according to a confident rationality. Freud reminds us, however, that the confidence is misplaced; the noticeable arrogance of politically motivated groups is one more sign of an origin whose force has to be suppressed at all times. Defenses and reaction formations are constant necessities. The more the religious is suppressed, the more it continues to operate; and with greater power and impunity, unconsciously, through energetic channels with their own inner logic and ends.

The force of one aspect of suppression, most especially in the last half-century of liberal confidence, has been ongoing and vigorous. Liberal societies have consciously determined themselves according to a self-declared detachment from religion; by doing so, they have retained (unconsciously and in the very workings of the super-ego) the very worst of the religious imagination and its absolutism. The present conditions can be given one more theoretical explanation, once more to recall the *Introductory Lectures* and one specifically on "Some Thoughts on Development and Regression – Aetiology." We continue to emphasize, in a way that seems to me of utmost importance, how Freud's views are leading towards the discontents of civilization and due to one specific transference. "Hysteria and obsessional neurosis are, as you know, the two chief representatives of transference neuroses" (16:343). The transference shown, in *The Future of an Illusion*, will be unequivocal.

The political has become unconsciously metaphysical, supported by one absolute drive – a morality that has now begun to show its most disquieting aspects: its orthodoxy has been driving at a totality, and that is the reason

Freud often used the word *danger*. The suppression of the religious has been unsuccessful. The political exhibits its religious remnants. It may have displaced and/or condensed the religious element of everyday life. In doing so, it has unwittingly ensured that it would remain as a perpetual presence and dominate consciousness to such a degree that the psychical repository of the religious suppressed would eventually become overpowering. The development of the idea of the screen memory was not to be restrained to the problem of forgetting and remembering. The same mechanism extended itself to other psychical operations. A screen memory, as such, "owes its value to a memory not to its own content, but to the relation existing between that content and some other, that has been suppressed" (3:320). One can feel confident in now altering the concepts and writing, via Freud, that a *screen politics* is one that can be perceived not only by its content (the moral) but to the traditional religious that has been suppressed. The diminished sense of the religious in our secular society of liberal democracies has made it possible for an absolutist and authoritarian political movement to emerge and with a drive far more powerful than any previously known when the theological and the political could still be discerned in its conscious relation.

Anticipating the first conclusion, Freud writes: "Education freed from the burden of religious doctrines will not, it may be, effect much change in men's psychological nature" (21:54). Education, religious doctrine, and human nature. Freud is under no illusion: ridding oneself of one foundational element of social life in the world would not abolish the psychological dynamics of the human. The *apparent* freedom would prove to have much more disastrous effects; the *cognitive* education – to be free from religion – did not have an equal effect on the depth-psychological because the transference was wholly unconscious. Once the religious and the political came into contact, unconsciously and precisely due to the pretensions of secularity, the effects would prove to be powerful. Freud warned us that the waning of religion would actually increase neurotic afflictions. The statement, far from being in any way connected to an either/or, defense or critique (which Freud knew would ultimately change nothing in the unconscious disposition of human beings individually, in groups, or in an entire society) led his reader to a much more important realization. While many read the work as, simply, anti-religious, Freud was far more intricate and went a long way in reminding everyone how secularity would have its own unexpected consequences. Freud's analysis could only be recognized when the historical conditions reached a state where his writings, from a century ago, arrived at their proper destination – that is, the future and the present of our illusion.

Only because latencies, displacements, and screens are psychologically operative does the present time suffer from a state earlier described as a kind of contagion. The either/or is both too simplistic and too convenient. The difference is more nuanced than first appears, as Freud tells us when he communicates with his interlocutor. "You emerge as an enthusiast who allows himself to be carried away by illusions, and I stand for the claims of reason, the rights of scepticism" (21:51). Does the sentence, with a *free context*, allow for the interpretation of the enthusiast and the sceptic to be political opponents and therefore far different than in the analytic setting? Because, if the argument proposed here holds, the relationship Freud sets out between his two opponents (which are two individuals in the analytic setting – or, for Freud, a self-analytical soliloquy) is by no means the same as political opponents; or to use a stronger word that later will have to be placed beside the imperative of loving one's neighbor as oneself, *enemies*. Two preliminary arguments have been made: one, the illusion of a political secularity, two, the specifically analytical nature of the two "opponents" who are implicated in a binding transference. Once both are taken into consideration, and with a certain re-orientation to *The Future of an Illusion*, we can resist the facility of an either/or choice and, instead, think with Freud and other analysts who gave us sufficient subtlety to think for ourselves;[41] because if, in the preceding sections, the moral pretensions of our age have been correctly evaluated, then we can begin to highlight more observations that (in keeping with the force of psychoanalysis to make us skeptical about ourselves) will give everyone some thought as we move towards our conclusion on the discontents of civilizations. One statement from Neville Symington can serve as a transition to our next section. "Psychoanalysts have had patients who consciously affirm their commitment to truth, justice, and compassion but whose inner dispositions are utterly ruthless."[42] It appears indisputable that, among its other attributes, psychoanalysis has always had the courage to treat our most cherished ideals with a certain distance. Freud experienced the consequences of his courage firsthand and often. We are fortunate that Symington, for one, can give us a sense of how complex human beings can in fact be – and are, and in no area of human life perhaps more so than in that new conjunction of the moral and the political, there precisely where *truth and justice* meets the *ruthlessness* of the super-ego. Are we not historically familiar with political revolutions and the methods they have adopted to organize their ideals – at the expense of human beings who, as always, are made to suffer and die as the sacrificial subjects they have always been made to be? Is it any wonder that Freud, on more than one occasion, uses the Soviets as a specific example of moral ruthlessness to achieve its ends?

Freud's development in *The Future of an Illusion* reaches another important point when the relation (between Soviet ideology and unconscious religion) is finally made explicit as a historical phenomenon; its particularity should not make us complacent about its perpetual threat as a psychological disposition. The return to infantile defenses is once again a recollection of Freud's foundational argument in group psychology. The infantile nature of religious sensibilities, which has been so welcome by secularists, is no longer going to be as satisfying when the previous discussion of the infantile and the primitive in group psychology is brought forward to the future of our liberal illusions. Throughout this section, Freud has been regarded as someone who acted essentially as a translator between the creations of the psyche and its reality. To do so he had to become ever so conscious of what his writing, and its levels, could mean. To meet Freud, as it were, halfway (or as close as possible as a reader), Sarah Wood has given us a serviceable term, the *force of reading* and the "extraordinary act of attention to the idiom."[43] As we move to the next section, Freud can leave us with one more confirmation. There are numerous references we can rely on to consider how the manifest writing of *The Future of an Illusion* is only one aspect of its immediate presentation that requires a supplement in interpretation. There may be no better origin, with the ones already mentioned, than in one particular section of "The Claims of Psycho-Analysis to Scientific Interest" where he opens Part II with non-psychological sciences and philology. This one section, on language, gives us a kind of testimony that we are conscious of and yet forget when reading. Freud writes: "It may be pointed out that the interpretation made by psycho-analysis are first and foremost translations from an alien method of expression into the one which is familiar to us."[44] Since we *read* with a familiar consciousness, unless we are prepared to recognize unconscious intentions and the writings (and our own unrecognized assumptions), we risk losing an essential communication – as Freud conveys in this one writing in particular.

(k) The Revival of Infantile Defenses

Any satisfactory perception in the one-dimensional critique of religion in *The Future of an Illusion* should, by now, have become at least doubtful. Reviewing the premises of the work has made it possible to offer alternative interpretations; they are of sufficient importance to further suspend traditional judgments and to continue to examine Freud's presentation. The previously mentioned work on "The Claims of Psychoanalysis to Scientific Interest" did not fail to mention the theme of development (which has been central for us since regression) and how its findings were extensive. "From the very first psycho-analysis was directed towards tracing developmental processes. It began by discovering the genesis of neurotic symptoms, and was led, as time went on, to turn its attention to other psychical structures and to construct a genetic psychology which would apply to them too" (13:183). The expression "genetic psychology" presents us with a better sense of what to expect once we turn to one of the discussions in *The Future of an Illusion* on infantile defenses and their effect in any social reality where individuals, groups, or an entire society, are involved. The organization of his writing, structurally, continues to *activate* previous discoveries (foundational ones, on regression) and their relevance.

Recollecting the psychical process of regression and its tie to the revival of infantile and primitive defenses makes the condition of the contemporary adult filled with more than a few perpetual unconscious influences. The origins of a primary experience can be in part re-traced and for the many reasons Freud will give us as to the nature of human beings as they mature from the period of infantile vulnerability to the equally demanding life of the more or less mature adult; resiliency and the strength of the ego are conditions to be consciously developed in order to avoid relying on too many consolations, including assumptions made about the nature of reality. "For this situation," Freud tells us, "is nothing new. It has an infantile prototype, of which it is in fact only the continuation. For once before one has found oneself in a similar state of helplessness: as a small child, in relation to one's parents" (21:17). Since we have the *psychical* "prototype," the individual can avail himself of its remnants for *any* illusion. Once the helplessness has been experienced as a condition of infancy, the emotions attached to the state of being can be revived; or to be more precise, in some cases they have never been overcome and have persisted throughout the process of a stunted maturity and, if the regressive process has been particularly acute, paralyzed at an infantile and primitive level. The unconscious effects of the super-ego are predominant. The introduction of an infantile situation that *precedes* any conscious awareness of religious life, as consolation or anything else, can be expanded from one narrow focus. Freud's analysis is attempting to be comprehensive and to understand the entire force of the civilizing process, from the infant to the individual to the group, finally to all of the most important institutions of society that form the ego according to particular social standards. By returning to the infantile state of dependence, when autonomy is only possible in daydreams and fantasies and play, or in a mild or excessive refuge in neuroses, Freud has taken us back to a universal situation, one whose impact would be perpetual and, in many ways, never overcome except through *the work* of maturity and the awareness of the role of both compensatory fantasy and desire. Maturity, however, is not easily achieved; the psyche is tempted to abandon its difficult work of growing up and regress to a state of thought and being for security. The illusion of the gain from illness is one form of evasion. Group identity, and ideology, can take the place of the personal work of being conscious; the ego could lapse into a state of *double conscience* – to use an early psychoanalytic term – and take refuge in the collectivity of a group, more so if it shared patterned characteristics. The sense of a "doubled" consciousness, and in particular the division within the super-ego, can also be defined in terms of a splitting.

In "The Uncanny," Freud wrote: "The idea of the 'double' does not necessarily disappear with the passing of primary narcissism, for it can receive fresh meaning from the later stages of the ego's development. A special agency is slowly formed there, which is able to stand over against the rest of the ego, which has the function of observing and criticizing the self and of exercising a censorship within the mind."[45] The regression of the group and, when the coercive manipulations are powerful enough, for an entire society, return to a state of infantile vulnerability in order to access, once more, the archaic defenses deployed at the time when there was no other alternative. These "ego disturbances," as a splitting that we have traced more directly to the division within the super-ego, "are harking back to particular phases in the evolution of the self-regarding feeling, a regression to a time when the ego had not yet marked itself off sharply from the external world and from other people" (17:236).

The dependent child will make way for the imperious adult who, understandably reacting against a former anxiety, insecurity, and intense struggle, proclaims himself as autonomous without first attending to the transition – which proves to be an illusion and with noticeable effects on psychological health, for himself and those who are exposed to him. The demand for reflection is negated because of the drive towards the external world; the control of others, more so when exercised with power, is a compensatory acting out that, ultimately, will cause increased conflict. While one level of Freud's exposition in *The Future of an Illusion* concentrated on the manifest presentation of a religious infantilism, the transition he soon introduces, and that forms the unity of the theological-political realist, is inseparable from his psychological preoccupations. The transference may have been presented with careful nuance; the reader who has lingered and returned and examined what appeared to be inconsequential has found himself with the possibility of a new and complementary argument. The nexus of infantile defenses and religion is only one manifestation of a much wider condition of being.

His psychobiography of Leonardo da Vinci had, in part, laid another groundwork: "when at a later date he perceives how truly forlorn and weak he is when confronted with the great forces of life, he feels his condition as he did in childhood, and attempts to deny his own despondency by a *regressive revival* of the forces which protected his infancy."[46] The psychical mechanism is not, in itself, religious. The experiences of the infant are recurrences of a struggle between the multitude of impressions, especially in the first few months of life, and external objects, a reality which can only be intuited without clarity or proper perception. When *The Future of an Illusion* is read psychoanalytically, then the human vulnerability to illusion is not simply attributable to religion. If only we could give ourselves the self-satisfaction that religion, and religion alone, had been the one human tradition responsible for our susceptibility to the loss of freedom and the diminishing of intelligence, how much easier would our cultural work be; if only one social and historical institution could be isolated and given sole *blame* (that is to say, allegorically, if only religion alone was *sinful*) then its eradication would once again restore the possibility of human freedom. Aira Laine makes a unique observation; the reference to reading is, again, noted: "When reading the work of Freud, one is repeatedly astonished by how many modern 'new' insights already exist in his writings."[47] Their "newness" continues because we are, in many cases, only now mature enough, as readers, to understand the implications of his psychoanalytic thinking from a century ago. Although the sense, for the time being, may not yet be fully perceived, it seems to me that Freud has achieved an unprecedented level of new cultural significance because he has so exposed the machinations of regression and all the symptoms they have produced in our contemporary liberal reality.

As long as Freud's psychoanalysis of religion is conveniently understood as complete (in conformity to an easily held atheism) then its interpretative supplement is simply ignored and its political meanings are suppressed. The regression of our contemporary liberal politics exemplifies the modern state of infantilism within the group as conditions of a pathology that allows for the power of the super-ego to express itself without limits. Freud has been consistent in his regards for the human individual and the pressures, overall, of human existence in a world that is, on the whole, indifferent to its needs and desires – or its well-being. If we recollect the previous arguments on the regressions of the group, we can see how Freud was adding to earlier observations, both practical and conceptual, to the present argument on illusion as a human tendency. His earlier consideration of Leonardo da Vinci's relationship to his father, religion, and his society, was not incidental to his thinking in the 1920s.

> The protection against neurotic illness, which religion vouchsafes to those who believe in it, is easily explained: it removes their parental complex, on which the sense of guilt in individuals as well as in the whole human race depends, and disposes of it, while the unbeliever has to grapple with the problem on his own.
>
> (11:123)

Freud's analysis, beyond one individual, had brought him to the sense of *any* form of social thought that could make it possible to be free of a "parental complex" and therefore (this, then, is where illusions become political) no longer restrained by a genealogical inheritance and indebtedness to prior generations.

Freud has already made the argument and without so much as a hesitation. The analytic transference of his writing, by the end, becomes much more explicit for anyone who could not perceive the many-layered nature of his presentation. We have to remind ourselves of Freud, the creative individual, who has left us a legacy of thinking that exceeds our common attitude. His own relationship to a great work of art, like Michelangelo's Moses, should be (for us) equally applicable to the awareness of how to read Freud. In "The Moses of Michelangelo," he writes:

> What grips us so powerfully can only be the artist's *intention*, in so far as he has succeeded in expressing in his work and in getting us to understand it. I realize that this cannot be a matter of *intellectual* comprehension; what he aims at is to awaken in us the same emotional attitude, the same mental constellation as that which in him produced the impetus to create… … To discover his intention, though, I must first find out the meaning and content of what is represented in his work; I must, in other words, be able to *interpret* it.[48]

There are two points of importance: one is immediate and furthers my interpretation of *The Future of an Illusion*, the other is a preparation for isolating the role of art and creativity for the understanding of an essential aspect of human being. Our attention to the creativity of *Totem and Taboo*, and to the role of the mythic poet, remains dynamic for us as readers. The example of two artists whose impact on the creation of the Renaissance is beyond estimate has been intentional.

A moment of transition, from the diagnostic to the remedial, can be anticipated. For the time being, my reading can express one distinction – which has been mentioned before: the difference between what is merely perceived cognitively, and what is perceived as a part of what Freud called an "emotional attitude"; that is, the affect behind the perception and how feelings and intelligence are inseparable. Without emotions, the work of the intelligence is incomplete and, like the problems of theoretical thought, potentially distorted. The previous identification of the hysterical or obsessive political activist is re-affirmed; but rather than relying on the religious argument, it is necessary to turn from the religious to the political and to again present how the psychical religious is projected into the political to form the amalgamation of the main theme of my psychopolitical essay. Once we recognize how Freud transfers his manifest discourse on religion to a latent discourse on politics, like the dream and its thoughts, we can begin to open up a different perspective and to acknowledge how the defense mechanism of the infant, which preceded any conscious awareness of religion, is at once a regression and a revival of a previous experience that finds one outlet in the intense desire to change the nature of reality. Infantile defenses are the grounds for the consolation of religion and, more so, operative in the transference to the political. That the identity with a particular group makes the process all the easier is but one of the characteristics of our present-day phenomenon.

"There is no doubt that from 1926 onwards the study of the defense mechanisms is to become a major theme of psycho-analytic research."[49] In *The Future of an Illusion*, the power of the defense mechanisms were introduced to emphasize how they were operative in all kinds of personal experience and in the dynamic of group behavior. It will be our responsibility going forward to continue to outline all the ways Freud makes the question of the "theological-political" explained by psychoanalysis as the unconscious of our present. He gives us a much more in-depth connection when he presents how their relationship has been determined (*will be* determined) by the dual workings of the super-ego and the death drive. In our day, the first principle has been wilfully abolished, only to give the political actor apparent freedom about how to determine social and political life. While the unconscious dynamic of infantile helplessness and rage are one of the unacknowledged expressions of the political activist, there is the added power of the super-ego morality and its innumerable injunctions. The regression and revival expressed two formidable psychical forces: on the one hand, the defense mechanism of the frustrated and helpless child; on the other, the drive of the super-ego and the death drive that, together, are irrepressible because of the moral rationalizations of destroying the old and the traditional. The pathology of the political has no restraints. It can act out all its psychical fantasies, conscious and unconscious, with impunity. The calls by certain groups to either "defund" or "abolish" the police, as a consequences, precisely, of pathological super-ego behavior, is one indication of how excessive the delusions have become. One can only wonder what would happen to some of these politically minded groups once the police were no longer in existence and we returned to a "state of nature" where the only ruling authority would, simply, be the exercise of brutal power or, once again, make it necessary (as Thomas Hobbes believed) to introduce the sovereign as a saviour and who would be inevitably made legitimate by divine dispensation.

One commentator refers to a "perverted liberalism,"[50] to define the times, a perversion of a reality that is optimally instrumentalized to serve psychological ends. The perversion has become not a deviation but, rather, the norm and so all the more obvious for its moral perversion, an issue that could be supplemented with another argument that would have to take its bearing in the origins of hysteria and in Freud's first discussions of sexuality. For our purposes, which has for the most part excluded the discussion of our moribund sexuality, the transition here has added one more element to the analysis of our political condition. On the topic of sexuality, Margaret Clark has made an incisive comment – which also (as we can notice) pointing out the inadequacy of readers. "They also pick up in passing the notion that Freud was hostile to religion. This traditional understanding of Freud, usually unexamined and simplified as pro-sex and anti-religion, continues the opposition of sexuality to religion which goes back a long way."[51] As long as manifest truths are not examined from the perspective of their much deeper resonances, we continue to undermine Freud's inquiry. There are no shortages of examples. Another can be added because of the context; that is, in "'Civilized' Sexual Morality and Modern Nervous Illness." If the connection is tied by the sex/religion bind, so traditional it has, by today, outworn its relevance, then Freud's message will remain unnoticed. The long quote in many ways sums up the psychopolitical essay thus far and what remains to be analyzed.

> A chronic neurosis, even if it does not totally put an end to the subject's capacity for existence, represents a severe handicap in his life... ... The situation would even be tolerable if neurotic illness were to exclude from civilized activities only a number of individuals who were in any case of the weaker sort, and allowed the rest to play their part in it at the cost of troubles that were merely subjective. But, far from this being so, I must insist upon the view that neuroses, whatever their extent and wherever they occur, always succeed in frustrating the purposes of civilization, and in that way actually perform the work of the suppressed mental forces that are hostile to civilization. Thus, when society pays for obedience to its far-reaching regulations by an increase in nervous illness, it cannot claim to have purchased a gain at the price of sacrifices; it cannot claim a gain at all.[52]

The truth of Freud's statement is, today, substantially different than it was when first written; and radically different, in sense, that when it was read (say, in the 1960s, or when Herbert Marcuse's *Eros and Civilization* was widely read) and for us today. The regulations of liberal society is no longer preoccupied with *sexual* morality, except to remove every single restriction deemed in any way prohibitive or a matter of prejudice. The word *phobia* is, today, overused. It is not a diagnosis but, rather, an accusation. Read from the perspective of our liberal morality, Freud's statement takes on a meaning that again can warn us to the danger he has several times alerted us about. Our contemporary morality has indeed managed to make the majority *obey*; the consequences, of increased neuroses, are intrinsically part of the same process of moralizing.

While the analysis has been ongoing and has partly identified the issues, it seems more and more the case that only psychoanalysis can provide us with a deep enough assessment of our political situation. The ego of the everyday citizen is, understandably, overwhelmed by the vehemence of the political. We have moved a considerable way from a supposed critique of religion to a much more comprehensive psychoanalysis of Western civilization and our liberal democracies. What remains? It should come as no surprise, though it is relatively rare in the literature, to read about "Freud's explicit moral philosophy."[53] Are we to suggest that psychoanalytic morality, which Freud advances in an unmistakeable way both in the "Postscript" of *Group Psychology* and in the work of the 1920s all the way to *Civilization and its Discontents*, can be a therapeutic alternative to the current state of liberal societies? We have mentioned, and now repeat, how one antagonism has to become much more conscious at the individual and social level: unless the ego is given enough strength and support (to its freedom and intelligence, creativity, and ability to love) the super-ego and the death drive are going to continue their collaboration and with ever more dire impoverishment. If the revival of infantile defenses was brought up again in *The Future of an Illusion* and to underscore the psychical vulnerabilities of the child as their persistence in the regressed adult, can we (with Freud) begin to organize an antidote and one specifically devoted to *the ego*? Before doing so, one last preoccupation in this section can turn, once more, to the dialogue between Freud and his imaginary interlocutor.

"You emerge as an enthusiast who allows himself to be carried away by illusions, and I stand for the claims of reason, the rights of scepticism" (21:51). Freud's written words, and their conscious transference, have to be correctly heard. He has told his interlocutor, the "enthusiast," that his now fervent belief in the ability to be free from illusions, religious ones above all, is something he should think about much more deeply. The education to reality demands that psychical impulses are at least temporarily made inactive. The ingenious reversal, transferring positions to highlight a psychical disposition in his "opponent," portrays Freud as the *sceptic*. In other words, he proclaims himself sceptical about the ability of someone to so easily declare himself free from religious illusions and to then take consolation in secularity. Freud points out that the freedom from a religious illusion (indeed, *any illusion at all*) is in many ways "the influence of your wishes." When our desires are remnants from infantile frustration, the consequences, for the adult, are difficult to manage. He continues and reaches one conclusion.

"You pin your hope on the possibility that generations which have not experienced the influence of religious doctrines in early childhood will easily attain the desired primacy of the intelligence over the life of the instincts. This is surely an illusion" (21:51). The all-important relation – religious doctrines and early childhood, and our first theme of intelligence – can be read much too easily and without taking into consideration his previous argument on infantile defenses. The diagnosis of illusion is, finally, revealed with force. The secular illusion has been (and is): if only we can educate ourselves beyond the prejudices of our religious illusions, then we will be free and intelligent and ultimately happier. Freud does not indulge us on this critical matter. The message could not be clearer: our drives precede our illusions and if the primacy of the intelligence is every going to be reached, for society (because we know that individuals can and have done so) then the nature of the obsessive drives will have to be finally understood both for their origins and intended purpose. Making only one comment on Freud's "pessimism," Didier Anzieu responds with the following:

> I share Freud's serene realism and constructive pessimism about projects that claim to change the basis of human nature or to control evolution…
> … I only know one attitude in the face of the inevitable wear and tear to

> psychological, pedagogical, moral, and political systems, and in the face of their alteration and perversion – what Aristotle called their 'corruption': to maintain by what one says, what one writes, and what one does, the straight grain that others warp.[54]

The illusions created by the psyche precede any kind of religious exposure to its beliefs or its orthodoxy. The threat to human intelligence analyzed in the various symptoms of group identification has one of its origins in the debility of childhood. The defense mechanism of *the adult* maintains the individual in a regressive state; the infantile affects are perpetually revived, as are the defenses which are responsible for what Anzieu calls the "warp" of the human and of reality. Can we at this point be satisfied with a superficial critique of religion when Freud gives us a much more complete analysis of the psychical origins of illusions? Religion may have indeed become a form of consolation from everyday life; it can hardly be identified as the only one or, as we now see, the one with the most grievous outcomes. Is the 21st century going to reach a point of political excess that, after all, is hardly new or unexpected?

Freud gives no one any illusions. The future he so clearly envisioned was, in many ways, our own. Readers who have been so satisfied by a superficial reading of Freud's "critique" of religion did not give themselves the needed extra work, consistent with analytic therapy in the clinical situation between two people, the on-going, interminable work of pressing the issues day in, day out, until as many if not all of the components are taken into account and their complex inter-relation examined for its effects *on life*. The biggest illusion of all is to consider that a cognitive realization of any situation can be sufficient to somehow overcome or resolve the psychological impact of distress and with so many symptoms being a cause of misery and unhappiness. Freud expressed skepticism because, above all, he was attempting to mitigate human suffering and contribute to some sense of human happiness, which, as he will defend in *Civilization and its Discontents*, could be attainable with the fundamental aspects of human life – freedom, intelligence, creativity, love, and, finally, the possibility of happiness. In the 1920s, and as a further commitment to the well-being of individuals and society, Freud unified his therapeutic and social-theory ambitions into a comprehensive whole. He was writing for posterity.

Our three previous allusions to the latent argument is now fully revealed and through Freud's "collaborator." The previous statement, on the first page of the concluding section of *The Future of an Illusion*, can no longer be read with interpretative complacency. While the interlocutor is defending religion, we should not give ourselves the assurance of simply rejecting his arguments – not if we want to remain related to Freud as he presents us with the single most-important argument of the work. Another "system of "doctrines" has indeed been presented and increasingly so in the first two decades of our century. The religious has been suppressed according to all the programs of a political secularity; what has become all too evident is that the "psychological characteristics of religion," the ones associated with the super-ego and the death drive, have become predominant and more enduring because better concealed.

If we follow Freud's presentation of two arguments, side by side, what begins to become clear as the end is approached is the most appropriate decision for the sake of psychological health. There is no point in simply following the one argument that, of course (who would dispute this?) the child requires to be educated and in ways that have nothing to do with knowledge as such but with the limits to what social being expects if one is to live within certain acceptable parameters. In one way or another, the existence of the super-ego in society is both required and desired. The problem, as we are now experiencing it, has occurred because of human arrogance in the face of our need for the limits of being. Starting out from the presumption that we could live more than adequately without the idea of God (indeed, much better) we set ourselves to creating a secular society based on our own designs. We were not, however, prepared for the outcome we now have. The once moderate super-ego, developing normally and in conjunction with other psychical agencies that were given *their* limits, once it was freed to express itself as it saw fit in the making of a moral world order, its methods and self-possession were no longer hampered by anything. Moral desire could become absolute. Freud gives us nothing less than a warning. "What is characteristic of illusions is that they are derived from human wishes. In this respect they come near to psychiatric delusions" (21:31). Our illusions can no longer be conveniently limited to religion; by doing so, we will only give ourselves the illusion of concealing our own *psychiatric* delusions. Freud does indeed present himself as an *iatros* of the *psyche* (a doctor of the soul), one who saw that the civilization as a whole had to be diagnosed.

At the beginning of VII, Freud asks a question. If the previous argument has had any merit, then this is the definitive turning point that leads to several inter-related conclusions and, together, are completed in *Civilization and its Discontents*. "Having recognized religious doctrines as illusions, we are at once faced by a further question: may not other cultural assets of which we hold a high opinion and by which we let our lives be ruled be of similar nature. Must not the assumptions that determine our *political regulations* be called illusions as well?" (21:34). The statement has not received the attention it deserves. To stress its importance – the *political regulations* is my italics – would mean a revaluation of our desire to affirm our superficial and merely cognitive knowledge of the illusions of religion (which we can, with misguided confidence, dismiss as archaic or superstitious) and not recognize Freud's profound question. Our political life has also been determined by illusions, and today with an even more important transference between one and the other to constitute the making of our thesis: the unconscious of the theological-political. The question, if heard with a certain attunement, is not asking if religion and politics may *both* be illusions. Everyone can answer the question with relative ease. The more far-reaching sense of Freud's question has to do with how his "reasoning in scientific work" has now brought him to conclusion far more significant than our illusions about "external reality." "Nothing ought to keep us from directing our observation to our own selves or from applying our thought to criticism of itself" (21:34). Who has paid sufficient attention to Freud's advice? Academics? These may be subtle reminders and easily passed over by a less than attentive reader; for Freud they are essential, for himself and his self-analysis as he thinks and writes, and for anyone who has been conscious of both the levels of his communication. At this transitional moment, he tells the reader that he cannot confine his work to a critique of religion but relies on the omnipresent opponent to introduce the implications of what has been presented thus far and what his "comprehensive task" (Freud's words) may be. Nothing can replace self-observation; and nothing can be a substitute for the reflection necessary to make our thinking – and, especially, the tradition of "critical" thinking – the grounds of all the ideas we may create in the foreseeable future. Is Freud preparing to make an argument about our political illusions which are, for us today, much more serious than any illusions about the existence of God or faith or ecclesial orthodoxy? Everything going forward will be committed to this one psychoanalytic insight; for if he relieved us of our illusions about the ideals of politics and showed their origins and their power, then the present appears to be a time when the whole of the dedication of Freud's thought at the level of a social assessment reaches another important phase. The work on illusions is not, ultimately, confined to religion. A repetition for emphasis will not be wasted. "What is characteristic of illusions is that they are derived from human wishes. In this respect they come near to psychiatric delusions" (21:31). Can we then make the claim that the illusions of politics are examples of psychiatric delusions – and with consequences for social life that, despite the fulfillment of ideals, can also lead to the worst kinds of coercions and manipulations? Can we also make an unequivocal statement and recognize how the politics of the present are pathological and are displaying some of the more obvious characteristics of mental illness? We are, as we considered Freud's claim about all illusions, given the opportunity to extend the analysis and continue with the psychiatric delusions of politics. Freud's complementary analysis is not overt, except on the rare occasions when he provides the readers one sense of the argument as a whole. The question can be posed again. "Must not the assumptions that determine our political regulations be called illusions as well?" (21:34). The question effectively has two parts. The first one, in the affirmative, is for Freud simple. The human wishes of politics (as the illusions of idealism) have had considerable effects on the propagation of social ideas and, more importantly, the daily lives of everyone in society. The more difficult problem lies in what has been called the theological-political relation. When Freud recognized the problem to be analyzed – "we must ask where the inner force of those doctrines lies and to what it is that they owe their efficacy" (21:29), which is a question he has asked, three times, in the beginning – the foundation of the religious illusions, once it extended itself to other social forms, opened the way for an unprecedented knowledge of the "force" of the political. To make the case for religion being an obsessional neurosis is *not* the whole of Freud's argument or critique.

Unless the unconscious machinations of the super-ego are not more precisely defined and without reference to any conscious sense of the religious, then the most insistent phenomenon of the times will continue to proceed without the slightest obstacles; the screen becomes the sole exhibition and so the only reality to witness and perpetuate. My interest in reading and interpreting Freud (from the standpoint of an analysand) is done for specific reasons; they are not, simply, methodological. When the secondary literature on Freud and religion is considered, one overwhelming conclusion presents itself. There is what appears to be a consensus and one based on a *first* reading – as if the first utterance (like one from an analysand) were heard as concluding remarks as opposed to the ongoing working of reaching an event beyond the limits that are always present. Another example can be cited for its focus, only, on religion.

> While religion is acknowledged as having a socially integrating function and fostering acculturation, its origins link it to regressive tendencies. Religion inscribes in cultural formations a repressive mechanism that restricts the drives while offering wishful substitute satisfactions. It thereby inhibits human potential for independence by sustaining an infantile psychical organization dependent on authority.[55]

Freud, however, makes the *exact same argument* about politics. He does not, simply, point out their many similarities. A comparative exercise, however informative, would remain superficial. Freud has been presenting a much more formidable problem – one that we can now begin to slowly sum up as the psychoanalysis of the theological-political in today's liberal society. Before doing so, and to provide one more point to my interpretation of reading Freud, an observation from one of the most perceptive of psychoanalysts can be relied upon. Janine Chasseguet-Smirgel is, once again, astute in her observations: "The process of creation, including literary creation, remains bound up first and foremost with verbal thought (daydreaming), but is also accompanied by the capacity of communicate with the most primitive layers of the unconscious."[56] Freud has set himself towards this communication, for our benefit, and to make us aware of how susceptible we could always be to our illusion and how they were maintained by a more or less disavowal of reality and a more serious, because more hidden, splitting within the dynamic of the psyche.

One opportunity will not be passed up. That the passage is written in prison, where reading takes on a quite different meaning, only makes Antonio Negri's statement all the more poignant. Introducing his engagement with Spinoza, he will "interrogate a true master with a method of reading the past that allows me to grasp the elements that today coalesce in a definition of *phenomenology or revolutionary praxis* constitutive of the future. Moreover, this method of reading allows me (and truly obliges us) to come to terms with all the confusion and mystification… … we have been taught."[57] For me, the choice has been made since the beginning: phenomenology, or the awareness of what human consciousness can achieve, is infinitely preferrable to the idea of "revolutionary praxis" and the consequences Freud will diagnose, again, in *Civilization and its Discontents* as the worst form of political acting out.

(I) The Disavowal of Reality and Splitting

The foundational ideas from *Group Psychology* and the inter-related ones he developed in the years after are indispensable for a proper assessment of Freud's thinking about religion and the psychological processes of the gradual conversion towards secularism. The symptoms of contagion, susceptibility, and imitation, as first examples of social influence, remain operative and essential as the ground for also understanding the predicament of the contemporary individual. Freud makes sure to incorporate the findings of the 1921 work into the thinking about the nature of any illusion (in origin and outcome) and how they can easily spread. "Through some kind of diffusion or infection, the character of sanctity and inviolability," Freud writes, "has spread from a few major prohibitions on to every other cultural regulation, law and ordinance" (21: 41). In *The Future of an Illusion*, the morality of the super-ego has been present throughout the different parts of his analysis. The culmination of one argument needs to be more completely appreciated: the "diffusion" has led to a totalizing obsession with "every other cultural regulation," including how the law is perceived and enacted. This is the point at which Freud adds to his singular argument; for once the unhampered political illusions are one of the outcomes of the loss of the religious, then one has to add one further and essential point: the transference from the religious to the political has occurred without, it seems, any awareness. The transference has been elusive. The psychological effects of such a social transformation have not been fully recognized as to their effects. To be liberated from a historical set of binding ideas (thought to be wholly negative by liberal

consensus) did not create ideal conditions of either freedom or intelligence; the transference towards a theological-political totality made it possible to relieve oneself, self-consciously, of religious illusions only to transform them into social and political illusions – and with one devastating outcome; they had, as Freud tells us, the characteristics of psychiatric delusions. Ideals had become pathological. Due to some of the mechanism analyzed previously, the religious was far from abolished and superseded; if anything, its psychical power became more effective as it made itself morally inviolable by separating itself from religious symbolism and the specificity of ecclesial dogmas; the effects of one institutional set of regulations and self-understanding could pass from one to the other. The psychical mechanism at work could be analyzed more deeply and from a dynamic Freud had witnessed firsthand when the morality of the super-ego and the destruction of the death drive were, first, identified according to the masochism-sadism relation and, finally, with the development of one of the earliest of psychoanalytic concepts (the French *double conscience*) and its manifestation in splitting.

In general terms, the concept of "a splitting of consciousness" (3:47) was already present in the 1894 "The Neuro-Psychoses of Defense." The development of the concept, which would preoccupy Freud until the end and in one of his last publications,[58] became more intricate once it was introduced in the 1920s and as one way (as I've presented here) to understand the splitting *within the super-ego*. Splitting can be added to the analysis of group psychology, and more particularly to the neuroses of politics, and how it manifests itself in two ways. The political implications continues to be our main focus. "Splitting is seen clearly in groups that define themselves in opposition to other groups… … rivalry may disintegrate into pathological splitting and retributive frenzy."[59] Splitting has become pervasive and one more indication of the vagaries of the super-ego – which, for us now, displays itself (betrays itself and its motives) in the social and political sphere.

The contributions made by Rachel Blass are going to be relied upon more than once to give us one more support to the whole of my psychopolitical essay. She writes: "Splitting as the manifestation or consequence of disavowal is introduced primarily in some of Freud's writings in the 1920s."[60] The connection, between splitting and Freud's writings at this particular time, are for me an ongoing presentation of the development of psychoanalysis as he dedicated himself to the problems of culture or civilization. We've had the occasion to put forward several concepts thus far. Blass places disavowal and splitting side by side while reminding us of the presence of these ideas in Freud's writing going back as far as the *Studies on Hysteria* and, for example, the previously mentioned idea of a "*double conscience*," which the French allows us to interpret in two ways: as the splitting of *consciousness* and the splitting of *conscience*. The latter is especially important because it allows us to understand the split between the super-ego of care, solicitude, compassion, and the much more vengeful super-ego of judgment and condemnation and persecution. The political neurotic has no need to disavow the difference; judgement is rationalized in the name of an inviolable justice. The splitting, however, becomes much more difficult when the super-ego and the death drive are collaborating towards one end that is contradictory.

A familiar problem can be mentioned: that some others believe that splitting should be "banned from the psychoanalytical vocabulary"[61] will not dissuade us, not when we've reached a concept that allows us to continue and to insist that nothing from Freud's thinking and writing can be expunged. The call to *ban* a psychoanalytic concept is more a sign of a personal motive than a proposal that can be taken seriously. It is not hard to be suspicious of editorializing. As for Pruyser's question – "what splits in splitting? – my answer has been, hopefully, clearly presented since *Group Psychology*: the split within the super-ego, which still does not accurately depict its character since a split simply implies two. Previous descriptions have attempted to show the super-ego as infantile, primitive, and highly fragmented.

One of the difficulties faced by anyone thinking about splitting had to answer several related questions; that the psyche is indeed split has to be more specifically defined and in order to now come to a preliminary conclusion before turning to Freud's *Civilization and its Discontents*. We can, with sufficient confidence, think about the split between the "super-morality" of the super-ego and how it has been implemented in liberal democracies from the sadistic compulsion towards the destruction of Western civilization – both as a reality, in society, and an idea. Although we do not want to conflate disavowal from splitting, they both serve to keep a particular defense mechanism in place. For one, the split between the illusion of moral goodness and political rage, each enacted for entirely different purposes, is disavowed; whether disavowal is essentially different from repression need not be addressed for our purposes, except to indicate how the political neurotic is not remote, detached, or isolated. On the contrary, and to recall an earlier comment in relation to *Group Psychology*, the primary identification with the group allows for a public participation in the transformation of unsatisfying reality at the cultural and biological level. One way to conceive of the disavowal and the split, as a state of "inbetweenness,"[62] does not consider another option, which for me is more illustrative of the agonistic relation. Splitting creates psychical extremes, disavowal nullifies their relation and so allows for the continuity of the illusion. I am not, in principle, in disagreement with R. D. Hinshelwood and the sense of repression and splitting being intimately related.[63] However, given how *repression* and *forgetting* are bound to each other, and compared to my previous arguments on the absolute need for the omni-presence of historical trauma, and the identification, introjection, and projection of the dead victim, any idea of repression in the process has to be aware of what memory *means* and how, and to what ends, it becomes instrumental. Memory, when serving ideological traumatism, can be extremely selective or exaggerated; and it can be *invented.* Splitting may have some relation to repression; as a whole mechanism, it may be more serviceable (clinically and practically) to conceive it in terms of two concepts Freud made use of in his short essay "Negation"; that is, affirmation and negation.

Recalling the three operations of hysterical identification, introjection, and projection, theological remnants of all kinds re-appeared in disguised forms. The suppression of the religious allowed other forms of the *perverted sacred* and the holy and the idolatrous to become manifest, beginning with the dead victim of history who could both be infinitely mourned and used as a rationalization for reactions in the present. While Richard Fenn, for example, has described the situation and "societies subject to both sacrilege and secularity,"[64] the concept of sacrilege can be set aside in order to choose others that are more evident and less likely to be ignored because of their religious underpinnings. A politics driven by the effects and rationalizations of mourning were not going to be easily dissuaded from their aims; the grief of mourning-politics would be both an outpouring of sentiment and an equal expression of the aggression now all too common for anyone who lack these finer feelings. The double nature of modern politics can be presented as the repetition, in disguised form, of religion, one that "brings with it obsessional restrictions, exactly as an individual obsessional neurosis does" which at the same time "it comprises a system of wishful illusions together with a disavowal of reality" (21:43). Restrictions and illusions: the two go hand in hand and as one more symptom to recognize in our contemporary liberal reality.

If *The Future of an Illusion* is interpreted as one more feature of our psychopolitics, and as a foundation soon to be completed in his *unbehagen* of civilization, then it takes on much more important characteristics. To interpret the work psychopolitically, the whole of Freud's thinking from the 1920s has to be thought about comprehensively and towards one conclusion – which is, in the end, a warning of an impending possibility. One consequence of splitting was described this way; introjection and projection are mutually serving forces and are explicitly split between the two drives Freud has recently created in his new system of psychical reality.

> Judging is a continuation, along lines of expediency, of the original process by which the ego took things into itself or expelled them from itself, according to the pleasure principle. The polarity of judgment appears to correspond to the opposition of the two groups of instincts which we have supposed to exist, Affirmation – as a substitute for uniting – belongs to Eros; negation – the successor to expulsion – belongs to the instinct of destruction.[65]

Are we willing to extend our argument even further and, consistent with the entirety of the work and interpret one statement in more than one of its dimensions? For when Freud says that "we are telling the truth in symbolic clothing" (21:44), are we at all justified in thinking that the analyst has spoken in such a way as to be interpreted *doubly* by his listener? We've come to a conclusion that, if indeed it is the case, would force us to re-think the nature of *The Future of an Illusion* and yet with a reflection that should be more than familiar. Has Freud's critique of religion been a displaced foundation for the psychopolitical analysis that both ends the work and prepares for the conclusion of a decade of work and *Civilization and its Discontents*? To add to the question, we have had – most recently, and with more frequency – an awareness by non-psychoanalytic thinkers of the oppressive power of negation and the need to turn in another direction for thought and life. Freud's word *affirmation* can be one term for what appears to be a growing *philosophical* ideal. Although the university has been portrayed with some measure of scepticism, there are individuals who are, by virtue of their work, offering their own alternatives to what passes for thought today. Alain Badiou has been mentioned on several occasions.

Psychoanalysis added one more responsibility to its therapeutic endeavors: its clinical work would have to devote itself more and more to assisting the analysand in working through the manipulations of the superego and to become strong enough, independent enough, autonomous enough, to resist the coercions of moral imperatives and to avoid falling into a compliance that, today, has become such a characteristic of the life within liberal democracies. Coercion, compliance, and consensus; they operate as relational and with one goal in mind: to force the individual to submit to the ideals of a group who, by force of will has driven itself to one supreme influence. Freud's insistent reminders, since *Group Psychology*, on the importance of intelligence and freedom, was everywhere present in the declarations he makes about the psychical effects of religion and how they can be so easily transformed and, as displacements, more effective than ever when politicized.

One could, with sufficient time and concentration, focus exclusively on the dialogue between Freud and his "opponent" (that is, with himself as an analysand and with himself as an analyst – which makes the dialogue a four-part one) and come to more than a few conclusions that would leave us with the most interesting kind of doubts. On summing up, coming as it does at the end of the penultimate section, is supposed to be, in a sense, final. Freud appears to tell his opponent that, once freed from the religious illusion of another world and now "concentrating all their liberated energies into their life on earth, they will probably succeed in achieving a state of things in which life will become tolerable for everyone and civilization no longer oppressive to anyone" (21:50). Is there *anyone* with a firm understanding of Freud and psychoanalysis who could possibly believe in such an idealistic future, one that is completely out of the question and due to the conclusions Freud will soon present? *Civilization no longer oppressive to anyone*? Surely this is an illusion Freud has never for one moment entertained as a realistic possibility. To define this as some kind of "pessimism" (a word often used to describe Freud) ends up lacking all meaning. "I know how difficult it is to avoid illusions; perhaps the hopes I have confessed are of an illusory nature, too" (21:53). The statement, then, was only made from one and by no means total idealistic position. At the start of this work, the argument stated that it was an error to proceed with an either/or focus – either the faith of religion or the reason of secularity. At the end and in the transition towards our last chapter, the choice between one and the other has never seemed more inadequate. The facile opposition between the one and the other is itself responsible for creating a closed structure and from where alternatives are excluded. Once more, and with more conviction, the argument Freud has been outlining is one focused on a civilization he recognized to be neurotic. Reading him makes it impossible, and inadvisable, to continue to believe in the illusion of a religious critique and the convenient attribution of social neurosis to religion. After all, as he will tell us soon, science was no less capable of being pathological. The atrocities of Thanatos would only be more numerous and with ever more barbarism. For us to assess Freud the thinker a century after one of his most long-lasting contributions towards an analysis of civilization requires us to extend ourselves and our own thinking and so recognize his ambitions. If we were to lead to one conclusion, which allows for a continuity in Freud's assessments of the malaise of civilization, it would be this: "education freed from the burden of religious doctrine will not, it may be, effect much change in men's psychological nature" (21:54). Freud came to the conclusion that it was not religion, in itself, that led to all kinds of human debilitations. There was, it seemed, a "psychological nature" that at the same time as creating consolations for the difficulties of human existence also made the situation no better and, perhaps, even worse. When Freud began his work in the 1920s, the overwhelming sense of the nature of civilization forced him in certain directions. By the time he reaches the end of the decade and sets himself to writing on the malaise of civilization, one suspicion has not been relinquished. His psychopolitical investigation reaches a culmination and one that consolidates his position as a realist and without adopting a facile either/or choice between two positions that were, in themselves, psychologically inadequate; neither faith nor reason (alone) could account for the growing problems of social life. Only by recognizing the psychological aberrations of both could it be possible to fully understand the role of the moral super-ego and the death drive in society. Can we go as far as presenting an argument based on the good/bad object relation and establish what may very well be a unique phenomenon in our time: the preservation of the dead victim of history as the good object and to be introjected and perpetually mourned at the same time as the most intense expression of contempt for the bad object splintered, everywhere, in culture? His concept of negation has become particularly relevant. We can now add how there is "an important relationship between splitting"[66] and our previous triad of identification, introjection, and projection. The splitting, as a psychical description, must also remain viable as an operation that occurs in the real world, of human beings and ideas, and as the separation of groups. Melvin Lansky's contribution to our argument overall can be repeated here. "Splitting is seen clearly in groups that define themselves in opposition to other groups... ... Rivalry may disintegrate into pathological splitting and retributive frenzy."[67] Lansky's concern with forgiveness makes us aware, and with troubling implications, that a fundamentally religious virtue has been repudiated, like others, in order to forcefully abolish any sentiments that might interfere with the implementation of a new social and political order. The psychoanalytic writers who have been most consequential, and who have contributed to the present psycho-political essay, have been those who have carried their research towards this one severe problem. Heinz Weiss has said that the concept of splitting is still "in progress." Be that as it may, its progress is, for us, more than sufficient for its analytic conclusions. Weiss' "brief introduction" to three different perspectives allows us to choose the most important and one he adopts from the ideas of Tomas Plänkers. "If splitting comes to dominate large groups within society, it may give rise to violence and totalitarianism. The same process, he supposes, may be operating in a more hidden way in the complex dynamism of postmodern, neoliberal economy."[68] My only objection to the above would be on the concentration on the "neoliberal economy." We are today no longer able to isolate the socioeconomic conditions of a society, as has been consistent in one analysis since the 19th century and Marxism, when the dynamics of our theological-political liberalism has so altered society as a whole. Our *psychical* economy has made itself predominant.

From the beginning of my interpretation, one argument has been central: Freud's writing on the future of an illusion, could be read (at its manifest level) as a work of moderate interest on a critique of religion. Another installment was necessary before the future was presented. In the meantime, in preparation for the culmination of an argument, Freud's ultimate concern was not with the effects of religious belief, faith, or piety. His thinking was much more ambitious and expressed most especially for *future analysts* who were going to be faced, more and more, with a different kind of analysand and social individual. So, when Freud's interlocutor again raises objections (whether we identify him or her as an analyst or an analysand) and asks him why he is intent "to upset that faith" when he knows that it won't make any difference to be believer, another reason can found. Does Freud want to undermine faith? Or does he have a much more important reason for his apparent critique of religion? The rhetorical question, which has been answered, opens one last argument. The last two sections of *The Future of an Illusion* are conclusions in more ways than one; because if we maintain the structural integrity of the whole and now connect the re-emphasis of the super-ego at the beginning with the turn towards speculations about ideals and political utopias, then we are in a better position to evaluate the specificity of the work and, in the next chapter, its relation to *Civilization and its Discontents*. If we acknowledge the work of the previous years on group psychology and the emergence of the power of the superego, then Freud's ultimate purpose for his analysis of religion does not actually concern himself with the nature of belief or faith or religious illusions – of which there are, of course, many beside the religious ones; rather, he is motivated, as he has been all along, to trace how the religious characteristics of the superego, once deracinated from their origins, are able to be displaced and projected onto a much wider field.

The last sections of the work once again take up the "discussion" between Freud and his interlocutor. One repetition can bring the chapter to a provisional conclusion. If we keep in mind our method of interpretation, the question Freud asks: "must not the assumptions that determine our political regulations be called illusions as well?" (21: 34) is, in itself, incomplete. It is, first of all, *rhetorical*. The answer is obvious; what needs to be more fully explained (this, now, is where our real interest has been) is how our religious illusions have been internalized by political aspirations and therefore revealed an old relation, one stated in modern terms as the theological-political. To politically evaluate the relation, however, is always going to prove inadequate. It's my contention that only Freud's analysis is fully capable of revealing how the unconscious internalization of religious principles, once they become dynamically active and powerful in the psyche, have untold consequences, many that have become all-too evident in our present. The prevailing ideals of the times (justice, equality, rights), for all their merit and necessity, have proven to be directed by a morality that seems, as Freud argued, in the guise of reaction formations and split by a myriad of group initiatives. The highest values of society have become so perverted as to be no longer recognizable and, indeed, tending towards the very opposite of their intention.

There are many ways to understand Freud's suggestion that "the relationship between civilization and religion must undergo a fundamental revision" (21:39). If we do so superficially, according to the rational or even scientific arguments of the atheist and the secularist, we will be no closer to understanding the super-ego effects of our contemporary situation and so run the danger of being misled. Freud's self-analysis allows us to interpret how subtle and far from one-dimensional his arguments are. There are numerous instances of his thought being fully evident and not as straightforward as secularists would have it; because if we see him contributing to the abolition of God and religion as a regulative idea, we at the same time fail to acknowledge a prime psychoanalytic insight. Our certainties and convictions come at a high cost to our intelligence and freedom of thought. "Our plea for ascribing purely rational reasons to the precepts of civilization – that is to say, for deriving them from social necessity – is interrupted by sudden doubt" (21:41). The doubt may not be so sudden after all. The apprehension has been present all along; now is simply the opportune time to express it once again, and to the readers who themselves have had doubts about the new secular constitution of society and the effects it has had on their thinking, their freedom, their life.

We are not at all surprised when, in the penultimate section, Freud turns to the illusions of politics and the example of revolution. The whole purpose of the work has been heading towards this one end. The displacement he has been conscious of for quite some time has, finally, come to pass, and with a historical actuality that would run its course and with untold misery in its wake. Freud announces the end of political revolutions.

> Once before an attempt of this kind was made to substitute reason for religion, officially and in the grand manner. Surely you remember the French Revolution and Robespierre? And you must also remember how short-lived and miserably ineffectual the experiment was? The same experiment is being repeated in Russia at the present time, and we need not feel curious as to its outcome. (21:46)

The anticipation, in 1927, of how the Soviet revolution would be a repetition was no secret for Freud. His creative myth in *Totem and Taboo* left no doubts about the consequences of a decisive event of transforming society: the ensuing society of the most repressive laws, controls, and self-surveillance were inevitable. And yet the historical knowledge of a prior situation, the French or the Soviet, will not do us any good at all if we simply analyze it as history and not as Freud intended it – that is, as the possibility of our present and as a psychical disposition always prepared to be re-activated. The psychoanalytic demand, then, involves us in much more than a symmetrical situation, the political initiative as the abolition of religion. For us today, the demand is much more consequential. If we give ourselves the illusion of secularity without realizing how the religious has been internalized in our psyches, in the dynamic of the super-ego, and powerfully projected into the transformation of reality, we will not be aware of how the ideals of our culture have been inverted into political perversions, the same ones which led the communist experiments to be so atrocious for human beings. The punitive cruelty of the super-ego and the distortions of a politically motivated psyche driven by sadistic and masochistic inclinations should no longer be as unconscious as they have been. The splitting has been exposed and analyzed in a number of different ways. We can postpone, for a little longer, the associated problem of what Nietzsche called nihilism and Freud defined with the term *Thanatos*; but the super-ego and the death drive are no longer as strange as they may have once appeared when the latter was considered from the perspective of the biologism of constancy. The task ahead remains and to be defined no longer as a much too simple either/or, the rationality of secularism and the illusion of religion. The illusion, in effect, was to believe in such a simplistic reality, one that had to ignore the complex insights of psychoanalysis for it to be believed. What Freud calls his "*education to reality*" and as the whole purpose of *The Future of an Illusion* becomes more clearly seen when the political argument (for a revolution, and a secular one at that) is no longer tenable. The conclusion is unequivocal. Freud writes:

> If you want to expel religion from our European civilization, you can only do it by means of another system of doctrines; and such a system would from the outset take over all the psychological characteristics of religion – the same sanctity, rigidity, intolerance, the same prohibition of thought – for its own defence.
>
> (21:51)

The present situation is perfectly reflected in Freud's analysis. While secularity has given itself the confidence of freedom from religious influence, it has completely failed to realize how deeply it had been formed by "the psychological characteristics of religion" and how its effects have been exacerbated by the growing demand for moral perfection. We are not only left with one impression – "education freed from the burden of religious doctrines will not, it may be, effect much change in men's psychological nature." Freud's last work as the summation of a decade of psychoanalytic work on civilization and, for us today, how the religious dynamic of the super-ego has come to dominate the social and political life of liberal democracies. Freud again asks: "How can we expect people who are under the dominance of prohibitions of thought to attain the psychological ideal, the primacy of the intelligence?" (21:48). *Intelligence*: Freud returns again to one of his most impassioned concerns and one that exceeds our understanding of rationality. Intelligence, including how intense our emotions can be, and for the origin and expression of obsessions, remains the one human attribute most in need of support because of how the ideal of love requires the relation of emotions and intelligence to flourish. The question has to be asked with several meanings simultaneously: they have been with us the entire time, for nothing has been more preeminent than the ability to use human intelligence in and for freedom and for love. Have we now arrived at a strange though not wholly unexpected juncture? Is Freud and psychoanalysis to be again so maligned by our culture because, as we move on with increasing speed and urgency, his writings can force us to pause and reflect on our contemporary situation and if we are individually (and perhaps collectively) capable to re-thinking the nature of the human and so our future? The question is posed while recalling the "Postscript" of *Group Psychology* and the proposal for at least an awareness of re-affirming our erotic nature, as essentially creative, devoted to life, and capable to holding off the temptations of the death drive. In *Civilization and its Discontents*, Freud will be even more thorough and, as the culmination of a lifetime of thinking, lead his readers not to any supposed "pessimistic" conclusion, but on the contrary a commitment to the very ideals he has always supported. The conclusion of section VI can be carefully re-read and its apparent meaning altered. "Either these dangerous masses must be held down most severely and kept most carefully away from any chance of intellectual awakening, or else the relationship between civilization and religion must undergo a fundamental revision" (21:39). Indeed, but when we read Freud's statements with the whole of our preceding arguments in mind, then the "intellectual awakening" (which is, precisely, the rhetoric used today) will not be possible until the theological-political nature of our liberal democracy is exposed and the present-day complicity between secular civilization and unconscious religion is recognized to be a now momentous movement that is both moral and nihilistic. The analysis of many of the symptoms have resulted in a severe portrait of the present times. Any notion of "pessimism," for us or Freud, is misplaced. In *Civilization and its Discontents*, he will provide a sustained analysis and defense of culture and put forward, finally and unambiguously, his own ideals of intelligence and freedom, creativity and love and psychological health. The analysis of our many discontents will not be resolved; they will, however, be confronted by the spirited affirmation of the values of the human and their persistence, as a matter of necessity, in human life and by psychoanalysis. Although we can share a certain sympathy with John Steiner and his analysis of "psychic retreats," his conclusion will be resisted. "Projective identification is used in ways which makes it more or less irreversible. Parts of the self are split off and projected unto objects where they permanently reside, remaining unavailable to the self."[69] The diagnosis, for extreme cases, appears hopeless; and yet to resign oneself to an observable state of affairs will not be dissuasive enough to continue with the responsibility at hand and to turn to *Civilization and its Discontents* to find a series of achievable remedies for individuals and, perhaps, for societies as a whole.

Notes

1 Rempel, Morgan Henry. "Understanding Freud's Philosophy of Religion," 215–242 *Canadian Journal of Psychoanalysis*, Vol. 5, No. 2 (Nov. 1997), 222.

2 Mills, Jon. "Preface" to his edited *Rereading Freud: Psychoanalysis through Philosophy*. Albany: SUNY, 2004, x.

3 Dougherty, Jude P. *The Logic of Religion*. Washington, D.C.: The Catholic University of America Press, 2003, 110. Dougherty gives 4 pages to Freud.

4 Bataille, Georges. *Visions of Excess: Selected Writings, 1927–1939*. Ed. With an Introduction by Allan Stoekl. Tr. Allan Stoekl, with Carl R. Lovitt and Donald M. Leslie, Jr. Minneapolis: University of Minnesota Press, 1985, 15–16.
5 LaMothe, Ryan. "Freud, Religion, and the Presence of Projective Identification," 287–302 *Psychoanalytic Quarterly*, Vol. 20, No. 2, 2003, 287. "Antipathy" is a very strong emotion. "Preoccupation," on the other hand, has many different meanings, including a deep interest.
6 Gay, Volney. "Sigmund Freud on Religion," in *Religion, Theory, Critique: Classic and Contemporary Approaches and Methodologies*. Ed. Richard King. New York: Columbia University Press, 2017, 121.
7 Baranger, Willy. "The Ego and the Function of Ideology," 217–228 in *The Work of Confluence: Listening and Interpreting in the Psychoanalytic Field*. Madeleine and Willy Baranger. Ed. Leticia Glocer Fiorini. London: Karnac, 2009, 218.
8 Kahn, Victoria. *The Future of Illusion: Political Theology and Early Modern Texts*. Chicago: The University of Chicago Press, 2014, 147.
9 Hewitt, Marsha Aileen. *Freud on Religion*. Durham, UK: Acumen, 2014, 21.
10 Freud, Sigmund. "The Future Prospects of Psycho-Analytic Therapy." SE 11:141.
11 Lear, Jonathan. "The Illusion of a Future: the rhetoric of Freud's critique of religion," 83–97 in *On Freud's "The Future of an Illusion."* Ed. Mary Kay O'Neal and Salman Akhtar. London: Karnac, 2009, 85.
12 Frie, Roger. "Psychoanalysis, religion, philosophy and the possibility of dialogue: Freud, Binswanger and Pfister. 106–116 *International Forum of Psychoanalysis* 21, 2012, 106.
13 Novak, David. "On Freud's theory of law and religion," 24–34 *International Journal of Law and Psychiatry*, 48 (2016), 33.
14 Eagleton, Terry. *Reason, Faith, and Revolution: Reflections on the God Debate*. New Haven: Yale University Press, 2009, 140-1. The question is posed: in what follows, one answer (given to us by Freud) will be presented.
15 Johnston, Adrian. "The Triumph of Theological Economics: God goes underground," 3–50 *Philosophy Today*, Vol. 64, Issue 1 (Winter 2020), 9.
16 Bollas, Christopher. "Introduction" to Jonathan Sklar's *Landscapes of the Dark: History, Trauma, Psychoanalysis*. London: Karnac, 2011, xvi.
17 Richards, Arnold. "The Need not to believe: Freud's Godlessness Remembered," *Psychoanalytic Review*, Vol. 96, issue 4 (Aug. 2009), 561–578, 563. The more one is attentive to the language of his readers, the more one attitude becomes evident: despite recognizing the "stylistic" difference in the prose (which is not aesthetic but, rather, *transferential*, and consciously so) Richards does not go the necessary next step and ask himself the reason for Freud lacking in "graces" and why he is so fierce he writes as if *with a hammer*.
18 Kronemyer, David E. "Freud's Illusion: New Approaches to Intractable Issues," 249–275 *International Journal for the Psychology of Religion*, Vol. 24, No. 4, 2011.
19 Hardt, Michael and Negri, Antonio. *Assembly*. Oxford: Oxford University Press, 2017, 8. In lieu of a longer response, which in any case has, I think, more than evident throughout the whole of the psycho-political essay so far, these two representatives of "radical" thought (of the Left wing kind) are no farther along than the thinkers associated with the Frankfurt School. As long as traditional thinkers continue to identify, for example, what Hardt and Negri call "the dark mirror of right-wing movements," then we incur two risks: one, simply continuing to identify the problems that are already (and have been) more than obvious to us without turning the analysis back on ourselves to see how all the pretensions of liberation, as are so promoted in liberal democracies today, are also the cause of significant problems for individuals no less than for society. We can continue to direct our attention to "the violence of religious identities," but until such time as the

religious identifies are discovered to be unconscious and at the heart of liberal democratic idealism then the problems of the 21st century are going to become infinitely worse than they already are.

20 Wahl, William H. "Pathologies of Desire and Duty: Freud, Ricoeur and Castoriadis on Transforming Religious Culture," 398–414 *Journal of Religion and Health*, Vol. 47, No. 3 (Sep 2008), 398.

21 Clark, Margaret. *Understanding Religion and Spirituality in Clinical Practice*. London: Karnac, 2012, 2.

22 Reijzer, Hans. *A Dangerous Legacy: Judaism and the Psychoanalytic Movement*. Tr. Jeannette K. Ringold. London: Karnac, 2011, 57.

23 Freud, Sigmund. *Fragment of an Analysis of a Case of Hysteria*. SE 7:59–60.

24 Canestri, Jorge. "The Logic of Freudian Research," 117–129 *Freud and Judaism*. Ed. David Meghnegi. London: Karnac, 1993, 120.

25 Frankland, Graham. *Freud's Literary Culture*. Cambridge: Cambridge University Press, 2000. A section of a chapter is titled "Freud as stylist: Artful Revelations

26 Jacobs, Michael. *Sigmund Freud*. Second Edition. London: Sage Publications, 2003, 153.

27 Foresti, Giovanni. "Freud's writing in the twenties: theory and constructs and clinical research in Inhibitions, Symptoms and Anxiety," 200–218 *On Freud's "Inhibitions, Symptoms and Anxiety."* Ed. Samuel Arbiser and Jorge Schneider. London: Karnac, 2013, 205.

28 Mahony, Patrick J. *Freud as a Writer*. New Haven: Yale University Press, 1987, 2.

29 Sauvayre, Pascal and Vegas, Monica. "An even hover-reading of Freud: The work of metaphor," 1343–1367 in *International Journal of Psychoanalysis*, Vol. 97, No. 5, 1362.

30 Freud, Sigmund. *The Interpretation of Dreams*. SE 4:305.

31 Ricoeur, Paul. *Freud and Philosophy: An Essay on Interpretation*. Tr. Denis Savage: New Haven: Yale University Press, 1970. The Section is in Book II: Analytic: Reading of Freud.

32 Kristeva, Julia. *The Incredible Need to Believe*. Tr. New York: Columbia University Press, 2009, 4.

33 Grubrich-Simitis, Ilse. *Back to Freud's Texts: Making Silent Documents Speak*. Tr. Philip Slotkin. New Haven: Yale University Press, 1993.

34 Akhtar, Salman. "Introduction" to *On Freud's "The Future of an Illusion."* Ed. Mary Kay O'Neil and Salman Akhtar. London: Karnac, 2009.

35 The reference is to Peter Gay's work of the same name, which in turn was adopted from an expression used by Freud to describe himself to Oskar Pfister. His position on the matter has been well-noted. In Gay's introduction to *The Future of an Illusion* in the edited collection (*The Freud Reader*) he writes: "his professional interest in the phenomenon of religion was anything but abstract. It was fueled by his principled, highly aggressive, anti-religious stance," 685. "Highly aggressive." How such a strong emotion can be noticed is not at all clear. One notices the work to be not at all aggressive; on the contrary, the complexity of his presentation cannot include the emotion of anger, hostility, or aggression. Gay continues: "one of its devices, familiar from several other writings of Freud's, is the use of dialogue to make some crucial points. This underscores Freud's deliberate informality, the wish to reach a broader public than sheer technical papers ever could." As my argument will show, the appearance of a dialogue, for a broader public, is not as straightforward as Gay would have us believe.

36 Kenny, Dianna T. *God, Freud and Religion: The Origins of Faith, Fear and Fundamentalism*. London: Routledge, 2015, 70.

37 Freud, Sigmund. "The Goethe Prize." SE 21:212.

38 Strauss, Leo. *What is Political Philosophy? And Other Studies.* Chicago: The University of Chicago Press, 1959, 222. The chapter in question is "On a Forgotten Kind of Writing," in part a response to his critics and the recent publication of his *Persecution and the Art of Writing*. While esoteric writing is alluded to by Freud, he does not, in the end, make a habit of the practice. Quite the contrary; the statement was made as a reminder not so much of a conscious withholding or a technique of writing but rather as a reminder of our divided psyche and how we are always tempted to hide elements from within ourselves and then find all kinds of pretext to keep ourselves well concealed, guarded, and secure.
39 Freud, Sigmund. "Screen Memories." SE 3:306.
40 Farrell, John C. *Freud's Paranoid Quest: Psychoanalysis and Modern Suspicion.* New York: New York University Press, 1996, 2. The reader drawn to this work will have to evaluate the argument that follows. According to Farrell, it is Freud who is, like other moderns, paranoid.
41 In her review of recent publications at the time, Nurit Novis-Deutsch discussed "Psychoanalysis and Religion in the 21st Century: Competitors or Collaborators?" (616–623 *American Imago*, Vol. 65, Number 4, Winter 2008). Phrased this way, the question may still be significant and with a new-found *collaboration* between psychoanalysis and religion (and philosophy) as one response to the moralizing politics of our times.
42 Symington, Neville. *Emotion and Spirit: Questioning the Claims of Psychoanalysis of Religion.* London: Karnac, 1998, 58.
43 Wood, Sarah. *Without Mastery: Reading and Other Forces.* Edinburgh: Edinburgh University Press, 2014, 126. Her added sense of "the beyond of language" is, for me, understood to be the truth of the analysand's speech when confirmed, several times, by affect; and then complemented, again by the truth of analysis, in the consciousness of the transference.
44 Freud, Sigmund. "The Claims of Psycho-Analysis to Scientific Interest." SE 13:176.
45 Freud, Sigmund. "The Uncanny." SE 17:235.
46 Freud, Sigmund. *Leonardo da Vinci and a Memory of his Childhood.* SE 11:123.
47 Laine, Aira. "On the edge: the psychoanalyst's transference," 1171–1183 *International Journal of Psychoanalysis*, Vol. 88 (Oct. 2007), 1172.
48 Freud, Sigmund. "The Moses of Michelangelo." SE 13:212.
49 Laplance, J. and Pontalis, J.B. *The Language of Psycho-Analysis.* Tr. Donald Nicholson-Smith. New York: W.W. Norton & Company, 1973, 109–110.
50 Fleming, Bruce. "Conservative, Liberal, Perverted Liberal," 532–537 *Society*, Vol. 56, No. 6 (Dec. 2019).
51 Clark, Margaret. *Understanding Religion and Spirituality in Clinical Practice.* London: Karnac, 2012.
52 Freud, Sigmund. "'Civilized' Sexual Morality and Modern Nervous Illness." SE 9:202–203.
53 Eriksson, Johan. "Freud's Psychoanalysis: A moral cure," 663–675 *International Journal of Psychoanalysis*, Vol. 95, No. 4, 2014, 666.
54 Anzieu, Didier. *A Skin for Thought: Interviews with Gilbert Tarrab on Psychology and Psychoanalysis.* London: Karnac, 1990, 84–85.
55 Di Censo, James J. *The Other Freud: Religion, Culture and Psychoanalysis.* London: Routledge, 1999, 31.
56 Chasseguet-Smirgel, Janine. ""Creative Writers and Day-dreaming": A commentary," 107–121 *On Freud's "Creative Writers and Day-Dreaming."* Ed. Ethel Spector Person, Peter Fonagy, Servull Augusto Figueira. London: Karnac, 2013, 113.

57 Negri, Antonio. *The Savage Anomaly: The Power of Spinoza's Metaphysics and Politics*. Tr. Michael Hardt. Minneapolis: University of Minnesota Press, 1991, xxi, my emphasis.
58 In the posthumously published "Splitting of the Ego in the Process of Defense." SE 23:271–278.
59 Lanksy, Melvin. R. "Forgiveness as the working through of splitting," 374–385 *Psychoanalytic Inquiry*. Vol. 29, No. 5, 2009, 379.
60 Blass, Rachel B. "Conceptualizing splitting: on the different meanings of splitting and their implications for the understanding of the person and the psychoanalytic process," 123–*129 International Journal of Psychoanalysis*, Vol. 96, No. 1, 2015, 128. Rachel Blass' essay (which outlines four different kinds of splitting) will be read specifically in relation to disavowal. To do so gives me the opportunity to add to the psychical characteristics that allows for the collaboration (which should be completely antithetical) between the super-ego and the death drive.
61 Pruyser, P. "What Splits in 'splitting'?" 1–46 *Bulletin of the Menninger Clinic* 39.
62 See, for one example, Stephen Blumenthal's "A State of Inbetweenness: The Challenge of Working with Disavowal," 4–16 *British Journal of Psychotherapy*, 38, 1, (2022).
63 See his "Repression and Splitting: Towards a method of conceptual comparison," 503–521 *International Journal of Psychoanalysis*, 89.3, 2008.
64 Fenn, Richard K. "Soul-loss, the Sacred and Secularity," 181–197 *Religious Studies and Theology*, Vol. 31, No. 2 (2012), 182.
65 Freud, Sigmund. "Negation." SE 19:239.
66 Soreanu, Raluca. "The Psychic Life of Fragments: Splitting from Ferenczi to Klein," 421–444 *The American Journal of Psychoanalysis*, 78, 2018, 422. She makes an additional comment on the manner in which "fragments of the psyche become depleted in a lasting manner." The idea of "depletion" can be compared to Freud's consistent concern with the sense of human *impoverishment*. By bringing the two together, we are adding one more psychoanalytic concern to our original and guiding concepts with the loss of intelligence and the diminishing of freedom.
67 Lansky, Melvin R. "Forgiveness as the Working Through of Splitting, " 374–385 *Psychoanalytic Inquiry* 29, 2009, 379. The contribution is important for our argument overall because Lansky makes a proposal about the need to forgive in order to become psychologically healthy. The theological virtue of forgiveness has been socially and politically abolished because the obsessive imperative of judging have become predominant.
68 Weiss, Heinz. "Three Papers on Splitting: A Brief Introduction," 119–122 *International Journal of Psychoanalysis* 96, 2015.
69 Steiner, John. *Psychic Retreats: Pathological Organization in Psychotic, Neurotic and Borderline Patients*. London: Routledge, 1993, 54.

4

THE MORAL COERCIONS OF LIBERALISM

> The cultural super-ego has developed its ideals and set up its demands. Among the latter, those which deal with the relations of human beings to one another are comprised under the heading of ethics. People have at all times set the greater value on ethics, as though they expected that it in particular would produce especially important results. And it does in fact deal with a subject which can easily be recognized as the sorest spot in civilization.
>
> *Civilization and its Discontents*

(m) "The Sorest Spot in Civilization"

The attention of our reading to Freud's work on the nature of one illusion has led us, after noting the transference from the religious to a political and the human propensity for relying on idealistic supports for our existential difficulties, to one more consolidation of the theological-political argument and to the work that serves us as the culmination of a series of inter-related projects in the 1920s. Freud's systematic shift, from the religious to political illusions, and their mutual intertwinement, has made it necessary to bring his thinking on the nature of civilization towards a change in focus and to examine how the nature of contemporary liberalism had been fundamentally altered. Recalling the introduction of the primal myth of *Totem and Taboo*, we are now nearer to our summing up. The symptoms of a psychopolitical movement have been, at least partly, detailed over the course of my essay. Reading Freud as he represents the many connections of the analyst/analysand relationship has made it necessary to avoid any turn to a one-dimensional interpretation, most especially if it

DOI: 10.4324/9781003410911-5

confirmed desires rather than facts, assumptions taken to be real, and all the ways to perpetuate illusions and fantasies. One perception can be emphasized once again. "Repeatedly society makes tragic decisions based on a mythology that emanates from wishful thinking and ideology."[1] Freud has given us an analysis of our self-congratulatory indulgences on the nature of secularity and, by doing so, ensured we would not be so readily susceptible to false beliefs about ourselves or the world. Our inability to recognize the nature of our super-ego unconscious has made it easier to believe we were abolishing one historical facet of life and replacing it with another, better, more enlightened one. The illusion of a substitution has been (and is) showing a number of adverse social effects; how long the epochal drive lasts cannot at this time be anticipated. The beginning of a new decade does make a transition foreseeable. Despite the force of the super-ego and the death drive, there are hopeful signs for a break, or perhaps a more easily achieved pause, in the current persistence of an entire worldview.

Freud's psychoanalysis of the theological-political order of our liberal society was the focus of a comprehensive project that, for us, comes to a conclusion with *Civilization and its Discontents*. The *personal* analysis is more inadequate than ever. One has to be presumptuous to turn to "Freud's final ten years" and define the period this way: "a portrait of exposure, shame, and anxiety takes form as the decade grinds into 1930."[2] Leaving aside any reductive appeal to history, or, worse of all, *ad hominem* comments, one illusion turned out to be, for us, part of a much more in-depth analysis of the nature of human self-deception. In *Civilization and its Discontents*, and beginning with Freud's exchange of letters with Romain Rolland, we can begin to close one presentation of our contemporary psychopolitical reality. As Freud admits, "the task is an immense one, and it is natural to feel diffidence in the face of it. But here are such conjectures as I have been able to make" (21:99). The immensity of the project certainly did not prevent him from the task ahead; so many obstacles had already been overcome.

The reference to love, in the context of his 1926 letter to Roman Rolland, can re-affirm Freud's commitments – for future analysands and readers. Does Freud's language of *apostolic love* surprise us? What are we to make of his self-description as "a disciple of the love of mankind"? Do any of his past writings prepare us for this one-time declaration? And can we disagree with Alfred Tauber when he calls Freud "an apostle of humanism"?[3] The commitment has been clear from the beginning. Love, as opposed to the bind of libidinal groups and the hatred it has shown, will be primary and once more connected to the other psychoanalytic ego-ideals: intelligence, freedom, creativity, and psychological health. The analysis of our contemporary situation has made our human antidotes necessary. Freud writes to Rolland and tells him.

> Long before I saw you, I had honoured you as an artist and as an apostle of the love of mankind, I was myself a disciple of the love of mankind, not from sentimental motives or in pursuit of an ideal, but for sober, economic reasons, because, our inborn instincts and the world around us being what they are, I could not but regard that love as no less essential for the survival of the human race than such things as technology.[4]

Freud identifies with characteristics he himself has maintained throughout his life: *art and love*. In his "Afterword" to *Political Freud*, Eli Zaretsky asks: "Is Freud, in any real sense, still our contemporary?"[5] Although the question has been answered without any hesitation at all, this might be an opportune time to once again stress the extent of Freud's relationship to us today, which is both meaningful and necessary and, if we can sustain the whole of the preceding argument, once again timely. Can we, analysands and readers, recommit to the work of both interpreting our contemporary situation and finding alternatives to its systematic order? No thinker, with very few exceptions, has better prepared us for our present. We can regard morality as the "sorest spot" of our liberal civilization and, today, as something much more serious. The moral and the nihilistic have been presented as wilful partners. Analysis has been succinct and unapologetic. In *Atheist Delusions*, David Bentley Hart writes: "the ethics of modernity is – be perfectly precise – nihilism."[6] The most intense opposition can once again be stated; but now in a way that is more startling. Can the love of psychoanalysis oppose the hatred and nihilism of our modern morality? This one opposition seems to be unavoidable. Has our projected commitment to equality and justice and rights (due to the unavoidable resentment and vengeance associated with its goals) in fact suppressed *authentic* love and have liberal ideals, when supported by critique and negation, made many people far worse than discontented? Hypochondria and traumatisms have been organized to serve the ends and of a specifically political gain from illness. Are we at a historical juncture when the critical and the moral, so tied, so restrictive, can be rethought as a particular malaise of our time? Has Freud allowed us to more readily perceive a reality that threatens to be overwhelming in its totality?

By opening with a reflection on religiosity, the "feeling" of something beyond the mundane and the everyday and the wholly material, Freud took the reader back to a fundamental relation with *his* consciousness as well as the courage and originality of the mythic poet who dared to introduce a different interpretation of tradition. After all, what can be more "oceanic" than the unconscious – including its imagination and creativity when properly understood and in an intimate, and conscious, relations with the healthy ego capable of recognizing the difference between pathology and intelligence, neurotic regression and dynamic creativity? Has Freud presented us with a conscious displacement of the oceanic feeling and transferred it from the traditionally religious and towards much more expansive, the human insofar as capable of love and creativity? His unique understanding of dreams left him with permanent insight to human knowledge and, more importantly, to the inter-play of interpretation and intelligence, which was far more important than the belief in "progressivism." *Progressive*: that word has become conspicuous as a political identification and to oppose it to the *conservative* – which is to say, cultural values worthy of being preserved, defended, and *lived* as they have been since our classical foundations in the four pillars of Western civilization: Judaism, Greece, Rome, and Christianity. That our "progressivism" is cowardly is only one of its more egregious characteristics. The assumption of progress does nothing to alter anything previously discussed about regression; the propaganda of the former can only be understood by the latter.

Relying on the work of Theodore Adorno and the Frankfurt School and the contribution they tried to make for psychoanalysis in the sphere of politics, Jamieson Webster writes of "Freud's critique of the idea of progress as a secular liberal theology in *Civilization and its Discontents*."[7] The important critique of science (or, better, scientism) and technology by Freud was not as important, and certainly not as thorough, as his analysis of the individual psyche. Webster rightly emphasizes *cure* along with critique; the latter may turn out to be a more important ideal, for our future, than any merely critical evaluation of reality. *Technological* progress has not been our issue in the essay; nor are the creations of capital and techno-scientism – for these deserve their own separate analysis. In any case, the word and phenomenon has been so taken for granted that it has been normalized to the point of being empty of meaning. There has never been a greater chasm between our objective inventions and our subjective condition as individuals or as a liberal society. Technological innovations are ubiquitous and expected; whether they are all-too-often trivial (and injurious) is another matter. Intelligence and freedom: Freud never lost sight of what he was defending and, if need be, against the complacency of society's material progress. While it is true that "Freud's text places itself on the borderline between a tempered, sceptical liberalism and a much profound disillusion with the possibility of community and the ideals of progressive growth,"[8] the noted pessimism must be considered by the reader as an association not easily sustained when the ideals of psychoanalysis are considered.

Élisabeth Roudinesco not only calls the 1929 work on *Kultur* a sequel to *The Future of an Illusion*, she describes it as "the darkest no doubt but also the most luminous, the most lyrical, the most poetic of all his books."[9] Luminous, lyrical, poetic: these descriptions (noticeable by their tendency towards the aesthetic) are in contrast to other appraisals that are, if not opposite because of the metaphors of "dark," fully aware of the always *possible* direction of civilization and the conflict between Eros and Thanatos.

Comments here and there will be mentioned to highlight certain responses and their place in our ongoing conversation with others. "Freud has a tragic view of civilization… … much individual and social neurosis and misery derives from the creation of civilization… … Freud's psychoanalysis is therefore politics."[10] The relationship, between the "poetic" and the "tragic," is at least one possible connection. When we then add love (as well as, in another section, a problem not to be minimized and for us as a conclusion – that attainment of *happiness*) the last of our works leaves us with more than sufficient suggestions for a possible future. Is Freud really the pessimist many believe him to be? Or can he be seen in an entirely different light once we recall, for one, the "Postscript" of *Group Psychology* and the now explicit relationship between all of his psychoanalytic ideals? Whether the all-important love of psychoanalytic therapy is enough cannot, today, be completely secured except in the clinical setting; any influence outside has to be a supplement provided as, also, a necessity. Clinical work has to be also intrinsic to our *everyday reality*. Analysands live the obligation on a daily basis. The internalization of a psychoanalyst, who *lives* and *works* towards a healthy psyche, is surely preferrable than the introjection of dead ego-ideal who is mourned and remains in a state of perpetual decomposition. Freud is indeed a political writer, as long as the definition, for us, is augmented by everything we have thus far presented. To be more precise, Freud is a psychoanalyst of the theological-political. His love is sober, neither sentimental nor idealistic, felt for the continuing support of *the ego* (the individual) against all instrumentalization. There is to be no "requiem for the ego," as Tauber writes with a warning. On the contrary. The work will have to focus on minimizing the effects of the super-ego and the death drive and doing so by assimilating the consciousness of psychoanalytic insights back into the ego and for the purpose of making it resilient and strong. One argument can be stated and to introduce another one of Freud's answers to an objection. "What is not made explicit by Freud is that mankind also needs to confront the *ethical choices* made in resorting to aggression and violence as a solution to social and political problems."[11] The problem, as Freud presents it, is much more complicated than the *conscious* decision about thoughts and actions; if only "choices" were the only problem. In any case, no one can accuse Freud of evading choices, ethical or otherwise; he had plenty to make in his own lifetime and without being timid about possible reactions. Many were hardly easy. On the contrary, that is precisely what he has been doing all along, and without any self-congratulatory attitude that would confirm a certain status for him except the independence of mind necessary for anyone who finds himself with original and disturbing ideas for the status quo.

Ethical choices are making aggression (if not out-and-out "violence," because there are many forms of coercion, including the now prevalent moral "training workshops" in the private and public sector) perfectly acceptable since policies are done for the "greater good." Institutional guidelines are intent on promoting our moral inadequacy. The catastrophes of the last century were lessons; because today two of the principal methods of the fascist and totalitarian mind – the leader and the state – have become, in liberal democracies, irrelevant. The group psychology of the present has divested itself of one leader; and it has circumvented the power of the state by enforcing its policies on governmental bureaucrats who are more than happy to implement policies that make the state *appear* moral and gives them the illusion of relevance and superiority. Deborah Prentice asks us: "what gives *liberal norms* – or any norms – the *power* to shape social reality? To put it simply, the power resides in people's *desire* to be right – to see the world *correctly*."[12] The currency of the last word has been noticeable. "To be right." The *need* to feel a certain kind of justification has been widely shared, which can be more clearly understood in light of the growing propaganda of everyone's (and civilization's) moral inadequacy. The number of our most perceptive commentators have, hopefully by now, resulted in a necessity for readers: to re-evaluate their thinking – about themselves, others, and the world.

This is the situation we find ourselves in – and as anticipated by Freud in the final work of the decade, with the exchange of letters with Romain Rolland, in effect not markedly different from the relationship he developed with his interlocutor in *The Future of an Illusion* in what he called "Conversations with an Impartial Person."[13] Freud's relationship to Rolland has been interpreted by Joseph Avery who, in reading the letter titled "A Disturbance of Memory on the Acropolis," writes that it is "a psychoanalytic essay, an exercise in self-analysis."[14] Freud's *self-analysis* has been constant since the very beginning. In the work that opens with a response to Romain Rolland, who had sent him a letter about his religious views, Freud mentions the *sense* of an "oceanic" feeling that he feels wholly without. He does not deny its existence and acknowledges its place in human life. "The only question is whether it is being correctly interpreted and whether it ought to be regarded as the *fons et origo* of the whole need for religion" (21:65). Once Freud has given momentary attention to the religious feeling expressed to him by his friend, he turns his attention to the "need for religion," a need that will be seen to extend beyond its usual categories (of "faith," for example, *pistis*, a certain kind of "trust" and conviction) and profoundly effect social life. Is this Freud's "only question?" Or does his depth-psychological understanding of the oceanic feeling not extend itself towards other human thoughts and acts – for example, in terms of love and art? The psychoanalysis of religion and its conclusion that it represents one of the many illusions in human life will hardly be the whole story; and if, in reading Freud, we can come to other observations, the malaise of civilization will be given other analyses more relevant for our contemporary situation. The power of our contemporary super-ego can no longer be ignored; the pretensions of its goodness have been exposed. Are we justified in analyzing our moral drive as potentially *evil* and therefore rely on theological language, no different than Freud's characterization of the repetition compulsion as "demonic." A recent publication, on the problem of freedom, has analyzed "the diabolical character of modern liberty."[15] Does Freud offer us a therapeutic answer to the moral super-ego and death drive of the theological-political by turning towards love and, for him, one of its most profound effects? Are we prepared to extend Freud's argument as it leads to the most intimate relationship between love and creativity – that is, the erotic insofar as it enhances human being in its aesthetic appreciation of existence.

While *Civilization and its Discontents* opens with the continuation of an earlier argument, Freud soon moves into an even more comprehensive analysis than before; the direction was pressing, as can be seen by the repetition. "The further question then arises, what claims this feeling has to be regarded as the source of religious needs" (SE 21:72). The stated question has already been answered. The repetition is expressed in order to introduce an argument as to the social nature of the religious *need* and how the oceanic feeling experienced by an individual is not at all how one aspect of religion is felt, and imposed, socially. On the one hand, Freud presents us, again, with the analytic belief that the religious feeling is nothing more than the persistent trace of the child's helplessness and the need for a father's protection. On the other, the origin of one human need may also be related to one that, in this work, reached a place of unmatched prominence: the artistic and, with one description that should make us double-aware of "the intoxicating quality of feeling" (21:83) of aesthetics, the *aisthesis* as the sensual appreciation of the world. Does Freud rehabilitate the capacity for a certain "quality of feeling" by transforming it from one reality to another? Does the feeling of the expansive not make us intimately connected with the ability to create and, equally as important, the reverence for life and creation? One should take note of Freud's expository organization. The composition presented earlier as a form of displacement can also be recognized in the conscious order of his arguments: the discussion of love is followed by one on art. The "oceanic feeling" does not originate, nor is it confined, to religion. It is, as we all *feel*, essential to the experience of both love and art. There is, then, a profound feeling that is necessary for us to live as fully developed human beings; the antidote to the regression to the infantile and the primitive in the super-ego can be transformed by the work of love and the aesthetic.

Freud opened Chapter IV of *Totem and Taboo* with this statement: "there are no grounds for fearing that psycho-analysis, which first discovered that psychical facts and structures are invariably overdetermined, will be tempted to trace the origin of anything so complicated as religion to a single source" (13:100). *Overdetermined*: when, in the work on civilization, he sets out from a well-known origin, Freud expects the reader to be less than convinced by the first argument. He concludes with a classical evaluation. But, also, with a doubt easy to ignore for some; he has not given up on his suggestive language and continues to be conscious of the nature of his composition no less than on his reader's *analytic* responsibility. "The origin of the religious attitude can be traced back in clear outlines as far as the feeling of infantile helplessness. There may be something further behind that, but for the present it is wrapped in obscurity" (SE 21:72). The *origin* is mentioned no less than three times; the last stands out, for its "obscurity." At the present time, Freud admits without hesitation, how the origin of the feeling is still mysterious. "But for the present its is wrapped in obscurity." Is he referring to the present of his era? Or is there a meaning, and an implicit one, concealed in part by a screen that can only be removed by remembering previous arguments in *The Future of an Illusion*? Freud might make it seem as if this "obscurity" cannot be in some way be illuminated and therefore will remain outside his investigations. Not at all. There is something "behind," obscure and hidden from this first analytic insight; and he has already identified it. As soon as Freud devotes himself to clarifying the problem further, he comes upon psychoanalytic insights that are far more important than childhood traces because these, more seriously, are fully mature and hidden with even more repressive tenacity – as they need to be if the religious unconscious is going to be hidden from the morality of a newly-founded theological-political society. One possibility stands out. The "infantile-helplessness" thesis has been made; any "obscurity," however, as can be expected from a psychoanalyst no less from an analysand and reader, remains to be investigated. Any notion of something "behind," out of view but nonetheless present, is one of the motivations of the analytic inquiry. The first classical thesis can be stated: the need for religion is analogous to the child needing protection from the father. The foundations are only the beginning of consequences that extend from the objective dependence of the child to the development of mechanisms of defense that, as an adult, will continue to be effective and, because unconscious, all the more debilitating. Are we justified in once again being circumspect about our approach to Freud's writing and to remember how, in *The Future of an Illusion*, the manifest declarations were not always as transparent as they have been interpreted? Guy Stroumsa, someone who has distinguished himself as an exceptional *reader*, tells us that "Freud perceived himself as the leader of a revolutionary movement threatened by persecution, and required to act with great caution, sometimes even hide his views on highly contentious topics."[16] The previous "obscurity," then, might be one more marker for analytic reader even though going as far as "hiding" his views would be counter-productive. Uniquely representing them is by no means a concealment. Can the infantilism of a political morality, with all its weakness and vulnerability, be overcome by the mature recollection of eros? Could the super-ego morality of the present be a reaction against the "memory" (or a piece of historical reconstruction) of a past history experienced as traumatic that, in itself, precludes any love and certainly no creativity since it depends on an absolute interpretation safeguarded by morality which judges the past one-dimensionally? Are we faced with a difficult imperative and one so antithetical to the moral fantasies of the times and what has been called, with some regularity and no longer as jarring as it once was, "a culture victimhood"? We can, of course, continue with the bind of trauma and victimhood; or we can begin to think about whether an "active forgetting"[17] might not be in our best social interest. One forgetting would free us for a pause and a re-examination of what Freud himself proposed as possible remedies.

"The psychological significance of religious ideas" (SE 21:25) taken up in *The Future of an Illusion* left Freud with a sense of incompletion; because he knew, once he forced himself beyond the familial relations (of father and son, God and his children) that there were other latent meanings to be analyzed. The reality of religion in its infancy was not at all the same as its manifestation later – in the coming-to-be of modernity and for the adult. Once the thesis of the dependent child on the all-caring love of God is displaced and religion, for all intents and purposes, is relegated to nothing more than an archaic superstition, one should become extremely aware of what takes its place. Voids can be filled much too quickly and without sufficient preparation for consequences. Freud made a distinction in *On Narcissism* that has added meaning; our beginning with the bind of love and hate finds its most intense expression after Freud leaves us with a staggering insight. "The highest phase of development of which object-libido is capable is seen in the state of being in love… … while we have the opposite condition in the paranoic's phantasy (or self-perception) of the 'end of the world'" (14:76). Our inability to acknowledge Freud's *metaphysical* insights have at times prevented us from recognizing how profound his analysis was, in fact, capable of revealing. Is there a more stark difference than the one supporting love (including procreation) and what Freud calls, without ambiguity, the *paranoid desire* for the end of the world? The nihilism of the death drive has been impelled towards this one catastrophic ambition: to destroy life as represented by the history of our Western civilization. We can now repeat earlier notes, in the Introduction, on the disposition to obsessional neurosis.

> The characteristics peculiar to both of them – megalomania, turning away from the world of objects, increased difficulty in transference – have obliged us to conclude that their dispositional fixation is to be looked for in a stage of libidinal development *before* object-choice has been established – that is, in the phase of auto-eroticism and of narcissism. Thus these forms of illness, which make their appearance so late, go back to very early inhibitions and fixations.[18]

Megalomania, aversion to reality, negative transferences: the latter is especially important given our arguments about the introjection of a dead ego-ideal and, therefore, as a consequence, the development of a deep hatred for the living.

We have, for Freud, the return to an extreme relation: the "love" and the paranoia of a systematic political madness. The psychopolitical essay has been divided between love and the current obsessions of the politically minded moralists. A note from *Totem and Taboo* – in effect, our starting-point, and written in 1913, the same year as the essay above on the disposition to obsessions – brought together two relations. "An obsessional neurosis is a caricature of religion and that a paranoic delusion is a caricature of a philosophical system" (13:73). The obsession and paranoia of the present has resulted from an uneasy alliance. Our very first and still most important term, "the return of the religious," can be recalled. Since religion has been – so it has been presumed to be – obliterated and superseded by secularism, with the emancipation of the saeculum presumed to be real, the reality of a psychical dynamism is able to more effectively be influential. In effect, there are two layers in Freud's writing. Making the layers more visible is not arduous, not once the interpretation of how dreams are made and then interpreted is, indeed, the "royal road to the unconscious." To a certain individual – the analysand as a reader – Freud's writing presents itself dynamically. His political sensibilities are not going to be eclipsed; they are as important as they are pronounced when he commits himself, without apologia, to discussing the formation of the cultural super-ego. A century on, Freud can still remarkably be someone who can offend and upend all the niceties of our most trusted ideals. One can expect that exposing the unconscious nature of our morality today will be met with the same kind of outrage as when Freud made us aware of our hidden nature and we suffered from the same narcissistic disappointments as in the previous changes in the realities of the world. In many ways, our unconscious is more ignored today now that Freud (ironically, like religion) has been culturally repudiated.

In the past, when religion had influence on social life (in part, through its work on conscience) it could still regulate extremes. Today, the order has been replaced. In doing so, other forces have come to be hyperactive.

> Religion restricts this play of choice an adaptation, since it imposes equally on everyone its own path to the acquisition of happiness and protection from suffering. Its technique consists in depressing the value of life and distorting the picture of the real world in a delusional manner – which presupposes an intimidation of the intelligence. At this price, by forcibly fixing them in a state of psychical infantilism and by drawing them into a mass-delusion, religion succeeds in sparing many people an individual neurosis.
>
> (21:84)

Group psychology and *mass delusion*. One word can easily be substituted; in place of "religion," another can be joined for a double-relation. If, in the past, religion served to spare the individual from being neurotically afflicted alone, the demise of conscious religiosity and its replacement by a self-possessed secularity has resulted in a similar reproduction in the political. Is it not evident that today it is precisely politics that has undermined "the value of life" and through its distortions about the moral inadequacy of the world – most especially in the past, in the whole of history – given itself the unparalleled power to correct all the flaws committed by Western civilization. Freud's language is specific and unmistakable. It echoes *Group Psychology* and once again makes it incumbent on the reader not to be so self-satisfied with the critique of religion and instead reflect his argument and how the "intimidation of intelligence," analyzed as a symptom of group psychology, is today widespread. Depression, distortion, infantilism, and mass-delusion: *Civilization and its Discontents* repeats the analysis of the symptoms of group psychology; and with an addition that, now, cannot be ignored or dismissed. A word is now conspicuous: *happiness*. In what way does Freud attempt to confront the malaise of civilization and, still, despite everything, make the claim that it is still possible to achieve a measure of happiness as long as the desire to correct the world is abandoned for a much more reachable end? Freud's antidote to the symptoms and root causes of our social neuroses will only be overcome, he believes, by once again re-committing ourselves to the principles of culture he has been defending for his entire life: love, freedom, intelligence, and creativity, all of them necessary to attain at least a level of happiness or what the ancient Greeks called *eudaimonia*, the happiness of a self-flourishing human being.

One experiment in reading – substituting the manifest of the religious for the latent of the political – reveals a completely different way to both conceive of the political and understand its effects. Psychoanalysts who are as committed to reading as they are to listening have added an incomparable insight for us – in two ways. Danielle Quinodoz tells us that "Freud himself signposted the new paths" and also expressed a certain relation by being "faithful to Freud's heritage." How does she do this? "I shall take care of his heritage by discovering new developments," she writes, adding "however minimal they may be – the discoveries I make in contact with Freud's."[19] His work in *Civilization and its Discontents* turns into one all-important direction when the theme of the religious is no longer isolated into itself but the dynamic indication of a psychical disposition of the human. "It is asserted," he writes:

> that each one of us behaves in some respect like a paranoic, corrects some aspect of the world which is unbearable to him by the construction of a wish and introduces his delusion into reality. A special importance attaches to the case in which this attempt to procure a certainty of happiness and a protection against suffering through a delusional remoulding of reality is

> made by a considerable number of people in common. The religions of mankind must be classed among the mass delusions of this kind. No one, needless to say, who shares a delusion ever recognizes it as such.
>
> (21:81)

Paranoia, correction of reality, construction of a wish, delusional remoulding of reality. All of them are quintessentially political and, also, the negative of the oceanic. Surely no one is so self-confident in the singularity of their reading that they all-too readily accept Freud's statement (on religion) and not recognize its reality for a great many number of other human endeavors. If politics – especially today – is not "a delusional remolding of reality," then our psychopolitical essay can no longer be defended and the reader has a decision to make. But if our main thesis can be maintained and Freud has adopted both an "opponent" in *The Future of an Illusion* and an interlocutor through the writing of letters in his work on civilization, then we can continue and bring the project to a provisional conclusion. Supplements will be added in due time. If Freud has been concerned all along, as a psychoanalyst, and as a humanist, with a "technique in the art of living," the work on civilization will allow him to carry the whole project forward and make a series of proposals on how to best avoid the most stringent demands of social prohibitions and make love, first of all, the first response for a moderate human health in the face of growing pressures from neurotic and paranoid alternatives. While Freud does not resign himself to the analysis to come, in part because of his defense of his psychoanalytic ideals, he also does not avoid considering the most difficult problems confronting individuals. Our "social regulations" are not only, in his words, inadequate; they have become part of the problem itself. They are now so prevalent that the antidotes to their forceful reality are no mere ideals to be, simply, thought about but conceived for what Freud has called the art of living. We are ever more skeptical about the prospect of what Elizabeth Young-Bruehl calls a "psychoanalysis-socialism synthesis."[20] It would be much more preferable to allow psychoanalysis to continue to develop on its own and without extraneous interference – because how "socialism" and all its political theories sees the reality of our social existence much differently, and with different sets of principles, than Freud and all those who have decided to remain faithful to his discoveries. If psychoanalysis is to develop, in this century, it will not be through an already-attempted experiment. The results are no secret. The alignment of one version of psychoanalysis and politics may have been, for some, intellectually productive. Have they been psychologically beneficial?

(n) The Inadequacy of Our Social Regulations

Freud's analysis of the discontents of civilization began, on one level, with the consolation of religion and on a still mysterious feeling, the "oceanic" one invoked by Rolland and associated, also, to art and love; on another and simultaneous level, he was to examine the many regulations of social life which, consciously, were intended to contribute to its stability and order; the examples were innumerable and, also, necessary. *Civilization and its Discontents* could be read with this one purpose in mind, to see how Freud evaluated various cultural achievements, the demands they made on us, and some of the ways created to deal with the inexorable nature of reality. There is, however, one concern that, if not expressed for the first time, receives Freud's most committed attention in a work on the *unbehagen* of culture: the always-present ideals of human creativity, love and, finally, the challenge of *attaining happiness*. For someone as sober-minded as Freud to raise the problem of human happiness in the context of the aims and ends of civilization, the preoccupation was not one among others. In whatever we may conceive of this one paramount human *condition* – which is not to be merely fleeting and associated with a moment or a solitary experience – as a therapist Freud was committed to pursuing it as an attainable possibility, for life and as the end goal he had always been promoting in terms of overall psychological health. Witnessing unhappiness and misery in his neurotic patients was, we should not forget, a daily experience from the earliest days of psychoanalysis that had left a deep impression on him; his social and political analysis had done nothing to minimize an unshakeable awareness. We cannot neglect Freud's sympathies (and his sensitivity) for the everyday hardships of human life, both the irreducible ones and the ones we often subject ourselves to.[21] The many declarations in *An Autobiographical Study* and other writings of a personal nature may be guarded and only revealing during moments Freud is careful to choose, yet one senses that his memory of his earliest motivations were humanistic and that is the reason he became, after his medical and scientific studies, "a specialist in nervous diseases."[22] Human misery could be lessened and alleviated. The scientist in him had always been keenly aware of human suffering. The more perplexing problem must have motivated him all the more; for if there was one inescapable piece of psychoanalytic knowledge gained over a lifetime of work, one had yet to be solved even though he had witnessed it time and time again, for individuals and no less for society: all the ways in which suffering had been confronted, with different methods for a remedy, none had been effective enough to minimize the suffering. More seriously (and this is one of the main themes of a society of discontent) many of the efforts intended to make life more bearable had, in fact, contributed to making it far worse. Problems were often compounded during the effort to solve them. That has been the most obvious problem of the political initiatives taken during the processes of this century.

Howard Kaye would like to make a proposal: "what happens if we read Freud as the philosopher and social theorist he always aspired to be, rather than the medical scientist he often claimed to be?"[23] The question can be answered, unequivocally and, if necessary, polemically: if Kaye's question was taken seriously, then we would simply have a Freud that is convenient because we would have *only one* of the dimensions of psychoanalysis, one confined to sociology. He would be among *many other* social thinkers instead of the one individual who created psychoanalysis and therefore inaugurated a new way of thinking about the depth and complexity of human beings. The analysis of the individual and culture are inseparable; his social theory, if denied therapeutic aims, is only half as meaningful and, in fact, is deprived of its more unique motivations. Academic theories are inadequate because, aside from *reducing* Freud to be better managed, Kaye forgets one other essential individual who is rarely noticed – certainly by the academic community – but who has been, throughout this psychopolitical essays, indispensable. The analysand has been a constant in everything presented thus far, and on many different levels – which can never be *principally* theoretical. Alfred Tauber has been one of the few to acknowledge one aspect of the post-termination analysand. "In regarding *the analysand's insight as an ethical project*, we appreciate how Freud fulfilled his earlier humanistic aspirations, which in turn opens new pathways into this thought."[24] There seems to me no more important argument, for the whole of psychoanalysis, than to appeal not only to the analysand as a neglected individual, but, more specifically, to the inseparable relation between the analysand and the morality promoted with such conviction above all by academics and political activists. The ethos of the analysand has been the sense of an interminable responsibility towards the ego and society and to continually make the attempt to expose how the supposed morality of liberal society has been a source of deprivation and, to recall an earlier description, "impoverishment"; hence, the ego and the strength of the self-regarding analysand. Freud has been managed most especially when he has been disciplined by academics; the attitude stands out. "Towards the end of his life Freud was less optimistic about the prospects of addressing this pain through individual therapy, and saw psychoanalysis as an approach to understanding the cultural-historical nature of human beings."[25] Reading the work of non-analysts, which has been included as illustrative, allowed for some subdued responses, even to commonplaces. "Freud remained a nineteenth-century thinker in many respects."[26] That the sentence comes in a work entitled *Postmodern Theory and Progressive Politics* gives the reader another sense of a continuing relation – from a divided polarity. *My fidelity* remains, as does the obligation to continue to defend his transmission and conscious transference, which is more important today than it was in the 19th century. Any thinking about Freud and the "post-modern," much less what passed for "progressive politics" today, is highly inappropriate and risks confounding Freud, making him into what he has never been. A personal suggestion, made on more than one occasion, has been written by someone who, here, can be quoted very succinctly. Richard

Chessick's title *The Future of Psychoanalysis* is answered with the need to re-read "the Freud of the entire *Standard Edition*."[27] The insistence on reading Freud's writing, in its entirety, remains in effect; anything less will be incomplete and potentially distorted.

One thinker, and who has singled himself out by his ability to *read*, and to do so without prejudice, has made a suggestion (above all, to read once again) that will strike most with mixed feelings. This is the only time the "religious" and the psychoanalytic have come into contact, more than in passing.

> So: Begin anew to interpret Paul! I want also to add one last sentence, that I believe that Freud, so to speak, enters into the role of Paul, of the Paul who supposedly brings redemption only phantasmatically, while Freud realizes it through this new method of *healing*, which is not only an individual method, but also a theory of culture. Freud is a doctor not only of the individual, but a doctor of culture.[28]

It is because Freud has also been a "doctor of culture" that we have been given the opportunity to think about our social and political situation with a new way of thinking and of interpreting the phenomena of our collective life. If neurotic illness has become worse and for the reasons thus far examined, achievable remedies have been prepared – by Freud himself, repeatedly and consistently. No academic theorizing has ever been presented as in any way therapeutic, except from the illusory assumption that a changed social and political world is the *one* prerequisite for healthier individuals.

Freud noticed how the human attempts at making aspects of life bearable, endurable, liveable, had in many ways become *tragic* – prompted by furtive attempts to remedy a situation, only to add to the suffering. Only someone who was fundamentally concerned with the problem of human suffering, and who had dedicated himself to a practical project to alleviate it could then make the effort to offer a more wide-ranging proposal for society. The training of analysts was a practical project that had become essential for him. Does he write *Civilization and its Discontents* with resignation, or with the pessimistic frame of mind often attributed to him? Or does his thinking confront this one intractable problem with determination and precisely because he has known, for a long time, how the attempts to "regulate" social life for people's benefits had contributed negatively to the relationship of human beings to each other? The vulnerability of our bodies was an existential given, with death as the inevitable end; as was our relationship to nature, with its own identifiable rhythms, some easily anticipated, others much more sudden and unpredictable. All our attempts to deal with the adverse conditions of nature, we now know with even more certainty, have led us into a predicament that many believe will become worse in a century that may very well be decisive for the earth/world relation. As an organic whole, the world can only tolerate so much of its adverse conditions; the living conditions of a bio-sphere cannot be compromised without limits. Human beings are no different, except that the internal and external factors are so intrinsically related that coming to a resolution of conflicts requires painstaking attention. Failures are not uncommon. The presumption of "controlling" nature has led us to a situation that in our century may well come to a pressure-filled period – as scientists are now virtually unanimous in forecasting. As for our social suffering, Freud believes we have not yet become conscious of the will towards our own individual and collective pain – and, more importantly, admitted it to ourselves. We seem unable to confront one of our most enduring difficulties.

> We cannot see why the regulations made by ourselves should not, on the contrary, be a protection and a benefit for every one of us. And yet, when we consider how unsuccessful we have been in precisely this field of prevention of suffering, a suspicion dawns on us that here, too, a piece of unconquerable nature may lie behind – this time a piece of our own psychical constitution.
>
> (21:86)

Is Freud making a final announcement about our "psychical constitution" in some sense following a certain line of regression and making the outcome inevitable; or does he, because the issue seems so difficult, commit himself all the more rigorously to a set of proposals that extend beyond his analysis of group psychology, the super-ego, hysterical identification, the masochist-sadistic bind, and ultimately, the death drive, and offer us a project to consider and to realize? Does he, at the end of the decade and confident the work of the 1920s has been thorough, make a final statement? If so, we will see a particular unity in the re-affirmation of his psychoanalytic ideals. His support of love, freedom, intelligence, and creativity will, together and as conscious pursuits, make it possible to achieve a condition that has been elusive: happiness. My argument is antithetical to so many who have mistakenly defined Freud as a pessimist or as someone who had a tragic conception of human life. Psychoanalysis began as a form of therapy for the mental pain of patients; that it also believed itself capable of addressing larger questions of civilization was one mark of Freud as an individual and psychoanalyst who (completely differently than those who, like Marx, believed human misery could be alleviated if the material conditions of the world were changed) stressed the psychical over the material and the socio-economic. Before, then, accepting the makeup of our psyches as inevitably fated to suffer, it would be preferrable to first examine whether the particular forms of our "regulations" are not somehow responsible for at least some of the continued discontents. If they do originate, through a process of regression, in the infantile and the primitive psyche, psychoanalysis believes it is always possible to return to original conditions and find a way to free ourselves from a self-imposed condition, or at least prepare for the modification of its origins and effects. Our neurotic fixations can be given up. Maturity is possible because it is present as a possibility for the full-fledged human being. Freud has been committed to this one task – which is by no means easy: can we attend to the influence of our three-part psyche on the reality of the world and, with enough clarity and insight, be capable of altering even a small part of it for our benefit, that is, for our intelligence, our freedom, our creativity, and for our capacity to love and in ways that would not be compromised by the fateful aspirations of groups who, increasingly, are showing themselves more than willing to destroy other human beings and make their lives impossible? Have we, in the first decades of this century, exacerbated our situation and, apparently, with the best of moral intentions, only to reveal a terrible underside that is becoming more aggressive, hostile, and destructive? That would be a first necessary realization: for all our claims to be implementing all kinds of social policies intended to make the world a better place – more just, more equal, more right – it has been Freud who warned us both how its motives are not as clear as they are made out to be and, stronger still, may be leading us toward a social life much more *restrictive*, and painful, than has been anticipated. The prohibitions, on speech and writing, are becoming more noticeable. Life in liberal societies has in many ways become intolerable; how the smallest and most fragmented of minority views have been able to be so powerful is a question all of us will have to ask ourselves sooner than later. How much longer a moral acquiescence is accepted as the norm and perpetuated is an equally compelling question – for *all of us* and not only the few who have given themselves power and legitimacy. My psychopolitical essay has been concerned with this one fundamental problem. Freud gives us one incomparable idea. The "contention" has more force today than ever.

> We come upon a contention which is so astonishing that we must must dwell upon it. This contention holds that what we call our civilization is largely responsible for our misery… … It is a certain fact that all the things with which we seek to protect ourselves against the threats that emanate from the sources of suffering are part of that very civilization.
>
> (21:86)

If we are to look for an origin to Freud's thinking, there is one classical place for its emergence: it was only Oedipus' desire, a heroic one, to avoid fulfilling his fate that led him, precisely, to encounter the life situations that would make it possible for his catastrophic destiny to be realized. The structure of the Oedipal tragedy can be repeated for emphasis, as a matter pertinent for Sophocles' drama and our own contemporary reality. Is our situation in liberal democracies at the moment inevitable? Are we leading ourselves towards a tragic structure (loss of love, diminished intelligence, abolished freedom) and as a direct cause of our perverse and sadistic-masochistic morality?

If Freud does resign himself to a certain pessimism, because he recognizes how our attempts to remedy the difficulties of the human condition have too often resulted in the opposite of what was intended, the turn towards the transformation of the religious takes up his final concerns. The transference from the religious to the political is once again described – with the example of the Soviets paramount, just as it was in his work on illusions. His returns should appear to be conspicuous, and with precise intentions. One has to notice the structure of the whole of *Civilization and its Discontents*; its organization, and its relations, have not often been traced. It is important to follow how he constructs one presentation after another – from the inadequacy of our social regulations to the attempts to remedy them and, finally, how the drive towards secularism has revived the worst aspect of the psyche. The return to beginnings is necessary as it is programmatic. Has it, finally, become noticeable only today, when our social conditions allowed for a reading of Freud's century-old insights with sufficient acuity? There are insights made by psychoanalysis that have not been fully perceived, that could not have been revealed fully until such time as history prepared for their perception. Our own development, individually or as a civilization, still kept us removed from their truth; we were not yet prepared for the perceptions themselves and their meaning for us going forward. But this, to my mind, is the single most-relevant argument that can be made about Freud's thought: so much time spent on the interpretation of the psyche exposed him to the depth of human sense only reached by others of equal sensitivity. Nietzsche, as always, comes to mind. It is no wonder, then, how Freud's turn to secularity gives him the opportunity to revisit not only the illusion of religion but, more so for us, the illusion of its replacement. How the religious and the political are often discussed side by side, with examples, has been evident in previous work. The presentation in *The Future of an Illusion* is more exposed, given more breadth, placed beside the illusions that have been created from the pretensions of secularity.

> We shall therefore content ourselves with saying once more that the word 'civilization' describes the whole sum of the achievements and the regulations which distinguish our lives from those of our animal ancestors and which serve two purposes – namely to protect men against nature and to adjust their mutual relations.
>
> (21:89)

Freud might perhaps be surprised (or not) at how far our protection against nature has been "successful" and, at the same time, placed us in serious jeopardy. While the ecological sense might have been a distant problem, the idea of technological progress did not leave him with confidence. The "adjustment," or, more accurately, the maladjustments of our relations are as filled with challenges as they have always been; and in liberal democracies more so because the *regulations* have made *mutual relations* (that is, human relationships) filled with all kinds of rules and regulations and, more seriously, completely contradictory ones. The inquisitorial nature of liberal reality has not been at all hesitant in unleashing the worst kind of psychical violence on any individual deemed responsible for so much as *raising questions* or attempting to initiate a discussion where views can be freely expressed.

The back-to-back presentation in Chapter III deserves attention because, as he completes one consideration of the technological, he prepares for a significant transition. "With every tool man is perfecting his own organs, whether motor or sensory, or is removing the limits of their functioning" (21:90). One could pause on this comment alone and analyze its seriousness and how detrimental these "tools" have become. Marshall McLuhan has an unsettling word for it: "auto-amputation"[29] as well as presenting us with a picture of our *prosthetic* selves, the same metaphor Freud himself used when describing our drive towards "divinity." The medical metaphor will soon be used at a particularly important moment. Leaving the relation of scientism and technology and moving to Freud's transition serves our purposes since the prior sense of the inadequacy is now shown in relation to secularity. The species, as globalization becomes absolute, is being categorically divided: the psychological regression appears to receive its compensation (its consolation) by ever-new and renewable techno-narcissistic gadgets that are the only indication of our external progress. Our loss of love, loss of freedom, and loss of intelligence is compensated by lifeless matter and by facile interconnections. We are all too aware of how anonymous persecution has devastating effects on public opinion and individual lives. How has secularity not only been inadequate but detrimental and, ultimately, one more indication of our human failures? To the question Freud turns to the first intimations of the religious and its modern repudiation. How technology has become psychically idolatrous is not a separate issue. From the brief discussion, again, of the problems of technology, Freud moves seamlessly towards the religious. The psychical movement proceeds from the external to the internal, the material to the psychical. How the technological and the theological come into proximity is one more element of psychoanalysis that will only serve us as a background as we move toward our conclusions. To come to his summing up, Freud always returns to beginnings and the juxtaposition between the primal father and the divine.

"These gods were cultural ideals" (21:91), Freud writes, returning us to origins, its *fons* and *origo*, of religion and moving to our present response. His language, considering his earlier discussion of technology, is not accidental.

The perfection of organs through the use of technological tools, fully and almost unavoidable today is transferred into the realm of religion and the drive towards the secular. "To-day he has come very close to the attainment of this ideal, he has almost become a god himself." The announced "death of God" and the more general sense of his disappearance from society has given some the impression that they were now liberated from faith and superstition and, by doing so, could finally achieve the unimpeded possibilities of reason. The traditional authority of God was replaced by human ambition. The human took his place; and with a history that is, still, far from complete. When Freud tells us, in no way as a boast or an achievement, that "man has, as it were, become a kind of a prosthetic God" (21:91–92), the technological artificiality of a prosthetic appendage, or a whole body, is only one and not at all the most serious consequence of the rise of secularism. His example is specific and different than the ones in our Introduction and the many references to ghosts and specters and phantasms. If Freud's presentation in *The Future of an Illusion* left too many readers confident in the critique of religion and without also thinking about him as an analyst and therefore as a thinker who could not be easily reduced to a singular position, the transition from scientism and technology to secularism should leave little doubt. The attempt to transcend religion, and its commitments to avoiding a strictly materialist interpretation of the world and of human life, made secularity and technology the most intimate of collaborators, with consequences that, for the time being, are only incompletely perceived. The order to capital, scientism, and technology have been unified into a comprehensive worldview that has installed a one-dimensional determination of the world. How the morality of the super-ego has been a *collaborative* phenomenon can be witnessed in the frenetic attempt to reorder social relations and with the most demanding of bureaucratic initiatives. The attempt to safeguard the human from the obvious incursions may be more complicit than can be imagined.

The word *authentic* has not been used up until now; the real, the true, and the actual seems fitting when compared to the prosthetic and also to recall how, at one point, Freud exposed the mendacity of theological-political love and its divided commitment to equality, justice, and rights. Are our politically committed activists at all sure of their ideals and, more so, of the methods that have begun to be suspected and also perceived for their overbearing impositions? Our moral standards are becoming extreme, the methods to enforce them more so. We may be approaching the shifts of a decade that will not simply accept, passively, how much pain our moral activists have actually caused. Hyper-morality is causing harm that will take a significant amount of time to remedy. "In the interests of our investigations, we will not forget that present-day man does not feel happy in his Godlike character." Although we can acknowledge how the turn towards a self-possessed secularity has not produced any more happiness, the investigation remains incomplete if the attempt is not made to identify how the developments of society have created conditions that work against any sense of emotional stability and general contentment. One cannot easily forget a strong impression: liberal societies, some more than others, are not without a sense of a prevailing unhappiness, a cold and dour and severe disposition that has been created, artificially, to serve the ends of a propaganda directed by the super-ego.

When Freud then turns to the ideals of civilization, what he calls "his ideas of a possible perfection of individuals" (21:94), we come again to the problem of morals, and one which Freud has returned time and time again because its interest was, for him, inexhaustible and, more importantly for us, of "increasing the difficulty not only of describing them but of tracing their psychological derivation." To this problem he has been focused on for the better part of a decade and long before. The "psychological derivation" has had one origin in the murder of the primal father and many inter-related repercussions; whether it can, again, be explanatory when it is brought forward as a displacement will be a matter to be considered with time. The effort of *Civilization* will be decisive, and in a sense also cumulative because not only has Freud worked on noting the epiphenomenon of morals as they are manifested in politics, he also recollects his understanding of projection which he had already discussed in *Totem and Taboo*. The chronology he had constructed – from the primal horde to the herd, and for us the collectivity of liberal democracies, has led him to one inescapable conclusion. To the previous discussion of projection, we can recollect how, in his discussion in *Totem and Taboo*,

> the projection outwards of internal perceptions is a primitive mechanism, to which, for instance, our sense perceptions are subject, and which therefore play a very large part in determining the form taken by our external world. Under conditions whose nature has not been sufficiently established, internal perceptions of emotional and thought processes can be projected outwards in the same way as sense perceptions; they are thus employed for building up the external world, though they should by rights remain part of the *internal* world.
>
> (SE 13:64)

The *primitive* situation of the primal horde has not changed. The order to the social world seems to have continued from these origins and remained – even, or especially when, we pride ourselves on our many refinements. The analysis might be more severe than can be imagined. The external world has been constructed from the power of the internal machinations of the psyche and, today, driven by one obsession above all. Have we regressed to such a point that we are once again at a primitive stage of development *morally* while deluded into believing in our technological progress as a proper measure of ourselves. Are we now at a severe temporal disjunctions of the human? Freud remains the single most important thinker of the last century (along with one or two philosophers) because he left us with an inheritance – that is, a perpetual responsibility that is exemplified in the post-termination condition of the analysand who, despite the experience of a lifetime, as a whole, finds himself with a decision: to commit oneself to the individual responsibility of *working*, ceaselessly, day in and day out, to freedom and intelligence, creativity and love and psychological health.

"The last, but certainly not the least important, of the characteristic features of civilization remains to be assessed: the manner in which the relationship of men to another, their social relationships, are regulated" (21:94–95). If we began with the sense that our social regulations were "inadequate," how does Freud respond to this historical situation and, also, prepare us for its reality? "The task is an immense one," he admitted, for him as it is, no less, for us. Turning to the human confrontation between love and hate, affection and aggression, will be one of the final points to examine once again before concluding with the continued presence of guilt and death drive in Freud's ideas about society and, despite them, the possible work towards the attainment of happiness. The previous commentaries on the super-ego and the death drive will be carried forward. We are, now, much further along then before, and at quite a distance from one trend, mentioned earlier, when some analysts believed that the super-ego should be "laid to rest." The metaphor was not, for us, tangential, not when mourning and the dead, specters, ghosts, and hauntings have been constant references. We can agree with one of Alan Karbelnig's comments, in an essay called "laying the death drive to rest," that the "stubborn persistence" of the death drive, "especially because of the political problems associated with it, calls for further investigation."[30] Approaching the end of our psychopolitical investigation calls for a few more comments. A conclusion, after the diagnosis, remains. Whether the confluence of our relationship to nature, our own finite bodies, and our "social regulations" have become inescapably tragic is a problem that cannot be in any way neglected.

(o) Love, Aggression, and the Neighbour as Our Enemy

Throughout my psychopolitical essay, the discussion has revolved around the many issues of a super-ego morality and death drive hatred against civilization and how the impairment to intelligence, freedom, and creativity might now have to depend on Freud and his support of love as one of the ways we could bring ourselves to turn away, affirmatively, from our unconscious theological-political reality. Have we reached the point when Freud can offer us a number of essential and universal remedies as antidotes to the malice of our times and in the form of a *strong egoism* and, above all, the ability to once again love, authentically, without being compelled by no longer believable obsessions? The striking self-definition of someone who has made love a vocation (in the everyday therapeutic situation) may very well be one of the most poignant ways for psychoanalysis to renew its presence in culture and to once again make us conscious of our conflicts. We need not define Freud's transference love as "agapic."[31] His love was by no mean unconditional, as he makes (perfectly) clear in the antagonistic set-up between love and hate – and, at the risk of introducing another theological-political topic, neighbors, friends and *enemies*. At this moment nearing our conclusion, we can again refer to Freud's striking confidence to his friend Rolland. Love will be a consideration, as it has from the beginning when the binds of the group had altered the nature human feelings of love under the burden of theological-political symptoms.

In a chapter entitled "Responsibility beyond the Superego" and with the extraordinary consideration to a well-known attitude of the "ethical encounter" and one now over-used (and perhaps used up by the concept of "the Other") Eric Santner asks us to consider the ways in which "human beings register the impact of divine love."[32] How does one begin to address the chasm between the unconscious drive of destruction towards civilization and "divine love"? Freud has been nuanced and subtle in his presentation; adopting him for a theology of divine love is, simply, not possible given his personal sensibilities. His convictions are other than divine. They are wholly, and unapologetically, human; and so, when love has been introduced as a psychoanalytic ideal, how will it be presented and to raise to the level of its urgency beyond our accommodations to hate? Can we offer an alternative to the all the negative effects of the super-ego and the death drive and, to support and strengthen the ego, consider a necessary position of "aggressive self-assertion"[33] that would, *because healthy*, be neither narcissistic nor dominated by group psychology and therefore *individual*?

If, as Peter Sloterdijk tells us, "a titanic battle is being waged in our contemporary culture between the civilizing and bestializing impulses and *their associated media*,"[34] Freud has not hesitated to show us the extent of our own implications in the middle of the "battle." The awareness of such decisive confrontation in our time, which we have not ignored and tried to place at the center of our current reality, means a certain kind of perception will be necessary. Our psychoanalytic ways of seeing, through committed work, will have to supersede the drive of illusions; all the security and comfort devised by civilization to protect itself may have to be suspended or given up altogether. The ideologies of others will have to be denied. Exposure will have to be accepted as a risk, as a kind of disarming. A distinction made in the Introduction will not, hopefully, continue unabated. One might want to add, from a previous note, Christopher Bollas' concept of "perceptive identification," most especially because it points to a generosity of spirit and for affirming that the object is loved "for itself not for oneself."[35] We are, one fears, a long way from being capable of authentic love at all – whether it be framed as agapic, divine, or as transferential in the best sense of the word and, to become conscious of ourselves, as Freud made us aware from the nature of the analytic relationship. We have no choice but to be aware of the machinations of love as exhibited, politically, in the present; when love and vengeance are unified, one has lost all its sympathies. Once Freud introduced us to the phenomenon of transference-love, however, the consequences extended well beyond the analytic situation. Transferences were ubiquitous; and as soon as they no longer were analyzable because experienced as, simply true, their adverse effects had an extremely wide range. "Love consists of new editions of old traits and that it repeats infantile reactions... ... It is precisely from this infantile determination that it receives its compulsive character, verging as it does on the pathological."[36] To become conscious of transference love, outside the clinical situation, would go a long way in at least raising some awareness of our true *mutual relations*. Before identification can take place in the form of authentic love instead of the strictness of a group bind, and its limiting identity, we are still far from being capable of perception – of ourselves and our psyche as it has so determined our re-ordered reality today. The responsibility of an analysand, which has been constant in the psycho-political essay up until now, can be given one more impetus. The forms of hate and aggression outlined thus far have been many and inter-related; nearing our end, there will be the need to both recapitulate what has been presented and, finally, continue to stress the importance of our psychoanalytic ideals as counter-measures. The modern-day distortions of love and hate make it incumbent on any analysis to respond by being exemplary.

Despite Freud's sobering analysis, which cannot be defined according to incomplete standards of the optimistic/pessimistic relation, we can bring up two themes which were expressed in such clear terms – together: love and happiness as two human constants. When so much has been written about the pessimistic or the tragic or all the other definitions of his analysis of the malaise of civilization, the commitment to the human, despite so many obstacles, has never been abandoned. On the contrary. Freud did not resign himself, nor did he submit to an ethos of *adaptation*, which is nothing more than the conformism and lack of originality he disapproved of as an attitude to reality. His expectations, for analysands and readers, were not slight. How did he come to this ending, on love and happiness, when so much of his analysis of discontent made the reality at hand virtually inescapable? Not unlike the different measures of illusions, the *unbehagen* of culture did not leave him (he did not leave us) bereft of the possibility of a meaningful and healthy life.

In "Jensen's 'Gradiva,'" Freud writes: "Every psycho-analytic treatment is an attempt at liberating repressed love."[37] One word makes quite a difference. The repression is *not* sexual and is not associated with our standard assumptions about the meaning of the concept, which may have become over-saturated. The idea of "repression," so foundational for psychoanalysis, can in this one instance be given one interpretation that has been neglected in favour of a complete acceptance of repression as a specific response to an erotic (that is not simply a sexual) impulse. In this case, and to further my argument, *love has been repressed* by the moralizing super-ego and transformed by the demands made by groups in liberal society. The severity of judgment, condemnation, and punishment, analyzed earlier as sadistic, has therefore substituted love with its more intense drive towards a far harsher feeling. All the attention to sexuality, so exaggerated since we have been unable to view our human desires without moderation, has made it almost unnoticed, barely perceived, that love was going to be belittled once it came under the scrutiny of one side of the super-ego equation. We can, again and since our beginning, bring together the casualties of the power of the super-ego and death drive: the loss of freedom, the reduction of human intelligence, and the corruption of love are the three symptoms of our age with the most devastating effects. Are we to consider the reality of *the repression of love* by the super-ego a psychical relation that, in our world, has caused such infinite misery and continues to divide us in terms of our feelings and our objects of love? Repression, as a defense, has turned into something far more sinister because ideological and motivated by hostility and hate. As for the demand for recognition, those who are most vocal are destined to receive no acknowledgment and no sympathy. On the contrary, one of the effects will surely be indifference. Acknowledgment will surely (and have to) be denied if it is not based on reciprocity.

Freud's emphasis of love in *Civilization and its Discontents* is offered as an important counter measure to the psychical reality of our time. Those who have noted Freud's love are willing to introduce the sentiment, if, at times, with some prudence. "Our enquiry," Brian Clack writes, "retreats from the grandiose question about love's ability to heal and focuses instead upon a more modest one: how effective is love as a palliative?"[38] The ability of love to heal is not at all a "grandiose question," nor is its association with happiness. As for the palliative, the reduction of pain is no small matter; however, is there the possibility that a continuing commitment to Freud's thinking can lead us from our beginning in an infantile and primitive regression and reach a level of mature development? A palliative is not enough; the measure is insufficient because fatalistic. An analysand may want to introduce the startling difference between mortality and termination – which is, ultimately, a beginning and a psychoanalytic movement beyond both the theological and the, strictly, medical. Can the work towards termination lead us beyond the compromise of the palliative and towards a longer-term condition of healthy love and happiness as two essential and universal aims of being human? More than a palliative, love can be rehabilitated; to do so, however, all the obsessions with a narrow-minded sexuality (as the way towards "liberation") will have to come to an end in its ideological development and as one of the most forceful expressions of a clamorous propaganda over the last half century.

The earlier analysis, and therefore deep skepticism, of the "love" of group psychology, the super-ego, and the death drive, first made the passion closer to hatred. Despite Freud's knowledge about "the dark truth of love," which he has been more than forthright about when looking at masochism and sadism, the hope in the continued viability of a true, actual, and real love did not dispirit him. One truth is conceded. "The primacy of hatred as preceding love also implies a revelation of hatred as the dark truth of love," Jens De Vleminck begins. Despite the knowledge, he adds: "The human possibility of love is presented by Freud as a victory over hatred."[39] Is it possible to free the sentiments of love from its repression by the super-ego and its debasement by the death drive and turn our hatred, so intensified as a consequence of our urge to critique, and to negate with all the parallels known to us, historically, and in ourselves, towards its healthy and free expression? Does Freud offer us a psychoanalytic idea of love? If he does, its beginning will by no means rely on the strict definition of traditional models and will, moreover, not avoid a difficult dialogue. In "Instincts and their Vicissitudes," Freud writes: "It cannot be denied that hating, too, originally characterized the relation of the ego to the alien external world with the stimuli it introduces" (14:136).

Freud's turn to love and its highest representative in the Biblical ideal of the *love of one's neighbor* introduces one of the most persistent problems of civilization as handed down to us from antiquity: to the ideal of "loving one's neighbor as oneself," which is first expressed, in writing, in Deuteronomy and repeated in the Judeo-Christian tradition, Freud responds not only with "bewilderment," but also what we may call a healthy skepticism or, strongly put, some incredulity. His sensibility might even be harsher. His neighbor is, potentially, no friend at all; he may have to be declared an enemy and due to circumstances, so extreme, that no other declaration seems possible. A statement, from Carl Schmitt, strikes us forcefully in the present. "Any religious, moral, economic, ethnic or other antagonism will turn into a political antagonism if it is strong enough to effectively group people by friend and enemy."[40] Freud has his own way of expressing a human concern. Referring to the lofty idea of a "neighbor," his patience is short and unaccommodating. "If he is a stranger to me and if he cannot attract me by any worth of his own or any significance that he may already have acquired for my emotional life, it will be hard for me to love him" (21:109). Foregoing any idealism and taking a hard look at our human relations, Freud is not going to appeal to anything like our modern infatuation with "the other," and with a response that today can include more than skepticism but actually a note on its ideological hypocrisy. Pretenses are to be renounced. A stranger may prove to be less than worthy of care, more so when society continues to portray itself according to ideals of "inclusivity" when all indications tend towards much less than a confirmation; the displays of solicitude, for the other, have been done at someone else's expense and, often, with undisguised hostility. Freud's disturbing (or matter-of-fact) transition from the impossibility of fulfilling the love of one's neighbor to our intense capacity for hate and aggression prepares us for the conclusion to this work on civilization. How love will be preserved, and then accentuated, is one of the more remarkable features of the work. The honest appraisal by Freud is, for some, unnerving; he has more in store and due to everything he has come to discuss over the whole of the decade. He certainly has no delusions about the nature of love or influenced by wishes and ideals and has no desire to impose an ancient morality on anyone in his age – or our own. Freud does not give in to desires when thinking is demanded, not if illusions are going to be renounced. However counterintuitive it might at first appear, *giving up* on our group-ideals may prove to be highly beneficial and healthy. A *civil* society may be much better than a *moral* one. The renunciation of our moral obsessions may prove to be more healthy than anyone can imagine. Is it even conceivable, in our day and age, to stress duty over rights?

Freud's analytic work on reaction formation made ideals a matter of deliberation more than unquestioned acceptance and support. Not only does he withdraw from the first requirement; he is more than willing to take a realistic look at our natural feelings. "Not only is this stranger in general unworthy of my love; I must honestly confess that he has more claim to my hostility and even my hatred" (21:110). When a *particular stranger* takes refuge behind the language of trauma and victimhood to condemn others (in the name of justice) the responses can be expected, even if many people will express their thinking and feelings behind closed doors, in private and with the safety of not being monitored. One gets the sense that, at the present, many individuals in liberal democracies are splitting themselves between the truth of their private lives and the rigid acquiescence of their public existence. Once the moral and the accusatory are intrinsic to each other, not much empathy will ensue; indeed, an antipathy is now growing and in proportion to the incessant advertisement in liberal democracies about this or that issue that requires immediate attention. The empathic or "perceptive" identification called for by Bollas is not going to be possible if a small minority of activists, all with their own special and very personal agenda, continues to determine *everyone's* reality. *Enemies*: the sentiment can be expressed, and to think with Freud when strangers (who have amassed in groups, with narcissistic attention to themselves and their causes) have alienated any sense of a possible empathy; or to be simply moderate, tolerance. To avoid making enemies might require what is becoming almost impossible: who, today, is capable to questioning their most deeply-held political beliefs and moderating them in order to reduce the extreme divisions between ideas and the people who hold them? A prior argument, from our beginnings, in the Introduction and after, can be repeated: the "transformation of love into hate," which has been one of the most serious of our theological-political symptoms, has reached such an intensity that the consciousness of a disposition is no longer recognized; and yet, when it is "reinforced by a regression of love to the sadistic preliminary stage; so that the hate acquires an erotic character and the continuity of a love-relation is ensured" (14:139), the analysis clarifies so much of our predicament. Negation and critique has turned into a sublimated erotic pleasure of abhorring civilization.

Freud has no hesitation in discussing the opposite feeling of love – hatred – and so immediately preparing the reader for an assessment that challenges our ideals. When we recollect his analysis of group psychology, the present work on civilization is a continuation of a perpetual psychoanalytic concern. By then adding the imperative of loving one's neighbor with the even more impossible commandment to "love one's enemies," Freud reaches one more transitional point in his argument overall when he again introduces the concept of ethics into his discussion. One wonders how often we have overlooked some of Freud's more provocative ideas. It is understandable, if not excusable, to miss some; there have been so many of them. "Obedience to high ethical demands entails damage to the aims of civilization" (21:111). Freud has (perfectly) diagnosed our present. The demands of moral society have damaged civilization and continue to do so with such fervent commitment that one does doubt whether the damage is not irreparable. The more serious awareness has been in the intention of the damage. If Freud is saying what seems to be the case, is he (to be clear, for us) making the argument that our morality has been detrimental to civilization – and, more personally, to each one of us as individuals who are not necessarily members of a group and have no need or desire to be. The self-assertion by an individual is a prerequisite today, and with new personal imperatives: to *strengthen the ego* sufficiently to resist and be impervious to, and independent of, the moral manipulations of our age. Can we make a proposal about the self-possession of a healthy ego as one of the most stable of responses to the group psychology of today's morality? Is this Freud's argument, which here gets as close as it ever has to Nietzsche's extensive presentation, for one, of the genealogy of morals and which he complemented with his "Postscript"? Pursuing this one line of thought can be, for the many, unsettling. One has often heard a response that sounded like trepidation. To expose the origin of morals – as Freud has done since *Totem and Taboo* – makes many uncomfortable because of the moral implications for politics and, principally, for the reality of liberal democracies. After all, ethics and morality is supposed to be representative of our highest values. Is there a cause, for us, to wonder if at the beginning of the third millennia we are right to analyze how our moral drive at the moment may not be contributing to an unprecedented kind of social suffering and the degradation of the meaning of liberalism? The question has been already answered; that premise was foundational. Is idealism still possible when confronting enemies who have been given near-total authority and legitimacy? "The only thing than makes hope, repose, calm, and happiness possible is managing our relationships with others in a non-conflictual way."[41] The absence of conflict (in the self, with others) is one of the conditions of *calm* and *happiness*; these are *classical* ideals expressed, for example, by Epicurus. How can such a state be attained when so much of reality presents the most severe obstacles? The question is more in the nature of a summing up and following Freud towards the achievement of his ideals (at least, for individuals) and because he can so matter-of-factly reject impossible loves, of neighbor and, more so, of the enemy who has been given a stand-out definition by Alain Badiou. How appropriate that the statement comes in a dialogue called *In Praise of Love*.

> The issue is: do enemies exist? I mean by that, real enemies. A real enemy is not someone you are resigned to see take power periodically because lots of people voted for him. That is a person you are annoyed to see as head of State because you would have preferred his adversary . . . An enemy is something else: an individual you won't tolerate taking decisions on anything that impacts on yourself. So do real enemies exist or not? That should be our starting-point.[42]

Freud would not disagree. His assessment of morality in the universal aspiration of love (for everyone, without exception), and the even more demanding duty to love one's "enemies" is countered by Freud's discussion of aggression. "Men are not gentle creatures who want to be loved, and who at the most can defend themselves if they are attacked; they are, on the contrary, creatures among whose intellectual endowments is to be reckoned a powerful share of aggressiveness" (21:111). We can now point out how one element in the argument has been overlooked, and for reasons that tell us, as is usually the case, something far from complimentary about ourselves. Aggression, Freud tells us, is inseparable from our "intellectual endowments." In other words, and again recalling the argument from *Group Psychology*, the libido and loss of intelligence of the group is, in part, a consequence of the illusion of s *certain kind* of love. If he has been understood as intended, then it would seem as if our *ideas*, about the values we hold most highly, cannot be separated from our aggression. That one argument has been consistent; he has not wavered from identifying the most dangerous characteristics of the super-ego nor its most destructive compulsions when aligned with the death drive. "As a rule this cruel aggressiveness waits for some provocation or puts itself at the service of some other purpose, whose goal might also have been reached by milder measures." The aggressiveness is "cruel," a word that has been used several times before; which now brings us closer to the beginning of the argument, from the Introduction, and the path toward the conclusion given to us by Freud. The "inclination to aggression" has been accepted as a given. The historical examples, distant and all-too near, are enough for us not be in any way deluded about the capacities of the human animal to use his aggression on others and with a certain amount of satisfaction. Sadistic pleasure has its attractions and fulfillments. Can liberals give up the pleasure of moral sadism?

One of Freud's arguments is not new: the "mutual hostility" between human beings has been a constant threat to the stability of civilization. But if our sense has been right from the beginning, we are edging closer to a much more disturbing argument and one sustained by Freud himself in *Civilization and its Discontents*. How he responds to a fundamental nature of the human will be decisive, for him, for psychoanalysis, and potentially for us today. Intimately aware of the threat of this aggressiveness and hate, civilization has responded with all kinds of measures intended to ensure its safety. Is the engineered control of nature and the equally ordered modification of the human exactly part of the same human process? There was no need to live according to religious principles since human beings in liberal societies were rational enough to guide themselves; so it was assumed. The ideals of a secular society have been affirmed as an alternative to tradition. Have they been successful? Or are we increasingly noticing the consequences of a drive founded, in many ways, on something far worse than what Freud called a religious illusion, a more infantile and primitive one and enforcing its power on others with impunity? "The time comes when each one of us has to give up as illusions the expectations which, in his youth, he pinned upon his fellow-men, and when he may learn how much difficulty and pain has been added to his life by their ill-will." We can now even add something more disturbing: it has been, precisely, all their *good will* that is beginning to lead us more and more towards misery. Are "the good" making everyone, or at least many, unhappy? The use of the word *illusion* again is not accidental. Freud has returned us to a primordial human problem – the aspiration of our ideals over and above the reality of our situation. What happens, then, when the illusions are recognized but the psychical desire is so intense, so relentless, so obsessive, that it will not admit to the reality of the human condition but instead renews its effort and, despite any cost, will pursue the ideal to its own end? Have we reached such a situation today among the moralists of our liberal democracies who will go to any end to achieve their goals, no matter if the harm to our young is especially grievous? It is no wonder that the former discussion of illusion turns, now, towards politics and the example Freud is historically familiar with – formidably accurate and without the added insights of our 21st-century position. That he concentrates his analysis on the communists of the newly created Soviet Union has even more meaning for us today – that is, more meaning for our understanding of Freud's psychological perspective of movements that believe themselves to be guided by politics when they cannot give themselves such easy privilege. We should be doubly aware of the transitions in *Civilization* and the subtlety of Freud's presentation. The illusion of religion was one fact. The political is another. When they are brought together, Freud alerts us to a new phenomenon – that is, the theological-political morality of politics when it has become too idealistic. We are guided by one question: if Freud shared no illusion about ancient concepts on love, for the other, for the neighbor, because it was directed at an abstract object (who might, of course, also hate us, for their own reasons) is there nevertheless a fundamental principle of love, not separated from the *strength* of the ego, that can be both expressed and shared? Or, stated differently: does Freud offer us a concept of love that can be made real and actual and true? The arguments on love and hate have not been recognized for their ingenuity and most especially when – following up from the transition earlier traced in the future of an illusion from religion to politics – Freud turns to the unique example of the Soviet political experiment that, in principle and as their doctrines showed, was profoundly anti-religious and materialistic. His comments on the Soviets, when brought together, give us a stunning portrait.

The premise of the communist system is evaluated and set aside without difficulty for Freud because he has no illusions about one of its presuppositions, for one, the equitable distribution of property and wealth – that is, economic justice, a 19th century ideal (above all, Marxist) that has lost much of its relevance today. Class is no longer the category it used to be; other, more disparate groups, more self-righteous and much better organized than workers, have taken its place. Freud adds that he himself cannot determine whether the abolition of private property, for example, would change conditions for the better. "But I am able to recognize," he adds, "that the psychological premiss on which the system is based are an untenable illusion" (21:113). For the second time, he has used the word "illusion." The reminder is conscious, and specifically for his readers who can trace the origin to the word and where it was most prevalent, as a theme and as a title. The theological-political relation continues to be established. The illusion, for the Soviet communists, was a political one; the ideology of the collective served one of its purposes, as did one principal foundation in the economy of the state. We cannot avoid recalling its original analysis, in relation to religion, and how it has now returned in another, similar context: the premise of a "revolution," when its original meaning of a return and a repetition is understood to be an allegory of the celestial, a classical aspiration – "on earth as it is in heaven" – achieves one of its most noticeable illusions. The nature of our political ideals are no less decisive for both revealing our illusions and, more seriously, the ends we are prepared to follow for their attainment. No equitable distribution of private property and wealth will secure a more stable social system since the nature of human aggression will remain unchanged and still need to be expressed in one way or another. The infantile and primitive superego remains one irreducible problem. As for aggression, "it already shows itself in the nursery," Freud adds, in essence making aggressivity constitutional and characteristic of the human animal well before any socialization can take place. The infantile and the primitive super-ego can certainly be appeased and altered by healthier impulses; but not without first admitting how arduous the confrontation will actually be, in ourselves and in relation to others.

Just as Freud's analysis of the illusion of religion and how it could not be contained led him to make other, far-reaching statements on the nature of our social life, so in this case he continues the analysis and presses the issue further. The momentum of his argument can be appreciated if one reconstructs how the transition from love to hate happened in order to unify their relation. We have, as a species, and in our societies, adopted all kinds of ideas and methods to contain our aggression and violence. "It is clearly not easy for men to give up the satisfaction of this inclination to aggression" (21:114). Is this simply a statement of fact and a kind of resignation? More seriously for us, is morality and aggression inseparable today? "How the modern individual goes about destroying the new – and often in the very ways in which he tried to make it new – became Freud's abiding preoccupation: The past, he sometimes seems to be saying, is what we use now to destroy the future."[43] Individuals, groups, liberal society: the drive to create the new is leading to the destruction of any viable future and, in many cases, by reviving a completely mythological (that is, false) past.

The transition in *Civilization and its Discontents* from the ideal of the love of neighbor to a constitutive aggression begins the summing-up of the entire range of this thought in the 1920s and he does so by returning, once again, to the thesis of group psychology; the connections are explicit. "The advantage which a comparatively small cultural group offers of allowing this instinct [of aggression] an outlet in the form of hostility against intruders is not to be despised." The phrase itself is intriguing. We should not hate the *recognition* of an aspect of reality, even when it means accepting some form of hostility; acknowledging it will give us an advantage since we will not be disposed to easily being fooled by our illusions. Can *some* intolerance be acceptable and, perhaps, even healthy? The problem remains one of exclusivity and force. A "small cultural group" is best able to unify its identity – that is, first of all, the bind for itself – in order to better distinguish others who are not like them and therefore justify, politically, its hostility, its aggression, its hate. A healthy conscience is all the more necessary when the extremes have been noticed, enemies mentioned if not yet *declared.* When the political ideas of the group are turned into systematic propaganda, however, we have the conditions for a wider dissemination of its goals and the beginning of an excess of principles and methods, when *their decisions* becoming binding and intrusive. "It is always possible to bind together a considerable number of people in love, so long as there are other people left over to receive the manifestation of its aggressiveness." The insights from *Group Psychology* are carried forward and with an awareness that should be, for political idealism, devastating. If Freud was thought to be the secularist who devoted himself to exposing the illusions of religion, at the end of his examination of our social and political life at the end of the 1920s, he has arrived at a singular conclusion on the nature of civilization. It is surely not naïve. "When, with unsparing criticism, we try to uncover the roots of its imperfection, we are undoubtedly exercising a proper right and are not showing ourselves enemies of civilization." Freud finds no fault with the justifiable "criticism" of civilization insofar as it makes human life difficult and imposes restrictions that, for many, is a burden to endure. To our resistance he has no problems. His conclusions, however, leave no room for ideals when they lose a sense of themselves, their purposes, and how they will be achieved. "There are difficulties attaching to the nature of civilization which will not yield to any attempt at reform." Freud does not stop with this sober reminder. Imperfection is not going to be remedied. But there is a far worse problem to be faced. Why does he suddenly introduce the singular idea of "the psychological poverty of groups" – and we should keep in mind our first discussion of *ego impoverishment* – and re-emphasize, at the end of Chapter V, the danger posed by groups and their identification with each other? We are seemingly back at the original thesis, the one on the loss of freedom and the lessening of intelligence. The final addition, on love, completes his assessment of the problems of civilization as they were first presented in *Group Psychology*. He therefor offers a number of psychoanalytic principles which he has been organizing for the better part of a decade.

By Chapter VI, the problems he had outlined in group psychology and the illusion of ideals leads him, once again, to reminding us of the danger of the super-ego once it has exceeded its normal (and necessary) function and pathologically submitted to the impulse of aggression, sadism, and the death drive. We have long been accustomed to the acknowledgment of the instinctual desire around the erotic; once the sexually charged has been redirected towards a different set of desires, compelling as only idealist desires can be (to change the world, for the better) then a whole new set of problem are introduced into our social and political life. The moralistic developments of our time are giving us a sense of the intensity of political desires. One interjection has been suggestive, but not for the reasons intended by Douglas Hollan when he writes: "Life in communities is always challenging, if not hellish at times, and that at least some of this is related to the renunciation of desire."[44] We are more than aware of the ways civilization prohibits. However, if we spend some time thinking about the nature of the super-ego as a psychopolitical phenomenon, we are likely to see how the commands of the day are not only prohibitive ("thou shall not") but equally, and perhaps therefore more forcefully, with more compulsion, as matter of what will be *desired for all.* We are left with, for lack of a better word at the moment, an impasse: the drive of the culture in liberal democracies has been directed at the ideals of equality, justice, human rights – to highlight the trinity of the time. To achieve the three requires everyone to *desire the same ends*. But this is where the problems become something much more serious and unsolvable. The political masters of the moment insist on everyone having the same desire – which is unreasonable and one where many will, understandably, *refuse*. Desire cannot be dictated. To be commanded to desire the good, as presently conceived – as if our historical moment gave us the justification and legitimacy to judge the whole of the past – nullifies the judgment of the individual and demands nothing less than what has always been demanded from the individual: self-sacrifice. Today, the renunciation of desire has been replaced by the categorical imperative of everyone sharing the same desire and so forming an absolute consensus – totoal conformism and a consensus of the absolute. Many of us simply do not identify with the other or, more seriously, with the dead victims of history, in part because their present-day ancestors can draw on centuries of history to justify the demands, which are going to be infinite and where reconciliation will be nothing more than a slogan. There are so many dead that one would have to be highly selective about who, precisely, was going to be mourned. Everyone? No one has that much mourning or melancholia – unless one takes on the entire burdens of the world and interprets history according to only one perspective and simply turns away, selectively, from the making of civilization over the recorded history most known to us over the last three millennia.

Freud's return to the themes of aggression, sadism, and the death drive is necessary more so today when the force of our moral ideals has led to the two words he has stressed as major problems: coercion and domination. When the illusions of politics and the categorical imperative of the moral are combined into one total project for social life, we have the making of a restrictive situation that a justified authoritarianism will promote in the service of the good for all. What remains perplexing is how the highest ideals can be inverted and perverted into their opposite and to become, as Nietzsche analyzed prior to Freud, nihilistic. We can no longer be so self-assured about a growing menace and what François Villa has called the "disaster of totalitarianism." While many have been reluctant to take seriously the implications of a death-drive both in the individual and in society, others have made persuasive arguments. In the context of Freud's whole range of analysis, our psychical difficulties are more than ever necessary to confront. The death drive should be foremost in our minds. Villa, for example, believes we should not avoid "becoming *familiar* with the drive, admitting to its existence and full accepting its power in our daily lives."[45] If for no other reason than to be prudent and not exhaust any possibilities, the death drive should be kept in mind as we attempt to analyze social life today. Richard Rorty writes: "I think psychoanalysis needs to be used rather than transcended. We need to get closer to it than to distance it, to live with its terminology."[46] And no concept, for us, has been more immediate than the death drive and, as Rorty added, how psychoanalysis has made morality not one human theme among others but the one with, potentially, the most devastating effects as history has shown time and again.

As Freud continues with his exposition, he tells the reader that his current thought is "a matter of bringing into sharper focus *a turn of thought arrived at long ago* and of following out its consequences" (21:117). My italics serve to show how Freud presents an autobiographical statement for us. His own direction has not always been followed, to the spirit or the letter. His theory of aggression, sadism, and the death drive, once they have moved from the individual to the group and to society, begin to exhibit peculiar but identifiable characteristics. How they are unified into a psychopolitics is one of Freud's greatest achievements as a thinker. To have analyzed innumerable symptoms is one that requires more attention today than a century ago. How can we better notice how the most forceful drive "is diverted towards the external world and comes to light as an instinct of aggressiveness and destructiveness?" (21:119). Each is different: the aggressive impulse comes from the desire of the super-ego and its intent to impose its force on others through guilt and shame. This is the moralistic trend. The destructive part, however, is equally operative and is not content with the possible transformation of reality in terms of its moral improvement. The drive is not at all unified but at odds with itself; while the moralistic aggression attempts to coerce and dominate others, in part through the imposition of guilt, an equally forceful drive directs itself to the complete dissolution of reality – hence, the noticeable aversion to Western civilization increasingly exhibited by our political groups, the ones who have appointed themselves as the sole and legitimate judges of culture. Freud was well aware that "the assumption of the existence of an instinct of death or destruction has met with resistance even in analytic circles" (21:119). Previous references were sufficient to give us a sense of the resistance. To deny its reality would considerably lessen our ability to understand a contemporary phenomenon and attempt to think about possible ways to remedy its power. For our part, the death drive is accepted without hesitation since it has shown itself to be the only psychoanalytic idea complex enough to explain the tenet of our psychopolitical times. "I can no longer understand how we can have overlooked the ubiquity of non-erotic aggressivity and destructiveness and can have failed to give it its due place in our interpretation of life" (21:120). One addition remains as the conclusion to *Civilization and its Discontents* and the project of the 1920s. How does Freud, then, leave with us with something more promising than a constitutive aggression and hatred and, as he wrote to his friend Rolland, commit himself to the sense of himself being an apostle of love? The feeling of the oceanic as a profoundly human characteristic – and one inseparable, also, from an awareness of being terrestrial beings and embodied – can be intensified in order to accentuate the feelings of love, freedom, creativity, and intelligence. Freud's argument has been unsparing and free of any idealistic delusions. Is he still capable of leading us, after the complete diagnostic, toward a remedy? "Everything is derived from the vicissitudes of love," Michael Eigen writes. "This is the informal and final Freud, the man who, at the end, hooked up with his beginnings."[47] And so we too find ourselves at the beginning, in *Group Psychology*, with the "vicissitudes of love," but with a considerable difference: if the theological-political argument has been successful in showing how the morality of the super-ego and the double destruction of the death drive has been developing towards a nihilistic obsession, we are nevertheless left with an imperative and to once again re-affirm the ideals of the human and of psychoanalysis, the ones we have not for a moment forsaken. To the ideals of psychoanalysis, we can add one culminating value. Drawing upon the open-ended history of our classical past and at the origins of Western civilization can gives us (as it did Freud) one possible direction for our thinking no less than for the possibility of the attainment of the human happiness envisioned by psychoanalysis.

(p) Elusive but Not Impossible Happiness

That Freud begins the last chapter of *Civilization and its Discontents* with the problem of guilt should be an indication of how the many ideas of the 1920s led him to isolate one particular experience and the effects it can have on the psychopathology of everyday life. Our original thesis, on the transference between the murder of the primal father and the killing of God in our attempt to become modern is re-emphasized – with one crucial difference. For Freud, the killing of the primal father was decisive and led to the transformation of archaic societies in terms of installing a moral imperative, strict (defensive) laws, and the burden of a guilt with overwhelming power; the consequences of an act led to a new conception of a group, as a "band of brothers," that altered their self-consciousness and the limits of their future. One of our final questions can be raised, again in a different way, when a traditional and healthy conscience is overcome by theological-political guilt (for the murder of God) and for the historically verifiable, and yet still delusional, death of a new ego-ideal of civilization. "When is guilt normal and what does it become abnormal?"[48] The recovery of a moderate conscience was, for Freud, one of the many necessary changes for the neuroses of a society to be minimized. One of our problems has been: *how* did guilt become abnormal and doing so when moderate conscience became excessive and pathological, with extensive consequences for our ability to love and think? The answers, throughout the essay, have been many and overlapping. In order to reflect on the death drive of liberal societies against its own civilization, we mentioned, several times, one origin and symptom. Guilt has been imposed. The social dissemination of guilt has led to the death drive's antipathy towards love because of its emphasis on an impossible because belated justice and its true character not as redemption but as sadistic vengeance against itself. The conclusion to one writing in particular, *On Narcissism*, would be expanded.

> Originally this sense of guilt was a fear of punishment by the parents, or, more correctly, the fear of losing their love; later the parents are replaced by an indefinite number of fellow-men. The frequent causation of paranoia by an injury to the ego, by a frustration of satisfaction within the sphere of the ego ideal, is thus made more intelligible.
>
> (14:102)

Since, in the view presented in *Group Psychology*, both the fear of punishment and the loss of love from the parents has been overcome and substituted with a more powerful ego-ideal (all who have been killed in the historical development of civilization), Freud's concern with the experience of paranoia became more explicit and no longer confined to the *extreme* cases of psychosis; schizoid and paranoid symptoms became normalized by the theological-political obsessions of groups and their one-dimensional interpretation of history. The defense against the extreme power of the introjected ego-ideal, and the injuries of masochism, could only be managed by a relentless projection against the reality of civilization and, more immediately, the human body. The theological-political production of guilt has led to a number of other phenomena. There was one reason why Freud continued to hold fast to one psychoanalytic foundation. Can it be acknowledged as an unconscious dynamic and inseparable from the death drive?

The discontents of civilization, for some, are reaching a peculiar intensity in 21st-century life. One statement can summarize our analysis of the malice of the super-ego and the destructive rage of the death drive. In a chapter that can now be read in a different way, with a heightened perception than in 1989, Janine Chassequet-Smirgel gives us a profound understanding of "Perversion and the Universal Law" when she presents several impressions that should strike us with distinct poignancy.

> Should we not associate historical ruptures, which give us an inkling of the advent of a new world, with the confusion between sexes and generations, peculiar to perversion, as if the hope for a new social and political reality went hand in hand with an attempt at destroying sexual reality and truth?[49]

The destruction of sexual reality and truth has been intimated throughout my psychopolitical essay and, first, by indicating how the Oedipus complex has never been more opposed, in principle, and in fact, and with methods that are attempting to overcome a structure of history, both culturally and biologically. She adds: "Perversions are intimately connected with actual sadism, as the need to abolish the (genital) universe of difference and thus subvert reality *means that perversion is inevitably sadistic*" (183). Sadism, perversion, and the abolition of sexual difference: this is one obsession of the death drive in liberal democracies today against Western civilization. Are we going to continue to accept the moral coercion of our social world or are we, with Freud, going to respond with the perennial ideals of the human and once again re-affirm our conviction in (and our struggle for the realization of) freedom, intelligence, creativity, love, and, ultimately, the attempt to remain psychologically healthy to the best of our ability? Doing so requires, first of all, the recognition of a certain desire and its true psychological character. The truth is not new. Christopher Bollas (in 1987, when a certain kind of drive was already evident) wrote:

> I think that extremist political movements indicate a collective certainty that their revolutionary ideology will effect a total environmental transformation that will deliver everyone from the gamut of basic faults: personal, familial, economic, social and moral. Again, it is not the revolutionary's desire for change, or the extremist's longing for change, but his certainty that the object (this this case the revolutionary ideology) will bring about change that is striking to the observer.[50]

As it happens, and not incidentally, one of the thinkers who first introduced us to the return of the religious has also made significant interjections into other, related problems; because when Sloterdijk, confirming Freud's thesis in the "Postscript" and without the niceties of half-measures, writes that "what has hitherto been called morality is the universalism of vengeance,"[51] the diagnosis is one more confirmation on top of all the other ones presented thus far. We cannot spare ourselves the truth of our serious condition, however much it will wound the pride of others, if the predicament of our times is to be faced with a measure of calm and yet with resolve. Introspection is called for much more than reaction and acting-out and the pushy insistence of propaganda.

Our earlier examination of Freud's concept of the super-ego and the complications of the psyche's characteristics are, in 1929, refined and given further support. If guilt was understood to be the internalization of the individual's aggression, our theological-political emphasis cannot remain with this first psychical effect. The individual reacts to the internalized aggression by defending itself and finds it necessary to project the guilt externally. The burden of one individual (and the group he identifies with) must be shared. The political sphere is an instance of the sadistic individual to project the aggression outwards but to rationalize as a moral imperative, turning one's internal guilt towards the many faults of others and, more comprehensively, to the idealistic inadequacy of a world that can only be repaired by moral judgment and condemnation. The easily passed-over statement – "the field of ethics, which is so full of problems" (21:126) – is one indication of Freud's ability to see through the appearances of moral life and to recognize its psychical origin and consequences. Its duplicities can no longer be covered up; they are overbearing. The return to the problems of "the severity of the super-ego," which has been preoccupying him for the better part of decade, receives its full confirmation as well as its re-affirmation insofar as it expresses the drive of Thanatos. The repetition of previous illustrations serve as a summing up and, equally as important, for the possibility of a remedy. The diagnosis will not be left without a possible change *in ourselves*. The theme of happiness is one of Freud's final aims. One essential thinker, who complemented Freud in my Introduction, can return here near the conclusion to make an *affirmation*. The diagnosis has been made; the commitment to a remedy is offered. Equating Bollas' Freudian moment with Badiou's *event* gives us one authentic answer to "'how to change the world'? ... ... in being faithful to an event, in creating an equivalence between freedom and discipline, in inventing a new form of happiness which is a victory over the dictatorship of satisfaction and the power of the death drive."[52] The sensibility of one philosopher gives us confidence to imagine a relationship between two kinds of thinking (and feeling) and never more important in their agreement in the hope for happiness.

The politically neurotic individual undergoes several inter-related experiences as an attempt to deal with internal conflicts. Faced with the threat of the loss of love, despite the pretensions of conscience, and with the always looming possibility of being punished, the individual makes the desperate attempt to preserve itself (its psychical wholeness, always so vulnerable) by giving itself the privilege of external authority and so acting out its judgments on others. While there is no time to pursue the matter of a current phenomenon – the widespread experience of anxiety, especially among the young, which is complicated by infatuations with technology and delusional self-images – one can notice how the heightening of moralistic demands, on the one hand, and the laissez-faire permissiveness as it relates to a fantasy-fulfillment, on the other, accounts for one foundational problem in our current situation. No wonder the ego has been made so forlorn; caught between completely antithetical drives, the ego feels overwhelmingly pressured from two sides. The combination can now be more fully recognized for its fatal incommensurability. The moralist aggression of the super-ego and the permissiveness of libidinal fantasies cannot both be sustained, not without a permanent and injurious effect on the psychical life of the individual who, nonetheless (unable to recognize his specific condition) continues with one compulsive solution. Freud's reference to infantile regression, as in *Group Psychology*, is further developed when he now notes how the "child's revengeful aggressiveness" (21:130), is turned towards the external world. We are no longer in a situation where it would be possible to respond with the highest of ideals. Freud rejected showing love to an enemy. The enemy cannot be trusted to come halfway for the benefit of all. The nature of the primitive infant, who has not been able to develop according to healthy ends, is mired in a fixation and an obsession that is understood, cognitively, from the standpoint of the present, but in fact has antecedent causes that have been forgotten and repressed. To insist, as Freud does, on the understanding of repression as much more complex than its relation to sexuality, allows us to appreciate how the political neurotic acts out. Have we believed in the delusion of a liberated sexuality only to find ourselves bereft of love, except in the forms prescribed by a destitute present?

The modern individual has reached a level of conflict previously suppressed by the acceptance of the *reality principle* in the past – that is, in the entire history of civilization and how it has been created. The objective facts of history are, in our present, no longer a relevant concern. The matter has reached such a state of emotion due to the intensity of the ideals and the desperate desire to alter the world, and its memory as a whole, for the sake of the good. So when Freud arrives at the last chapter and the attempt "to represent the sense of guilt as the most important problem in the development of civilization and to show that the price we pay for our advance in civilization is a loss of happiness through the heightening of the sense of guilt" (21:134), we will have to now wonder if the recent, half-century drive towards the moral rectification of the world is not, in fact, responsible for creating the conditions of a chronic misery that nothing will be able to alleviate unless we offer a few remedies. Freud t presents us with a choice that today is of paramount importance. He has stated our predicament in the most direct way possible: the sense of *guilt* has made us *unhappy* because, for one, we are no longer able to love, cannot think freely, or exercise our intelligence for the purpose of a traditional ideal, that of self-cultivation. The excessive guilt of our liberal society has impoverished us and our genuine ability to love – or to be free to make personal decisions that are not mandated by social consensus. Indeed, what the pathologies of the theological-political project have not been able to realize is how their ideologies have been responsible for more than unhappiness; they have created the conditions for a malaise that is no longer even recognized as such since it has become a matter of the *status quo*.

Freud's analysis should make us pause: guilt has been an irreplaceable need in the development of civilization. Our problem, today, amounts to this: how has the promotion of guilt, and the various symptoms of masochism and sadism against Western civilization, resulted in an almost unlimited self-criticism and, as a consequence, left society fixated and obsessed with one total view of civilization. For anyone who has forcefully instituted moral guilt, the responses at this point have to be sharper and with a vigorous rebuttal. The friend-enemy divide may have to be adopted. Guilt has become a tyrannical device; shame has been added as one more attack on Western civilization. Exposing it is now to be accepted as a task and a confrontation. In *The Tyranny of Guilt*, Pascal Bruckner writes: "The critical spirit rises up against itself and consumes its form. But instead of coming out of the process greater and purified, it devours itself in a kind of self-cannibalism and takes a morose pleasure in annihilating itself."[53] The cannibal, unfortunately, has the tendency to "eat" others, consume them to the point of subsuming them into the self as a kind of burial. Klein's observations on the primitive psyche of the infant are, in this case, made explicitly political. The individuals have been, thus far, few who have had the courage to confront the "truth" as it has been disseminated for now the better part of a half-century. Our own decade makes Freud our contemporary and, as he's always done (along with the few like Nietzsche) given us enough insight to prepare for a possible future. "Freud interprets the alliance of morality and destructiveness, the proverbial cruelty of the super-ego, as an alliance of culture and death. His unveiling of the constitutive unhappiness of culture is at the same time a warning."[54] The problem of happiness becomes more prevalent at this time, and indeed as a "warning" to the dangers he has consistently presented.

Leading ourselves to one conclusion, and a proposal, it will be a matter of not minimizing Freud's concern with human happiness and its possible (if partial) attainment, which will only be achievable if we individually confront the power of the super-ego and of restoring moral balance within the psyche, that is, preserving the importance of conscience while lessening the cruel effects of aggression and destructiveness. The effects of our contemporary super-ego can no longer be accepted or tolerated and so must be confronted for its reality and its detrimental consequences. The individual within the clinical situation is not like the political neurotic who remains convinced by the most fatal of illusions that the transformation of external reality, for the good, the better, the perfect, will result in the amelioration of psychological health. *That one* illusion has caused the world much more than its share of misery. The realization of any such social and political change, for all its incremental improvements continues to be offset by the more serious expressions of aggression, so much so that sadism, as "a synonym for severe punitive aggression,"[55] is today more than evident as one of the overwhelming symptoms of our age. We can only postpone the confrontation with the death drive for so long. If guilt was a fundamental problem in civilization, its most severe consequence will be once again unavoidable. "Freud's writings on 'civilisation', 'war', etc., remain attempts to think through the contributions that psychoanalysis could make to the development of social and political communities."[56] While there has been no lack of attention to "communities," one has to wonder about their makeup; because if we set out from our beginnings and the problems of group psychology, it may perhaps be prudent to begin first with attention to the individual. Friendship is still one way for individuals to share in the commonality of experience. We can, with hesitation, agree. "We believe he [Freud] could have made more of the fact that friendship is an example of the ideal community to which we humans aspire but which generally remains elusive and unrealized."[57] But friendship, while it does not exclude community, may perhaps be best understood in relation to individual relationships and, often, one-to-one. Friendship, as exclusive, avoids the diffuse collection of individuals in a group as well as the sense of belonging to society as a whole. We may very well have to begin there, with two, and make the attempt to encompass more. While friendship, as the philosophical Greeks realized, was the highest and unmatched good, we are going to be put in a position where *enemies* (who, while preaching tolerance and "inclusivity," are dominated themselves by the psychopolitics of hatred) are going to have to be taken into consideration as we remain committed to our principal psychoanalytic ideals. One statement, in another "Postscript" (to the question of lay analysis), is perhaps unmatched in the whole of his writings for so clearly rejecting the illusions of theological-political. "We who are analysts set before us as our aim the most complete and profoundest possible analysis of whoever may be our patient. *We do not seek to bring him relief by receiving him into the catholic, protestant or socialist community*" (20:256, my emphasis).

Parenthetically, the majority of writers who have been interested in happiness never fail to mention a quote that has been interpreted far too axiomatically instead of being incidental.[58] Freud does mention the task of turning "neurotic misery into everyday unhappiness," yet the quote's meaning can be lost on us if we interpret Freud too narrowly and fail to acknowledge many other arguments – for example, the necessity of understanding our important relation to the reality principle and to avoid, despite its allure, the often deceptive promise of the pleasure principle. "Everyday unhappiness," compared to chronic misery, would in fact feel like a significant ease in *suffering* and, therefore, much more desirable than the phrase seems to convey. An admission is important. "We psychoanalysts are a little wary of happiness: deeply influenced by the pessimistic world-view of the discipline's founder, Sigmund Freud, we approach moments of joy with trepidation."[59] Leaving aside the strongly worded "trepidation," an analysand and reader do not see the pessimism but, rather, all the times Freud mentions happiness in *Civilization and its Discontents* and how, throughout his work, from first to last, he does not concern himself with any fleeting moments of happiness but its attainment as an attitude of life and as a condition of being.

When Freud writes that anxiety and the sense of guilt are, ultimately, "*fear of the super-ego*" (21:135), one of our main preoccupations can again be stated. How can this fear be lessened? How can the intimidation, first, be minimized? Ferenczi believed that only by ridding oneself of the super-ego entirely could a cure be achieved. The elimination of the super-ego is, in my estimate, unnecessary and, actually, undesirable. One other question can also be suspended, in part because of its rhetoric. How does one go about "subverting the superego"?[60] Preferably, and as Freud believed, it is a matter of providing support to the morally overwhelmed individual so that the hatred of the super-ego can be returned to its proper function of a moderate conscience and thus allow for other sentiments to be felt and expressed by a healthy (and a strong) ego. My earlier thoughts on repression can be given one more emphasis. Today repression has been about controlling forms of love so as to place hatred and resentment at the forefront of our social sensibilities. This is when our moral narcissism and a "strong egoism" is, also, one of the differences Freud told to become aware of *for therapeutic reasons.* In *On Narcissism* he writes: "A strong egoism is a protection against falling ill, but in the last resort we must begin to love in order not to fall ill, and we are bound to fall ill if, in consequence of frustration, we are unable to love" (SE 14:84). Is the attainment of psychological health only possible when a strong egoism and love are consciously related for the ends of happiness? Is a strong ego (that is, a strong and uncompromising individuality against the high-minded demand of groups) one of the sure ways to overcome the impoverishment of our times?

We can add to the previous arguments by re-emphasizing how our modern political situation, so burdened with the moral imperatives made by those who are so forcefully attempting to create a good, a better, a perfect world, has been driven by many intersecting debilitating emotions and psychological characteristics. "The sense of guilt, the harshness of the super-ego, is thus the same thing as the severity of the conscience" (21:137). A distinction can once again be made, and as psychoanalysts (and a writer) like Donald Carveth have stressed: conscience does not necessarily have to be *severe*. Our psychological challenge has been to recognize the importance of conscience in social life (to prevent, for one, pathological acts) and to trace when it increases to the level where it becomes sadistic. The force and power of our politically produced guilt has been projected into the world, unto others, as the reaction of the guilt of the entire history of the West. History has thereby been *exploited* to produce a crushing guilt on the present and to rationalize, to make necessary, all the resulting initiatives about justice and equality and rights.

The internalization of aggression and its product as the sense of guilt has not remained within the individual's psyche; it has been projected outwards in an ever-greater hostility and punitive aggression intended to *transform the past* and to phantasmatically revive all the dead of history. The present has been made to suffer because of the judgments projected back into the past, to the whole of history and Western civilization, and with an infinite retribution that will never be satisfied. The aggression and punitive superego led Freud to once more take up a discussion of one of his most controversial concepts. The death drive, as we saw, has not been widely accepted and continues to be debated. In the present context, it has been central to the argument as a whole. Pleasure and happiness will not be attained by any political initiatives, and certainly not ones that use the power of the super-ego to force others to submit to ever more exacting standards of thought and behavior – to the point of domesticated uniformity. The two are, in Freud's account, incommensurable. Individual happiness and the development of society will sometimes intersect but, for the most part, be independently of each other. It would of course be tragic if the individual's happiness, or sense of being, was wholly dependent on the developments of society, which is one reason some individuals (artists, for one) often choose the path of withdrawal and isolation. The encroachment on artistic autonomy is but one more symptom of our age; art has been made to submit to political propaganda. "The precepts of the prevailing super-ego" (21:142) will be less invasive the more an individual has become independent, a difficult task most especially when the drive of society has been pushed towards one aim. Without saying so, in so many words, as it were, Freud defines one of the most obvious problems of civilization. He sums it up: when *ethics* believes itself to be *therapeutic*; when it has given itself the illusion that society could be made better by ethical force, the ends will be unfortunate, and painful.

> The cultural super-ego has developed its ideals and set up its demands. Among the latter, those which deal with the relations of human beings to one another are comprised under the heading of ethics. People have at all times set the greater value on ethics, as though they expected that it in particular would produce especially important results. And it does in fact deal with a subject which can easily be recognized as the sorest spot in civilization. Ethics is thus to be regarded as a therapeutic attempt – as an endeavour to achieve, by means of a command of the super-ego, something which has so far not been achieved by means of any other cultural activities.
>
> (21:142)

When Freud, as a psychoanalyst (as a therapist) writes that one of his responsibilities is to minimize the demands of the super-ego in the patient, then we can see how the social and political super-ego of our times is to be opposed with equal commitment. "We are very often obliged, for therapeutic purposes, to oppose the super-ego, and we endeavour to lower its demands" (21:143). We could not have reached a more fitting conclusion to our psychopolitical essay and with the endeavor to minimize the effects of the super-ego in our lives. There is, then, one conclusion to our psychopolitical essay: in order to restore our perpetual attempt to achieve a sense of moderate happiness – through the main acts in human life capable of doing so, the ones Freud outlined so often – it will be necessary to oppose the drive of the present and reduce it to the level of conscience.

> I hasten to come to a close. But there is one question which I can hardly evade. If the development of the individual has such far-reaching similarity to the development of the individual and if it employs the same methods, may we not be justified in reaching the diagnosis that, under the influence of cultural urges, some civilizations, or some epochs of civilization – possibly the whole of mankind – have become 'neurotic'." An analytic dissection of such neuroses might lead to therapeutic recommendations which could lay claim to great practical interest.
>
> (SE 21:144)

This was Freud's project: to provide, first, an analysis of the future conditions of a theological-political society within the liberal tradition and, second, lead us not to a permanent cure, but a sense of "therapeutic recommendations" to alleviate the effects of the contemporary super-ego. He did so, from his furtive beginnings in Vienna when first listening to the associations of his patients, and then arriving at a set of proposals to alleviate both personal and social suffering.

Jeffrey Abramson believes that *Civilization and its Discontents* ends on a note of resignation. "It is to be hoped that the tendency of Eros to hold persons together will overcome the countertrend towards destruction and dissolution of life. But the hope is precarious, the moral use of death to check aggression through guilt a perpetual danger."[61] Freud's "therapeutic recommendations," for society, are unlikely to be realized. The individual, however, always has a choice and a decision to make. One last reference to the word "illusion" comes at an appropriate time and to highlight how its appearance in the discussion *on the future* has led to our own historical time. "One thing only do I know for certain and that is that man's judgments of value follow directly his wishes for happiness – that, accordingly, they are an attempt to support his illusions with arguments" (21:145). Our morality as representative of our "judgments of value" has not created happiness; on the contrary, we are facing a situation of increasing discontent and one caused by the greatest illusion of all: that the individual could become happy if only society was perfected, if only we could finally achieve, once and for all, justice and equality and rights and *objective reality* fulfilled our desires. That remains our universal illusion and one that the purveyors of political life will not renounce; how much everyone else continues to be burdened with *their expectations* remains to be seen. It is now only up to individuals, first alone, then with friends, who can give up on the illusion and, perhaps, with enough renunciation for the illusion of *political* happiness, return to the moderation first intended by our thinkers of political democracy. However counter-intuitive it may at first appear, a lessening of our moral high-mindedness may turn out to be necessary for the return to social moderation and, ultimately, to individual and collective health.

Cornelius Castoriadis believes that "psychoanalysis aims at helping the individual to become autonomous, that is, capable of self-reflexive activity and deliberation. In this respect, it belongs fully to the great social-historical stream and struggle for autonomy, the emancipatory project to which democracy and philosophy also belong."[62] At the end of this psychopolitical essay, any idea of an "emancipatory project" as well as the assumptions we make about democracy during the remainder of the 21st century are going to be analyzed with more attention to our social dynamics. Any sense of an *aporia*, in Giorgio Agamben's sense, can be a cause for awareness but not resignation; being aware of an "enemy" should no longer be overlooked. "Modern democracy's decadence and gradual convergence with totalitarian states in post-democratic spectacular societies… … may well be rooted in the aporia, which marks the beginning of modern democracy and forces it into complicity with its most implacable enemy."[63] The complicity is now a reality, as many have noted. How we respond to it will be telling and will reveal to us just how enamored we are with our values and our ideals. Psychoanalysts are in a unique position to assess our predicament. And even as the attempt has been made to live up to one of Didier Anzieu's commitments, for the one and for the many – to "find a psychoanalytic answer to human malaise in our present civilization"[64] – one cannot exclude possibilities that history has been more than illustrative in showing us what Thanatos can drive towards.

The psychopolitical essay has taken us to a few concluding remarks. Freud's preoccupation with the Soviets was to remain with him, as can be seen in the opening of the third section in *Moses and Monotheism*.

> We are living in a specially remarkable period. We find to our astonishment that progress has allied itself with barbarism. In Soviet Russia they have set about improving the living conditions of some hundreds millions of people who were held firmly in subjection. They have been rash enough to withdraw the 'opium' of religion from them and have been wise enough to give them a reasonable amount of sexual liberty, but at the same time they have submitted them to the most cruel coercion and robbed them of any possibility of freedom of thought.[65]

Reading the passage in light of the present should not be a surprise. The word *barbarism* is not as hyperbolic as it sounds. One affirmation can be restated, as it has been from the beginning; the ideals of psychoanalysis have been constant. "Besides being an ethical project, psychoanalysis is also a social institution within the democratic project."[66] As such, are we at the peculiar place, today, of making one last affirmation – as a question: is psychoanalysis the one humanistic thought capable of fully analyzing our conditions at the present and offering an alternative to consensus and therefore a change in a status quo that threatens to be barbaric? Whether the persistence of a certain kind of love can contribute to helping us attain some sense of happiness remains to be seen. Freud worked relentlessly to show us the many facets of our internal life and in the way it shaped what he called the "real" and then giving us more than sufficient ideas (to live) that could help us alleviate the sense of a perpetual unhappiness that, in the last half-century, has been made infinite worse. From the Introduction, the manipulations and distortions of love have been a primary concerns; at my end I can only re-state the ideals given to us by Freud and psychoanalysis, the ability to reflect on our internal and external obstacles and, with effort and discipline, re-commit ourselves to the fundamental human values of love, freedom, intelligence, and creativity. Will we be able to re-think the nature of liberal democracies as an instance of a theological-political reality and, if so, can we re-commit ourselves not so much to human ideals as definitions of the human as we continue to aspire to intelligence, freedom, and love as the preconditions of psychological health within ourselves? In the Introduction, and in a few selected other places, two of our impeccable thinkers (despite their very different political sensibilities) have provided us with a thinking productive for our own psychoanalytic essay. Recalling them at our end is done to give ourselves some indication of the nature of my psychopolitical essay, as a diagnostic, and what remains in terms of work and sustained commitment.

It was one of Freud's greatest contribution to thought to make us aware of not allowing ourselves any complacency when it comes to the decisive ideas of a culture that has developed itself out of the tireless work of individuals and people and will not then so easily be displaced by reactive groups who believe themselves working towards emancipation and not for a moment recognizing how they are contributing to suffering. If Sloterdijk is right, and I think he is, then the psychological problem has to be confronted and no longer allowed to simply set the terms of a social engineering gone morally awry. What he alerts us to (and by appealing to the "alert individual") is the need to begin a potentially long process of "anti-political therapeutics." That the quote comes from a work on Nietzsche should not surprise us. "A self-aware antipolitical therapeutics is required – not to depoliticize individuals, but to deneuroticize politics."[67] The biting irony of Bruno Latour's reference to "the immense grandeur of our morality"[68] is open-ended enough for our consideration. In the Introduction, where Badiou recognized the shifts from religion to politics, and here near the end where he has been forthright about the nature of human happiness – more specifically, *the metaphysics of real happiness* – a few parting words can be added. It is only right for us to choose a quote with a reference to *hauntings*. The ghosts of the dead have been, since the Introduction, first a metaphor and then a psychical reality. Badiou's declaration about the future of philosophy is, for me personally, doubly-true for psychoanalysis.

> The consequence I draw for philosophy is that, contrary to the usual assertion according to which "the end of metaphysics" you know, is being accomplished, and all that, philosophy precisely can not have an end, because it is haunted, from within itself, by the necessity to take one more step within a problem that already exists. And I believe that this is its nature. The nature of philosophy is that something is eternally being bequeathed to it. It has the responsibility of this bequeathal. You are always treating the bequeathal itself, always taking one more step in the determination of what was thus bequeathed to you. As myself, in the most unconscious manner, I never did anything as a philosopher except respond to an appeal that I had not even heard."[69]

In the most unconscious manner, the analysand can make his presence felt once more and to concur with Badiou on the question of listening and hearing, reading and interpretation.

The psychoanalyst who has received by far the most attention among academics in recent years has left us with a statement: that truth is mentioned makes it, for me, all the more welcoming. My revision of Lacan's very suggestive "in you more than you" (which, as he well knows, is a formulation written by St. Paul) first involves the answer to his question: "*what is the order of truth that our praxis engenders?*"[70] The truth it engenders, if an analysand may be allowed not so much last words as ones intended to be followed up at another time is to once again commit oneself to the truths already mentioned on many occasions and which will hopefully serve the thinking to come. Neville Symington contributes to our last section when he returns us to our beginning. "It is the creative act that we come to know ourselves, for freedom and creation are inseparable twins."[71] Freedom and creativity can only originate in love and in the persistent belief in the human. Final words by a philosopher and a psychoanalyst are appropriate. From *In the Beginning was Love*, Julia Kristeva writes: "From being the subject of an amorous discourse during the years of my analysis (and, in the best of circumstances, beyond them), I discover my potential for psychical renewal," and of "intellectual renovation."[72] Love and intelligence: together they have the ability for making us, in principle, transformed enough to once again be capable of individuality and freedom. Given the destitution of the contemporary state of liberal democracies, can we again make a prior commitment and a necessary return to the past and make a decision, one that Nietzsche presented to us as the only fitting relation to our "ghosts." "I prefer to understand the rare human beings of an age as suddenly emerging late ghosts of past cultures and their powers" (GS 84). To avail ourselves of their powers, *for life*, not death and endless recrimination, may re-direct us towards a future much more free than is currently the case.

Notes

1 Werman, David. "Freud's "Civilization and its Discontents" – A Reappraisal" 239–254, *Psychoanalytic Review*, Vol. 7, No. 2 (Summer 1985), 253.
2 Spero, Moshe Halevi. "The Civilization of Discontent: Notes on the Hidden Sources of Unbehagen in Freud's Analysis of Civilization," 221–253 *The Psychoanalytic Study of the Child*, Vol. 63 (2008), 229.
3 Tauber, Alfred. *Requiem for the Ego: Freud and the Origins of Postmodernism*. Stanford: Stanford University Press, 2013, 55.
4 Freud, Sigmund. "To Romain Rolland." SE 20:279.
5 Zaretsky, Eli. *Political Freud: A History*. New York: Columbia University Press, 2015, 195.
6 Hart, David Bentley. *Atheist Delusions: The Christian Revolution and its Fashionable Enemies*. New Haven: Yale University Press, 2009, 21.
7 Webster, Jamieson. "Critique and Cure: A Dream of Uniting Psychoanalysis and Philosophy," 138–157 *American Journal of Psychoanalysis*. Vol. 73, No. 2 (Jun. 2013) 141.
8 Ffytche, Matt. "Freud and the Neocons: The Narrative of a Political Encounter from 1949–2000," 5–44 *Psychoanalysis and History*, Vol. 15, No. 1, 2013, 15.
9 Roudinesco, Élisabeth. *Freud: His Time and Ours*. Tr. Catherine Porter. Harvard: Harvard University Press, 2016, 346.
10 Kirsner, Douglas. "Freud, Civilization, Religion, and Stoicism," 354–366 *Psychoanalytic Psychology*, Vol. 23, No. 2, 2006, 355.
11 Lothane, Zvi. "Freud's *Civilization and its Discontents* and Related Works: A Reappraisal," 524–542 *Psychoanalytic Inquiry*, Vol. 32, Issue 6, 2012, 532.
12 Prentice., Deborah A. "Liberal Norms and their Discontents," 516–518 *Perspectives on Psychological Science*, 7(5), 2012, 517. All the italicized concepts are my emphases.
13 Freud, Sigmund. "The Question of Lay Analysis." (SE 20:179–258).
14 Avery, Joseph J. "Rethinking the Freud-Rolland Relationship: An Explication and translation of Freud's "Acropolis Letter," 99–122 *American Imago*, Vol. 76, No. 1, Spring 2019, 99.
15 The subtitle of D.C. Schindler's *Freedom from Reality*. South Bend: The University of Notre Dame Press, 2017.
16 Stroumsa, Guy G. "Myth Into Novel: The Late Freud on Early Religion," *New Perspectives on Freud's Moses and Monotheism*. Eds. Ruth Ginsburg and Ilana Pardes, 210.
17 The arguments and references provided by Paul Muldoon in "The Power of Forgetting: Ressentiment, Guilt, and Transformative Politics" (669–683 *Political Psychology*, Vol. 38, No. 4, 2017) can be consulted.
18 Freud, Sigmund. "The Disposition to Obsessional Neurosis." SE 12:318.
19 Quinodoz, Danielle. *Words that Touch: A Psychoanalyst Learns to Speak*. London: Karnac, 2003, 184. Chapter 13 is called "Listening to Freud and speaking to the psychoanalysts of the future."

20 Young-Bruehl, Elizabeth. *The Clinic and the Context: Historical Essays*. London: Karnac, 2013, 73. Her suggestion of a "therapeutics politics" may in part take up one of the possible lines of thought in Freud himself; but the two words, together, have never seemed more alien to each other.
21 The title of Anthony Elliot's *Subject to Ourselves: An Introduction to Freud, Psychoanalysis, and Social Theory*. London: Routledge, 2015 is, as intended, wholly ambiguous: on the one hand we are perpetually working towards becoming subjects (bona fide selves) and on the other we can subject ourselves to the most adverse conditions of being – sometimes as a perverse necessity. Although I'm not, in principle, concerned with one of the categories he has highlighted (postmodernity) he does raise a question that returns us to a first argument. Elliot's last chapter is called "Postmodernity, or Modernity in Reverse," which to me once again confirms what others have thought about the modern: if it has, in fact, existed, it has been inseparable from a regression and therefore has not yet achieved what may still be possible in the future.
22 Freud, Sigmund. *An Autobiographical Study*. SE 20:15.
23 Kaye, Howard L. "Was Freud a Medical Scientist or Social Theorist: The Mysterious "Development of the Hero"," 375–397 *Sociological Theory*, Vol. 21, Issue 4, 2003.
24 Tauber, Alfred I. *Freud, the Reluctant Philosopher*. Princeton: Princeton University Press, 2010, 198, my emphasis.
25 Parker, Ian. "Freud's Culture," 45–59 *Re(con(figuring Psychoanalysis: Critical Juxtapositions of the Philosophical, the Sociohistorical and the Political*. Ed. Aydan Gülerce. New York: Palgrave Macmillan, 2012, 46.
26 De Zengotita, Thomas. *Postmodern Theory and Progressive Politics: Toward a New Humanism*. New York: Palgrave, 2018, 117.
27 Chessick, Richard D. *The Future of Psychoanalysis*. Albany: SUNY, 2007, xii.
28 Taubes, Jacob. *The Political Theology of Paul*. Ed. By Aleida Assman and Jan Assman et al. Tr. Dana Hollander. Stanford: Stanford University Press, 2004, 95, my emphasis.
29 McLuhan, Marshall. *Understanding Media*. Cambridge: The MIT Press, 1994.
30 Karbelnig. Alan Michael. "Laying the death drive to rest," *International Forum of Psychoanalysis*, 2021. Despite the admission that the death drive does deserve further investigation, he nevertheless comes to the conclusion that it is an "archaic idea" best forgotten. One of his arguments stands out: "for a lack of better phrase, the death drive harms psychoanalysis' public relations." We are far too along to be concerned with "public relations." They were a problem in Freud's day and they are no less today, with the added sense of both social indifference and hostility – due, in no small measure, precisely because of the dynamism of the death drive that is acting against the therapeutic insights and initiatives of psychoanalysis. While this will not be well received, one imagines, outside the psychoanalytic community, might we not venture to say that part of the hostility against psychoanalysis is because of its suspicions about the pretensions of the super-ego and just how far it can compel those susceptible to its contagion to act out their political beliefs. Psychoanalysis can hardly be concerned about its reception; it is far too late for that.
31 As in Eugene J. Koprowski's "Freud, Psychoanalysis, and the Therapeutic Effect of Agapic Love," 314–315 *Issues in Mental Health Nursing*, 35, 2014.
32 Santner, Eric L. *On the Psychotheology of Everyday Life: Reflections on Freud and Rosenzweig*. Chicago: The University of Chicago Press, 2001, 90.
33 Rehm, Marc. "Meditation on Aggression, Loss, Discovery, and Influence in Psychoanalysis," 528–541 *Psychoanalytic Dialogues*, 23:5, 2013, 532.

34 Sloterdijk, Peter. "Rules for the Human Zoo: a response to the Letter on Humanism," 12–28 in *Environment and Planning*. Tr. Mary Varney Rorty, Vol. 27, 2009, 24. "Their associated media" is my emphasis.
35 Bollas, Christopher. *The Freudian Moment*. London: Karnac, 2013, 66.
36 Freud, Sigmund. "Observations on Transference Love." (SE 12:168)
37 Freud, Sigmund. *Delusions and Dreams in Jensen's 'Gradiva.'* SE 9:
38 Clack, Brian R. *Love, Drugs, Art, Religion: The Pains and Consolations of Existence*. London: Routledge, 2016, 140.
39 De Vleminck, Jens. "The Dark Truth of Love: A Freudian Phenomenology of Hatred," 365–387 *American Imago*, Vol. 75, No. 3 (Fall 2018), 383.
40 Schmitt, Carl. *The Concept of the Political.* Tr. C.J. Miller. Antelope Publishing House, 2020, 19.
41 Oughourlian, Jean-Michel. *Psychopolitics*. Tr. Trevor Cribben Merrill. East Lansing, Michigan: Michigan State University Press, 2012, 81.
42 Badiou, Alain. *In Praise of Love*, with Nicolas Truong. Tr. Peter Bush. New York: The New Press, 2012, 58.
43 Philips, Adam. "Waiting for Returns: Freud's New Love," 171–187 *Salmagundi*, No. 148–149, Fall (2005/2006), 178–179.
44 Hollan, Douglas. "Cultures and Their Discontents: On the Cultural Mediation of Shame and Guilt," 570–581 *Psychoanalytic Inquiry* 32, 2012, 571.
45 Villa, François. "The Psychoanalytical Method and Disaster of Totalitarianism," 267–287 *Critical Inquiry*, Vol. 40, No. 2 (Winter 2014), 279.
46 Rorty, Richard. "Freud, Morality, Hermeneutics," *New Literary History*, Vol. 12, No. 1, Autumn 1980, 177–185, 181.
47 Eigen, Michael. *The Psychotic Core*. London: Karnac, 2004, 170.
48 Katchadourian, Herant. *Guilt: The Bite of Conscience*. Stanford: Stanford General Books, 2010, 117.
49 Chassequet-Smirgel, Janine. "Perversion and the Universal Law," 177- *Dimensions of Psychoanalysis: A Selection of Papers Presented at the Freud Memorial Lectures*. Ed. Joseph Sandler. London: Karnac, 1989, 178.
50 Bollas, Christopher. *The Shadow of the Object: Psychoanalysis of the Unthought Known*. New York: Columbia University Press, 1987, 27–28.
51 Sloterdijk, Peter. *Nietzsche Apostle*. Tr. Steven Corcoran. South Pasadena, CA: Semiotext(e), 2013, 34.
52 Badiou, Alain. *Happiness*. Tr. A.J. Bartlett and Justin Clemens. London: Bloomsbury, 2019, 88.
53 Bruckner, Pascal. *The Tyranny of Guilt: An Essay on Western Masochism*. Tr. Steven Rendell. Princeton: Princeton University Press, 2012, 34.
54 Drassinower, Abraham. *Freud's Theory of Culture: Eros, Loss, and Politics*. Lanham: Rowman & Littlefield Publishers Inc., 2003, 13.
55 Leonoff, Arthur. "Destruo Ergo Sum: Towards a Psychoanalytic Understanding of Sadism," 95–112 *Canadian Journal of Psychoanalysis*, Vol. 5, No. 1 (May 1997), 96.
56 Benjamin, Andrew E. *Working with Walter Benjamin: Recovering a Political Philosophy*. Edinburgh: Edinburgh University Press, 2013, 250. The quote comes in Appendix C: "The Illusion of the Future: Notes on Benjamin and Freud."
57 Capps, Donald and Carlin, Nathan. "Human Chances of Happiness: A Review of Freud's Civilization and its Discontents," 271–289 *Pastoral Psychology*, Vol. 62, Iss, 3 (Jun. 2013), 286.
58 As an example, we can think about M. Guy Thompson's "Happiness and Chance: A Reappraisal of the Psychoanalytic Concept of Suffering," 134–153 *Psychoanalytic Psychology*, Vol. 21, No. 1, 2004.

59 Akhtar, Salman. *Matters of Life and Death: Psychoanalytic Reflections*. London: Karnac 2011, 29.
60 Schmidt-Hellerau, Cordelia. "How Demagogy Works: Reflections on Aggression in Politically Fraught Times," 234–242 Psychoanalytic Inquiry, Vol. 40, Issue 4, 2020.
61 Abramson, Jeffrey B. *Liberation and its Limits: The Moral and Political Thought of Freud*. Boston: Beacon Press, 1984, 47.
62 Castoridadis, Cornelius. "Psychoanalysis and Politics," in *Speculations after Freud: Psychoanalysis, Philosophy and Culture*. Ed. Michael Münchow and Sonu Shamdasani. London: Routledge, 1994, 7.
63 Agamben, Giorgio. *Homo Sacer: Sovereign Power and Bare Life*. Tr. Daniel Heller-Roazen. Stanford: Stanford University Press, 1998, 10.
64 Anzieu, Didier. "Psychoanalysis Still." Tr. Chris Vanderwess and Ian Birksted, 109–116 in *International Journal of Psychoanalysis*, Vol. 102, No. 1, 2021, 109.
65 Freud, Sigmund. *Moses and Monotheism*. SE 23:54.
66 Reeder, Jurgen. "The enigmatic "notion of the subject": With philosophy at the interface of psychoanalysis and society," 114–121 in *The Scandinavian Psychoanalytic Review* 31:2, 2008, 121.
67 Sloterdijk, Peter. *Nietzsche's Materialism*. Tr. Jamie Owen Daniel. Minneapolis: University of Minnesota Press, 1989, 90.
68 Latour, Bruno. "Life Among Conceptual Characters: A letter to conclude the special issue of New Literary History and "Recomposing the Humanities with Bruno Latour"," 463–476 *New Literary History*, Vol. 47 (2/3), 2016, 476.
69 Badiou, Alain. "Philosophy as Biography." *The Symptom: Online Journal for Lacan.com*. https://www.lacan.com/symptom9_articles/badiou19.html.
70 Lacan, Jacques. *The Four Fundamental Concepts of Psychoanalysis*. Ed. Jacques-Alain Miller. Tr. Alan Sheridan. New York: W.W. Norton, 1977, 263.
71 Symington, Neville. *The Blind Man Sees: Freud's Awakening and Other Essays*. London: Karnac, 2004, 176.
72 Kristeva, Julia. *In the Beginning was Love: Psychoanalysis and Faith*. Tr. Arthur Goldhammer. New York: Columbia University Press, 1987, 3.

AFTERWORD

In a short but nonetheless suggestive article, Freud ends with nothing more, though nothing less, than a piece of commonsense advice. *Analysands* have taken it to heart; readers might do so as well. The first part is well-known to analysts and, so too, a source of continuing grievance for others. In "On Psychoanalysis," when he considers how his ideas have been controversial and opposed and would continue to be a source of cultural discomfort, he writes: "the progress of psycho-analysis is further retarded by the dread felt by the average observer of seeing himself in his own mirror." We have no doubt that this one necessity has caused the most resentment against Freud as an individual and against psychoanalysis as a *discipline*. He concludes: "Whoever wishes not to ignore a truth will do well to distrust his antipathies, and, if he wishes to submit the theory of psycho-analysis to a critical examination, let him first analyze himself."[1] All the psychoanalysts who have been complementary and supportive in the endeavor to present a psycho-political essay have fulfilled this one responsibility. There can be no shortcut or alibi for the need to begin an individual and cultural self-examination if the most oppressive tactics of the super-ego and the destructive impulses of the death drive are to be permanently prevented from achieving their objectives. In any event, the choice is ours.

Note

1 Freud, Sigmund. "On Psychoanalysis." SE 12:210-211.

BIBLIOGRAPHY

Abraham, Karl. "Melancholia and Obsessional Neurosis: Two Stages of the Sadistic-Anal Phases of the Libido." (1924), in *Selected Papers on Psychoanalysis*. London: Karnac, 1988.

Abramson, Jeffrey B. *Liberation and its Limits: The Moral and Political Thought of Freud*. Boston: Beacon Press, 1984.

Adorno, Theodor. "Freudian Theory and the Pattern of Fascist Propaganda," 118–137 *The Essential Frankfurt School*. Ed. Andrew Arato and Elke Gerhardt. London: Continuum, 1982.

Agamben, Giorgio. *Homo Sacer: Sovereign Power and Bare Life*. Tr. Daniel Heller-Roazen. Stanford: Stanford University Press, 1998.

Akhtar, Salman. "Introduction" to *On Freud's "The Future of an Illusion."* Ed. Mary Kay O'Neil and Salman Akhtar. London: Karnac.

Akhtar, Salman. *Matters of Life and Death: Psychoanalytic Reflections*. London: Karnac, 2011.

Ansermet, François. "Freud's Death Drive: the paradox of destructiveness," 71–77 *Freud and War*. Ed. Marlène Belilos. London: Karnac, 2016.

Anzieu, Didier. *A Skin for Thought: Interviews with Gilbert Tarrab on Psychology and Psychoanalysis*. London: Karnac, 1990.

Anzieu, Didier. "Psychoanalysis Still." Tr. Chris Vanderwees and Ian Birksted, 109–116 in *International Journal of Psychoanalysis*, Vol. 102, Iss. 1, 2021.

Appel, S. "Freud on Civilization," 625–645 *Human Relations*, Vol. 48, Iss. 6, Jun 1995.

Arditi, Benamin. *Politics on the Edge of Liberalism: Difference, Populism, Revolution, Agitation*. Edinburgh: Edinburgh University Press, 2007.

Askay, Richard and Farquhar, Jensen. "On the Nature of the Human: Sigmund Freud," 73–88 *Contemporary Psychoanalytic Studies*, Vol. 12, 2011.

Avery, Joseph J. "Rethinking the Freud-Rolland Relationship: An Explication and translation of Freud's "Acropolis Letter," 99–122 *American Imago*, Vol. 76, Iss. 1, Spring 2019.

Bachelard, Gaston. *The Psychoanalysis of Fire*. Tr. Alan C.M. Ross. Boston: Beacon Press, 1964.

Badiou, Alain. *Briefings on Existence: A Short Treatise on Transitory Ontology*. Translated, edited, and with an introduction by Norman Madarasz. Albany: SUNY, 2006.

Badiou, Alain. *The Century*. Tr. Alberto Toscano. Cambridge, UK: Polity, 2007.

Badiou, Alain. *Happiness*. Tr. A.J. Bartlett and Justin Clemens. London: Bloomsbury, 2019.

Badiou, Alain. *In Praise of Love*, with Nicolas Truong. Tr. Peter Bush. New York: The New Press, 2012.

Badiou, Alain. *Philosophy and the Event*, with Fabien Tarby. Tr. Louise Burchill. Cambridge, UK: Polity, 2013.

Badiou, Alain. "Philosophy as Biography." *The Symptom: Online Journal for Lacan.com*. https://www.lacan.com/symptom9_articles/badiou19.html.

Badiou, Alain. *Theory of the Subject*. Tr., and with an introduction by Bruno Bosteels. London: Bloomsbury, 2013.

Balibar, Étienne. *Citizen Subject: Foundations for Philosophical Anthropology*.

Badiou, Alain. "Construction, and Deconstruction of the Universal," Tr. Melissa McMahon, 21–43 *Critical Horizons*, Vol. 7, Iss. 1, 2006.

Baranger, Willy. "The Ego and the Function of Ideology," 217–228 in *The Work of Confluence: Listening and Interpreting in the Psychoanalytic Field*. Madeleine and Willy Baranger. Ed. Leticia Glocer Fiorini. London: Karnac, 2009.

Bar-Haim, Shaul. "The return of the Political Freud? Some notes on the new historiography of Psychoanalysis," 121–139 *History of the Human Sciences*, Vol. 32, Iss. 2.

Barrett, Bernard. *You Ought to! A Psychoanalytic Study of the Superego and Conscience*. London: Karnac, 2007.

Bataille, Georges. *Visions of Excess: Selected Writings, 1927-1939*. Ed. With an Introduction by Allan Stoekl. Tr. Allan Stoekl, with Carl R. Lovitt and Donald M. Leslie Jr. Minneapolis: University of Minnesota Press, 1985.

Benjamin, Andrew E. *Working with Walter Benjamin: Recovering a Political Philosophy*. Edinburgh: Edinburgh University Press, 2013.

Benvenuto, Sergio. *What are Perversions? Sexuality, Ethics, Psychoanalysis*. London: Karnac, 2016.

Bergmann, Martin S. "The Dual Impact of Freud's Death and Freud's Death Instinct Theory on the History of Psychoanalysis," 664–686 *Psychoanalytic Review*, Vol. 98, Iss. 5, Oct. 2011.

Bion, W.R. *Experience in Groups: and other papers*. London: Brunner-Routledge, 1989.

Black, David M. "Mapping a Detour: Why did Freud Speak of a Death Drive?" 185–198 *British Journal of Psychotherapy*, Vol. 18, Iss. 2, 2011.

Blass, Rachel B. "Conceptualizing splitting: on the different meanings of splitting and their implications for the understanding of the person and the psychoanalytic process," 123–129 *International Journal of Psychoanalysis*, Vol. 96, Iss. 1, 2015.

Bokanovski, Thierry. "Variations on the concept of traumatism: traumatism, traumatic, trauma," 251–265 *International Journal of Psychoanalysis*, Vol. 86, 2008.

Blumenberg, Hans. *Work on Myth*. Tr. Robert M. Wallace. Cambridge, Massachusetts: The MIT Press, 1985.

Blumenthal, Stephen. "A State of Inbetweenness: The Challenge of Working with Disavowal," 4–16 *British Journal of Psychotherapy*, Vol. 38, Iss. 1, 2022.

Bollas, Christopher. "Introduction" to Jonathan Sklar's *Landscapes of the Dark: History, Trauma, Psychoanalysis*. London: Karnac, 2011.

Bollas, Christopher. "Psychoanalysis in the Age of Bewilderment: On the return of the oppressed," 535–551 *International Journal of Psychoanalysis*, Vol. 96, Iss. 3, 2015.

Bollas, Christopher. *The Shadow of the Object: Psychoanalysis of the Unthought Known*. New York: Columbia University Press, 1987.

Brague, Rémi. *Curing Mad Truths: Medieval Wisdom for the Modern Age*. Notre Dame: Notre Dame University Press, 2019.

Britton, Ronald. *Sex, Death, and the Superego: Experiences in Psychoanalysis*. London: Karnac, 2003.

Brown, Wendy. *Edgework: Critical Essay on Knowledge and Politics*. Princeton: Princeton University Press, 2005.

Bruckner, Pascal. *The Tyranny of Guilt: An Essay on Western Masochism*. Tr. Steven Rendell. Princeton: Princeton University Press, 2012.

Burzstein, Jean-Gerard. *The Topological Transformation of Freud's Theory*. Tr. Marie-Laure Bromley-Davenport. London: Karnac, 2016.

Camus, Albert. *The Rebel: An Essay on Man in Revolt*. New York: Vintage Books, 1956.

Canestri, Jorge. "The Logic of Freudian Research," 117–129 *Freud and Judaism*. Ed. David Meghnegi. London: Karnac, 1993.

Capps, Donald and Carlin, Nathan. "Human Chances of Happiness: A Review of Freud's Civilization and its Discontents," 271–289 *Pastoral Psychology*, Vol. 62, Iss, 3, Jun. 2013.

Carveth, Donald L. *The Still Small Voice: Psychoanalytic Reflections on Guilt and Conscience*. London: Karnac, 2013.

Carveth, Donald L. "Why we should stop conflating the superego with conscience," 15–32 *Psychoanalysis, Culture & Society*, Vol. 22, Iss. 1, Mar 2017.

Castoriadis, Cornelius. "Psychoanalysis and Politics," 1–12 *Speculations after Freud: Psychoanalysis, Philosophy and Culture*. Ed. Michael Munchow and Sonu Shamdasani. London: Routledge, 1994.

Chabert, Catherine. "Can we do without the death drive?" *International Journal of Psychoanalysis*, Vol. 100, Iss. 6, 2019.

Chasseguet-Smirgel, Janine. "The Body and the World," 13–27 *International Congress Series*, 2006.

Chasseguet-Smirgel, Janine. ""Creative Writers and Day-dreaming": A commentary," 107–121 *On Freud's "Creative Writers and Day-Dreaming"*. Ed. Ethel Spector Person, Peter Fonagy, Servull Augusto Figueira. London: Karnac, 2013.

Chasseguet-Smirgel, Janine. *The Ego-Ideal: A Psychoanalytic Study on the Malady of the Ideal*. Tr. Paul Burrows. New York: W.W. Norton, 1985.

Chasseguet-Smirgel, Janine. "Perversion and the Universal Law," 177- *Dimensions of Psychoanalysis: A Selection of Papers Presented at the Freud Memorial Lectures*. Ed. Joseph Sandler. London: Karnac, 1989.

Chasseguet-Smirgel, Janine. *Sexuality and Mind: The Role of the Mother and Father in the Psyche*. London: Karnac, 1989.

Chessick, Richard D. *The Future of Psychoanalysis*. Albany: SUNY, 2007.

Clack, Brian R. *Love, Drugs, Art, Religion: The Pains and Consolations of Existence.* London: Routledge, 2016.

Clark, Margaret. *Understanding Religion and Spirituality in Clinical Practice.* London: Karnac, 2012.

Covington, Coline. "Populism and the Danger of Illusion," *Contemporary Psychoanalysis*, Vol. 54, Iss. 2, 2018.

Damisch, Hubert. "Bridging the Gap Between Two Scenes," 93–95 *Whose Freud? The Place of Psychoanalysis in Contemporary Culture.* Ed. Peter Brooks and Alex Woloch. Ithaca: Cornell University Press, 2000, 95.

Dare, Christopher, Anna Ursula Dreher, Alex Holder, & Joseph Sandler. *Freud's Models of the Mind: An Introduction.* Routledge, 1997.

de La Boétie, Étienne. *The Politics of Obedience: The Discourse of Voluntary Servitude.* Tr. Harry Kurz. Auburn, AL: Mises Institute, 2015.

Delay, Tad. *God is Unconscious: Psychoanalysis and Theology.* Eugene, Oregon: Wipf & Stock, 2015.

De M'Uzan, Michael. *Death and Identity: Being and Psycho-Sexual Drama.* Tr. Andrew Weller. London: Karnac, 2013.

Deleuze, Gilles. *Pure Immanence: Essays on a Life.* Tr. Anne Boyman. New York: Zone Books, 2005.

de Masi, Franco. "The perverse and psychotic superego," 735–739 *International Journal of Psychoanalysis*, Vol. 101, Iss. 4, 2020.

de Masi, Franco. *Working with Difficult Patients: From Neurosis to Psychosis.* London: Karnac, 2015.

De Vleminck, Jens. "The Dark Truth of Love: A Freudian Phenomenology of Hatred," 365–387 *American Imago*, Vol. 75, Iss. 3, Fall 2018.

Di Censo, James J. *The Other Freud: Religion, Culture and Psychoanalysis.* London: Routledge, 1999.

Derrida, Jacques. *Specters of Marx: The State of Debt, the Work of Mourning and the New International.* Tr. Peggy Kamuf. New York: Routledge, 1994.

De Zengotita, Thomas. *Postmodern Theory and Progressive Politics: Toward a New Humanism.* New York: Palgrave, 2018.

Doidge, Norman. "Classics Revisited: Freud's *The Ego and the Id* and "Inhibitions, Symptoms and Anxiety," 281–294 *Journal of the American Psychoanalysis Association*, Vol. 50, Iss. 1, 2002.

Donnet, Jean-Luc. *The Analyzing Situation.* Tr. Andrew Weller. London: Karnac, 2009.

Dougherty, Jude P. *The Logic of Religion.* Washington, D.C.: The Catholic University of America Press, 2003.

Drassinower, Abraham. *Freud's Theory of Culture: Eros, Loss, and Politics.* Lanham: Rowman & Littlefield Publishers Inc., 2003.

Dupuy, Jean-Pierre. *The Mark of the Sacred.* Tr. M.B. DeBevoise. Stanford: Stanford University Press, 2013.

Eagleton, Terry. *Reason, Faith, and Revolution: Reflections on the God Debate.* New Haven: Yale University Press, 2009.

Eigen, Michael. *The Psychotic Core.* London: Karnac, 2004.

Elliott, Anthony. *Social Theory Since Freud: Traversing Social Imaginaries.* London: Routledge, 2004.

Elliott, Anthony. *Subject to Ourselves: An Introduction to Freud, Psychoanalysis, and Social Theory.* London: Routledge, 2015.

Ellul, Jacques. *Propaganda: The Formation of Man's Attitudes*. Tr. Konrad Kellen and Jean Lerner. New York: Vintage Books, 1965.

Eriksson, Johan. "Freud's Psychoanalysis: A moral cure," 663–675 *International Journal of Psychoanalysis*, Vol. 95, Iss. 4, 2014.

Falcão, Luciane. "Death drive, destructive drive and desobjectalizing functions in the analytic process," 459–476 *International Journal of Psychoanalysis*, Vol. 96, Iss. 2, 2015.

Farrell, John C. *Freud's Paranoid Quest: Psychoanalysis and Modern Suspicion*. New York: New York University Press, 1996.

Fenichel, Otto. *The Collected Papers of Otto Fenichel*. London: Routledge & Kegan Paul, 1954.

Fenn, Richard K. "Soul-loss, the Sacred and Secularity," 181–197 *Religious Studies and Theology*, Vol. 31, Iss. 2, 2012.

Ferenczi, Sandor. *First Contributions to Psychoanalysis*. Tr. Ernest Jones. London: Karnac, 1994.

Ferenczi, Sandor. "Freud's 'Group Psychology and the Analysis of the Ego': Its Contribution to the Psychology of the Individual," *Final Contributions to the Problems and Methods of Psycho-analysis*. Ed. Michael Balint. Tr. Erich Mosbacher and others. London: Karnac, 1994.

Ffytche, Matt. "Freud and the Neocons: The Narrative of a Political Encounter from 1949-2000," 5–44 *Psychoanalysis and History*, Vol. 15, Iss. 1, 2013.

Fleischer, Les. "The Corruptibility of the Superego Revisited," 86–106 in the *Canadian Journal of Psychoanalysis*, Vol. 28, Iss. 1, 2020.

Fleming, Bruce. "Conservative, Liberal, Perverted Liberal," 532–537 *Society*, Vol. 56, Iss. 6, Dec. 2019.

Foresti, Giovanni. "Freud's writing in the twenties: theory and constructs and clinical research in Inhibitions, Symptoms and Anxiety," 200–218 *On Freud's "Inhibitions, Symptoms and Anxiety."* Ed. Samuel Arbiser and Jorge Schneider. London: Karnac, 2013.

Foss, Torberg. "Freud 100 Years Ago: Totem and Taboo (1912-1913)," 1–4 *The Scandinavian Psychoanalytic Review*, Vol. 36, Iss. 12, 2013.

Frank, Claudia. "On the reception of the concept of the death drive in Germany: the terminological ambiguities of the concept of the 'death drive'," 425–444 *International Journal of Psychoanalysis*, Vol. 96, Iss. 2, 2015.

Frank, George. "Freud's Concept of the Super-ego: Review and Assessment," 448–463 in *Psychoanalytic Psychology*, Vol. 16, Iss. 3, 1999.

Frankland, Graham. *Freud's Literary Culture*. Cambridge: Cambridge University Press, 2000.

Frie, Roger. "Psychoanalysis, religion, philosophy and the possibility of dialogue: Freud, Binswanger and Pfister," 106–116 *International Forum of Psychoanalysis*, Vol. 21, 2012.

Fromm, Erich. *Psychoanalysis and Religion*. New Haven: Yale University Press, 1950.

Fukuyama, Francis. *Identity: The Demand for Dignity and the Politics of Resentment*. New York: Farrar, Straus and Giroux, 2018.

Gandesha, Samir. "The "Authoritarian Personality" Reconsidered: the Phantom of "Left Fascism"," 601–624 *American Journal of Psychoanalysis*, Vol. 79, Iss. 4, 2019.

Gay, Peter. (Ed.) *The Freud Reader*. New York: W. W. Norton & Company, 1989.

Gay, Volney. "Sigmund Freud on Religion," in *Religion, Theory, Critique: Classic and Contemporary Approaches and Methodologies*. Ed. Richard King. New York: Columbia University Press, 2017.

Ghisalberti, Giosuè. *Animal Sacrifice and the Death Penalty*. Eugene: Wipf & Stock, 2022.

Girard, René. *The Scapegoat*. Tr. Yvonne Freccero. Baltimore: The Johns Hopkins University Press, 1986.

Girard, René. *Violence and the Sacred*. Tr. Patrick Gregory. Baltimore: The Johns Hopkins University Press, 1977.

Girard, René. *When These Things Begin: Conversations with Michel Treguer*. Tr. Trevor Cribben Merrill. East Lansing: Michigan State University Press, 2014.

Gourgoris, Stathis. *The Perils of the One*. New York: Columbia University Press, 2019.

Goux, Jean-Joseph. "Freudian Unconscious and Secularization of Judaism," in *Disciplining Freud on Religion: Perspectives from the Humanities*. Ed. Greg Kaplan and William Parsons. Lanham: Lexington Books, 2010.

Graziano, Manlio. *Holy Wars and Holy Alliance: The Return of Religion to the Global Political Stage*. Tr. Brian Knowlton. New York: Columbia University Press, 2017.

Green, André. *Illusions and Disillusions in Psychoanalytic Work*. Tr. Andrew Weller. London: Karnac, 2011.

Grotstein, James S. "Notes on the Superego," 257–270 *Psychoanalytic Inquiry*, Vol. 24, Iss. 2, 2008.

Guntrip, Harry. *Schizoid Phenomena, Object Relations and the Self*. London: Karnac, 2001.

Grubrich-Simitis, Ilse. *Back to Freud's Texts: Making Silent Documents Speak*. Tr. Philip Slotkin. New Haven: Yale University Press, 1993.

Habermas, Jürgen. "The Rational Meaning of a Questionable Inheritance of Political Theology," in *The Power of Religion in the Public Sphere*. Ed. And Introduced by Eduardo Mendieta and Jonathan Vanantwerpen. New York: Columbia University Press, 2011.

Hageback, Niklas. *The Death Drive: Why Societies Self-Destruct*. Las Vegas: Gaudium, 2020.

Hammill, Graham and Lupton, Julia Reinhard (Eds). *Political Theology and Early Modernity*. Chicago: The University of Chicago Press, 2012.

Han, Byung-Chul. *The Agony of Eros*. Tr. Erik Butler. Cambridge, Massachusetts: The MIT Press, 2017.

Han, Byung-Chul. *Psychopolitics: NeoLiberalism and New Technologies of Power*. Tr. Erik Butler. London: Verso, 2017.

Hardt, Michael and Negri, Antonio. *Assembly*. Oxford: Oxford University Press, 2017.

Hart, David Dudley. *Atheist Delusions: The Christian Revolution and its Fashionable Enemies*. New Haven: Yale University Press, 2009.

Hewitt, Marsha Aileen. *Freud on Religion*. Durham, UK: Acumen, 2014.

Hinshelwood, R.D. "Ideology and Identity: A psychoanalytic investigation of a social phenomenon," 131–148 *Psychoanalysis, Culture & Society*, Vol. 14, Iss. 2, Jul. 2009.

Hinshelwood, R.D. "Repression and Splitting: Towards a method of conceptual comparison," 503–521 *International Journal of Psychoanalysis*, Vol. 89.3, 2008.

Hinshelwood, R.D. (Ed.) *Influential Papers of the 1920s*. London: Karnac, 2014, 2014, 218.

Hobbes, Thomas. *Leviathan*. New York: E.P. Dutton and Company, Inc., 1950.

Hollan, Douglas. "Cultures and Their Discontents: On the Cultural Mediation of Shame and Guilt," 570–581 *Psychoanalytic Inquiry*, Vol. 32, 2012.

Holmes, Jeremy. "Superego: An attachment perspective," 1221–1240 *International Journal of Psychoanalysis*, Vo. 92, Iss. 5, Oct 2011.

Horney, Karen. *New Ways in Psychoanalysis*. Oxford: Routledge, 1939.

Huntington, Samuel P. *The Clash of Civilizations and the Remaking of World Order*. New York: Simon & Schuster, 1996.

Isaac, Jeffrey. "Liberal Democracy in Question?" 1–5 *Perspectives on Politics*, Vol. 15, Iss. 1, Mar. 2017.

Jacobs, Michael. *Sigmund Freud*. Second Edition. London: Sage Publications, 2003.

Johnston, Adrian. *Adventures in Transcendental Materialism: Dialogues with Continental Thinkers*. Edinburgh: Edinburgh University Press, 2014.

Johnston, Adrian. "The Triumph of Theological Economics: God goes underground," 3–50 *Philosophy Today*, Vol. 64, Iss. 1, Winter 2020.

Jones, Ernest. "The origins and status of the super-ego," *Influential Papers from the 1920s*. Ed. H.R. Hinshelwood. London: Karnac, 2014.

Jonsson, Stephen. *Crowds and Democracy: The Idea and Image of the Masses from Revolution to Fascism*. New York: Columbia University Press, 2013.

Jurist, Elliot L. "Whatever happened to the superego? Loewald and the Future of Psychoanalysis," 489–501 *Psychoanalytic Psychology*, Vol. 31, Iss. 4, 2014.

Kahn, Masud. *The Privacy of the Self*. London: Karnac, 1996.

Kahn, Paul W. *Political Theology: Four New Chapters on the Concept of Sovereignty*. New York: Columbia University Press, 2012.

Karbelnig. Alan Michael. "Laying the death drive to rest," *International Forum of Psychoanalysis*, 2021.

Katchadourian, Herant. *Guilt: The Bite of Conscience*. Stanford: Stanford General Books, 2010.

Kaye, Howard L. *Freud as a Social and Cultural Theorist: On Human Nature and the Civilizing Process*. London: Routledge, 2018.

Kaye, Howard L. "Raising Freud from the Dead," 294–298 *Society*, Vol. 57, Iss. 3, Jun. 2020.

Kaye, Howard L. "Was Freud a Medical Scientist or Social Theorist: The Mysterious "Development of the Hero"," 375–397 *Sociological Theory*, Vol. 21, Iss. 4, 2003.

Kenny, Dianna T. *God, Freud and Religion: The Origins of Faith, Fear and Fundamentalism*. London: Routledge, 2015.

Kernberg, Otto. "The concept of the death drive: A clinical perspective," 1009–1023 *International Journal of Psychoanalysis*, Vol. 90, Iss. 5, 2009.

Kernberg, Otto. "Limitations to the Capacity to Love," 1501–1515 *International Journal of Psychoanalysis*, Vol. 92, 2011.

Kirsner, Douglas. "Freud, Civilization, Religion, and Stoicism," 354–366 *Psychoanalytic Psychology*, Vol. 23, Iss. 2, 2006.

Klein, Melanie. *Love, Guilt and Reparation and Other Works, 1921,1945*. London: Virago Press, 1988.

Klein, Melanie. "Notes on Some Schizoid Mechanism," 1–24 *Envy and Gratitude and Other Works, 1946-1963*. London: Virago Press, 1988.

Klein, Melanie. *The Psycho-Analysis of Children*. Tr. Alix Strachey. London: Virago Press, 1989.

Koprowski, Eugene J. "Freud, Psychoanalysis, and the Therapeutic Effect of Agapic Love," 314–315 *Issues in Mental Health Nursing*, Vol. 35, 2014.

Kristeva, Julia. *In the Beginning was Love. Psychoanalysis and Faith*. Tr. Arthur Goldhammer. New York: Columbia University Press, 1987.

Kristeva, Julia. *The Incredible Need to Believe*. Tr. New York: Columbia University Press, 2009.

Kristeva, Julia. *Passions of Our Time*. Tr. Constance Borde and Sheila Malovany-Chevallier. New York: Columbia University Press, 2013.

Kronemyer, David E. "Freud's Illusion: New Approaches to Intractable Issues," 249–275 *International Journal for the Psychology of Religion*, Vol. 24, Iss. 4, 2011.

Lacan, Jacques. "Discourse to Catholics," in *The Triumph of Religion*. Tr. Bruce Fink. Cambridge, UK: Polity Press, 2013.

Lacan, Jacques. *The Four Fundamental Concepts of Psychoanalysis*. Ed. Jacques-Alain Miller. Tr. Alan Sheridan. New York: W.W. Norton, 1977.

Laclau, Ernesto. "Politics and the Unconscious," 231–244 Interview by Jason Glynos and Yannis Stavrakakis in *Subjectivity*, Vol. 3, Iss. 3, Sep. 2010.

Laine, Aira. "On the edge: the psychoanalyst's transference," 1171–1183 *International Journal of Psychoanalysis*, Vol. 88, Oct. 2007.

Lambert, Greg. *Return Statements: The Return of Religion in Contemporary Philosophy*. Edinburgh: Edinburgh University Press, 2016.

LaMothe, Ryan. "Freud, Religion, and the Presence of Projective Identification," 287–302 *Psychoanalytic Quarterly*, Vol. 20, Iss. 2, 2003.

Lanksy, Melvin. R. "Forgiveness as the working through of splitting," 374–385 *Psychoanalytic Inquiry*. Vol. 29, Iss. 5, 2009.

Laplanche, Jean. *Essays on Otherness*. Ed. John Fletcher. London: Routledge, 1999.

Laplanche, Jean. *Life and Death in Psychoanalysis*. Tr. Jeffrey Mehlman. Baltimore: The Johns Hopkins University Press, 1976.

Laplance, J. and Pontalis, J.B. *The Language of Psycho-Analysis*. Tr. Donald Nicholson-Smith. New York: W.W. Norton & Company, 1973.

Lapsley, D.K. and Stey, P.C. "Id, Ego, and Superego," 393–399 *Encyclopedia of Human Behavior*. Second Edition, 2012.

Latour, Bruno. "Life Among Conceptual Characters: A letter to conclude the special issue of New Literary History and "Recomposing the Humanities with Bruno Latour"," 463–476 *New Literary History*, Vol. 47, Iss. 2/3, 2016.

Latour, Bruno. *We Have Never Been Modern*. Tr. Catherine Porter. Cambridge: Harvard University Press, 1993.

Latrie, Stijn, Van Herck, Walter and Vanheerwijck. (Eds.). *Radical Secularization? An Inquiry into the Religious Roots of Secular Culture*. London: Bloomsbury, 2015.

Lavin, Michael and Holowchak, M. Andrew. "Beyond the Death Drive: The Future of Repetition and "Compulsion to Repeat" in Psychopathology." 645–668 *Psychoanalytic Psychology*, Vol. 32, Iss. 4, 2015.

Lear, Jonathan. *Happiness, Death and the Remainder of Life*. Cambridge, Massachusetts: Harvard University Press, 2000.

Lear, Jonathan. "The Illusion of a Future: the rhetoric of Freud's critique of religion," 83–97 in *On Freud's "The Future of an Illusion."* Ed. Mary Kay O'Neal and Salman Akhtar. London: Karnac, 2009.

Lefort, Claude. "Permanence of the Theologico-Political" in *Democracy and Political Theory*. Tr. David Macey. Cambridge: Polity Press, 2000.

Leonoff, Arthur. "Destruo Ergo Sum: Towards a Psychoanalytic Understanding of Sadism," 95–112 *Canadian Journal of Psychoanalysis*, Vol. 5, Iss. 1, May 1997.

Levine, Howard B. "Aggression and Psychoanalysis: Reflections," 43–59 *Canadian Journal of Psychoanalysis*, Vol. 25, Iss. 2, July 1, 2017.

Lilla, Mark. *The Once and Future Liberal: After Identity Politics*. New York: Harper, 2017.

Lyotard, Jean-François. *The Postmodern Explained: Correspondence, 1982–1985*. Tr. and Ed. by Julian Pefanis and Morgan Thomas. Minneapolis: University of Minnesota Press, 1993.

Long, Susan. *The Perverse Organization and its Deadly Sins*. London: Routledge, 2008.

Lothane, Zvi. "Freud's *Civilization and its Discontents* and Related Works: A Reappraisal," 524–542 *Psychoanalytic Inquiry*, Vol. 32, Iss. 6, 2012.

Mahony, Patrick J. *Freud as a Writer*. New Haven: Yale University Press, 1987.

Malancharuvil, Joseph M. "Projection, Introjection, and Projective Identification: A Reformulation," 375- in *The American Journal of Psychoanalysis*, Vol. 64, Iss. 4, December 2004.

Manninen, Vesa. "The face of fear: castration and perversion," 193–215 *The Scandinavian Psychoanalytic Review*, Vol. 23, Iss. 2, 2000.

McLuhan, Marshall. *Understanding Media*. Cambridge: The MIT Press, 1994.

McGowan, Todd. *Enjoying What We Don't Have: The Political Project of Psychoanalysis*. Lincoln: The University of Nebraska Press, 2013.

Meillassoux, Quentin. *After Finitude: An Essay on the Necessity of Contingency*. Tr. Ray Brassier. London: Bloomsbury, 2008.

Merkur, Dan. "The Antinomy of Morality in Freud," in *Ethics of Evil: Psychoanalytic Investigations*. Ed. Jon Mills and Ronald C. Naso. London: Karnac, 2016.

Merkur, Dan. *Unconscious Wisdom: A Superego Function in Dreams, Conscience, and Inspiration*. Albany: SUNY, 2001.

Miller, Janet. "The Enemy Inside: An exploration of the defensive processes of introjecting and identifying with the aggressor," 55–70 *Psychodynamic counseling*, Vol. 4, Iss. 1, 1998.

Miller, J.F. *The Triumphant Victim: A Psychoanalytical Perspective on Sadomasochism and Perverse Thinking*. London: Karnac, 2013.

Mills, Jon. "Preface" to his edited *Rereading Freud: Psychoanalysis through Philosophy*. Albany: SUNY, 2004

Mills, Jon. "Reflections on the Death Drive," 373–382 *Psychoanalytic Psychology*, Vol. 23, Iss. 2, 2006.

Montgomery, Scott L. "A Case of (mis) taken Identity? II: Freudian Language in the Ego and the Id," 51–81 *Psychoanalytic Review*, Vol. 88, Iss. 1, Feb. 2001.

Muldoon, Paul. "The Power of Forgetting: Ressentiment, Guilt, and Transformative Politics," 669–683 *Political Psychology*, Vol. 38, Iss. 4, 2017.

Negri, Antonio. *The Savage Anomaly: The Power of Spinoza's Metaphysics and Politics*. Tr. Michael Hardt. Minneapolis: University of Minnesota Press, 1991.

Nietzsche, Friedrich. *Daybreak: Thoughts on the Prejudices of Morality*. Tr. R.J. Hollingdale. Cambridge: Cambridge University Press, 1982.

Nietzsche, Friedrich. *The Gay Science*. Tr. Walter Kaufmann. New York: Vintage Books, 1974.

Nietzsche, Friedrich. *On the Genealogy of Morals: A Polemic*. Tr. Walter Kaufmann and R.J. Hollingdale. New York: Vintage Books, 1989.

Nietzsche, Friedrich. *The Will to Power*. Tr. Walter Kaufmann and R.J. Hollingdale. New York: Vintage Books, 1967.

Nissim Momigliano, Luciana. *Continuity and Change in Psychoanalysis: Letters from Milan*. London: Karnac, 1992.

Nobus, Dany. "Freud's Infernal Trinity: On the Vicissitudes of the 'Tripartite Model'," *Drawing the Soul: Schemas and Models in Psychoanalysis*. Ed. Bernard Burgoyne. London: Karnac, 2000.

Novak, David. "On Freud's theory of law and religion," 24–34 *International Journal of Law and Psychiatry*, Vol. 48, 2016.

Novick, Jack and Novick, Kerry Kelly. "The Superego and the Two-System Model," 232–256 in *Psychoanalytic Inquiry*, Vol. 24, Iss. 2, 2008.

Novis-Deutsch, Nurit. "Psychoanalysis and Religion in the 21st Century: Competitors or Collaborators?," 616–623 *American Imago*, Vol. 65, Iss. 4, Winter 2008.

Ogden, Thomas H. *The Matrix of the Mind: Object Relations and the Psychoanalytic Dialogue*. London: Karnac, 1992.

Ogden, Thomas H. "Reading Loewald: Oedipus Reconceived," 651–666 *International Journal of Psychoanalysis*, Vol. 87, Iss. 3, June 2006.

Oughourlian, Jean-Michel. *Psychopolitics*. Tr. Trevor Cribben Merrill. East Lansing, Michigan: Michigan State University Press, 2012.

Paul, Robert A. "Yes, The Primal Crime Did Take Place: A Further Defense of Freud's Totem and Taboo," 230–249 *Ethos*, Vol. 38, Iss. 2, 2010.

Parker, Ian. "Freud's Culture," 45–59 *Re(con(figuring Psychoanalysis: Critical Juxtapositions of the Philosophical, the Sociohistorical and the Political*. Ed. Aydan Gülerce. New York: Palgrave Macmillan, 2012.

Penot, Bernard. "The socalled death drive, and indispensable force for any subjective life," 299–321 *International Journal of Psychoanalysis*, Vol. 98, Iss. 2, 2017.

Perelberg, Rosine Jozef. "Psychoanalysis and Social Violence: Civilization and its Discontents revisited," 1248–1263 *International Journal of Psychoanalysis*, Vol. 101, Iss. 6, 2020.

Pettman, Ralph. "Psychopathology and world politics," 49–75 *Cambridge Review of International Affairs*, Vol. 23, Iss. 3, September 2010.

Pieszanski, Alberto. "Hysteria, A Century Later: Post-Kleinian Theory and Techniques," 102–111 *Psychoanalytic Inquiry*, Vol. 37, Iss. 2, 2017.

Philips, Adam. "Waiting for Returns: Freud's New Love," 171–187 *Salmagundi*, Iss. 148-149, Fall (2005/2006).

Plato. *Symposium*. Tr. Alexander Nehemas. Indianapolis: Hackett Publishing Company, 1989.

Plattner, Marc F. presents in "Illiberal Democracy as the Struggle on the Right," 5–19 *Journal of Democracy*, Vol. 30, Iss. 1, 2019.

Prentice, Deborah A. "Liberal Norms and their Discontents," 516–518 *Perspectives on Psychological Science*, Vol. 7, Iss. 5, 2012.

Pruyser, P. "What Splits in 'splitting'?" 1–46 *Bulletin of the Menninger Clinic*, Vol. 39.

Quinodoz, Danielle. *Words that Touch: A Psychoanalyst Learns to Speak*. London: Karnac, 2003.

Racamier, Paul-Claude. "On Narcissistic Perversion," 119–132 *International Journal of Psychoanalysis*, Vol. 5, 2014.

Rank, Otto. *Don Juan Legend.* Ed. Tr, with an Introduction by David G. Winter. Princeton: Princeton University Press, 2015.

Raschke, Carl. *Postmodernism and the Revolution in Religious Theory: Toward a Semiotics of the Event*. Charlottesville: University of Virginia Press, 2012.

Razinsky, Liran. "Driving Death Away: Death and Freud, Theory of the Death Drive," 393–424 *Psychoanalytic Review*, Vol. 97, Iss. 3, Jun. 2010.

Reeder, Jurgen. "The enigmatic "notion of the subject": With philosophy at the interface of psychoanalysis and society," 114–121 in *The Scandinavian Psychoanalytic Review*, Vol. 31, Iss. 2, 2008.

Rehm, Marc. "Meditation on Aggression, Loss, Discovery, and Influence in Psychoanalysis," 528–541 *Psychoanalytic Dialogues*, Vol. 23, Iss. 5, 2013.

Reicher, Stephen. "Crowds, Agency and Passion: Reconsidering the Roots of the Social Bond," 67–85 in *The Psychology and Politics of the Collective*. Ed. Ruth Parkin-Gounelas. London: Routledge, 2012.

Reiner, Anni. *The Quest for Conscience and the Birth of the Mind.* London: Karnac, 2009.

Reijzer, Hans. *A Dangerous Legacy: Judaism and the Psychoanalytic Movement*. Tr. Jeannette K. Ringold. London: Karnac, 2011.

Rempel, Morgan Henry. "Understanding Freud's Philosophy of Religion," 215–242 *Canadian Journal of Psychoanalysis*, Vol. 5, Iss. 2, Nov. 1997.

Ribaut, Gilles. "The Two Sources of Morality in Freud's Work," 135–141 *Psychoanalysis, Monotheism, and Morality: The Sigmund Freud Symposia, 2009–2011*. Ed. Wolfgang Müller Funk, Inge Scholz Strasser and Herman Westerink. Leuven: Leuven University Press, 2013.

Richards, Arnold. "The Need not to believe: Freud's Godlessness Remembered," *Psychoanalytic Review*, Vol. 96, Iss. 4, Aug. 2009.

Ricoeur, Paul. *Freud and Philosophy: An Essay on Interpretation*. Tr. Denis Savage. New Haven: Yale University Press, 1970.

Rifkind, Gabrielle. *The Psychology of Political Extremism: What Would Sigmund Freud have Thought about Islamic State*. London: Routledge, 2018.

Rorty, Richard. *Achieving Our Country: Leftist Thought in Twentieth-Century America.* Cambridge, Massachusetts: Harvard University Press, 1998.

Rorty, Richard. "Freud, Morality, Hermeneutics," 177–185 *New Literary History*, Vol. 12, Iss. 1, Autumn 1980.

Ross, Nathaniel. "Man's struggle for freedom: A psychoanalytical inquiry into the individual and social dimensions of human autonomy," 209–221 *Bulletin of the Menninger Clinic*, Vol. 38, 1974.

Roudinesco, Élisabeth. *Freud: His Time and Ours*. Tr. Catherine Porter. Harvard: Harvard University Press, 2016.

Rothstein, Arnold. *Making Freud more Freudian*. London: Karnac, 2010.

Rubin, Jeffrey. *The Good Life: Psychoanalytic Reflections on Love, Ethics, Creativity and Spirituality*. Albany: SUNY, 2004.

Russell, Francey. "Unity and Synthesis in the Ego Ideal: Reading Freud's Concept through Kant's Philosophy." 353–383 in *American Imago*, Vol. 69, Iss. 3, Fall 2012.

Rustin, Michael. "Psychoanalysis and Culture in Secular Times," 58–73 in *Culture and the Unconscious*. Ed. Caroline Bainbridge et al. New York: Palgrave Macmillan, 2007.

Ruszynski, Stanley. "The problem of certain psychic realities: Aggression and Violence as perverse solutions," 23–42 *Lectures on Violence Perversion and Delinquency*. Ed. David Morgan and Stanley Ruszynski. London: Karnac, 2007.

Santner, Eric L. *On the Psychotheology of Everyday Life: Reflections on Freud and Rosenzweig*. Chicago: The University of Chicago Press, 2001.

Sarra, Nicholas. "Attachment and Trauma in Groups and Organizations," 263–272 in *British Journal of Psychotherapy*, Vol. 35, Iss. 2, 2019.

Sauvayre, Pascal and Vegas, Monica. "An even hover-reading of Freud: The work of metaphor," 1343–1367 in *International Journal of Psychoanalysis*, Vol. 97, Iss. 5.

Schafer, Roy. *Tragic Knots in Psychoanalysis*. New Papers on Psychoanalysis. London: Karnac, 2009.

Schaffner, Anna Katherina. *Exhaustion: A History*. New York: Columbia University Press, 2016.

Schaeffer, Jacqueline. *The Universal Refusal: Psychoanalytic Exploration of the Feminine Sphere and its Repudiation*. Tr. David Alcorn. London: Karnac, 2011.

Scheidlinger, Saul. "Group Psychology Revisited: An Opportunity Missed," 389–392, *Psychoanalytic Psychology*, Vol. 20, Iss. 2, 2003.

Schindler, D.C. *Freedom from Reality: The Diabolical Character of Modern Liberty*. South Bend: The University of Notre Dame Press, 2017.

Schmidt-Hellerau, Cordelia. "How Demagogy Works: Reflections on Aggression in Politically Fraught Times," 234–242 *Psychoanalytic Inquiry*, Vol. 40, Iss. 4, 2020.

Sedlak, Vic. "The psychoanalyst's normal and pathological superegos," 1499–1520 *International Journal of Psychoanalysis*, Vol. 97, Iss. 6, 2016.

Segal, Hanna. "Psychoanalysis and Freedom of Thought," 51–63 *Dimensions of Psychoanalysis: Selected Papers Presented at the Freud Memorial Lectures*. Ed. Joseph Sandler. London: Karnac, 1989.

Schmitt, Carl. *The Concept of the Political*. Tr. C.J. Miller. Antelope Hill Publishing, 2020.

Schmitt, Carl. *Political Theology: Four Chapters on the Concept of Sovereignty*. Tr. George Schwab. Chicago: The University of Chicago Press, 1985.

Schwartz, Howard S. *Society Against Itself: Political Correctness and Organizational Self-Destruction*. London: Karnac, 2010.

Sherick, Ivan. "Hysterical Identification in an Eleven-Year Old Girl," 675- in *Psychoanalytic Review*, Vol. 101, Iss. 5, Oct., 2014.

Shmuel Erlich, H. *The Couch in the Marketplace: Psychoanalysis and Social Reality*. London: Karnac, 2013.

Sighele, Scipio. *The Criminal Crowd and Other Writings*. Edited, with an Introduction and Notes, by Nicoletta Pireddu. Translated by Nicoletta Pireddu and Andrew Robbins. With a Foreword by Tom Huhn. Toronto: University of Toronto Press, 2018.

Sklar, Jonathan. *Dark Times: Psychoanalytic Perspectives on Politics, History and Mourning*. Oxfordshire: Phoenix Publishing House, 2019.

Sloterdijk, Peter. "Cynicism – The Thought of False Consciousness." Tr. Michael Eldred and Leslie A. Adelson, 190–206 *New German Critique*, Iss. 33, Autumn 1984.

Sloterdijk, Peter. *In the Shadow of Mount Sinai: A Footnote on the Origins and Changing Forms of Total Membership*. Tr. Wieland Hoban. Cambridge, UK: Polity Press, 2016.

Sloterdijk, Peter. *Nietzsche Apostle*. Tr. Steven Corcoran. South Pasadena, CA: Semiotext(e), 2013.

Sloterdijk, Peter. *Rage and Time: A Psychopolitical Investigation*. Tr. Mario Wenning. New York: Columbia University Press, 2010.

Sloterdijk, Peter. "Rules for the Human Zoo: a response to the Letter on Humanism," 12–28 in *Environment and Planning*. Tr. Mary Varney Rorty, Vol. 27, 2009.

Sloterdijk, Peter. *Thinker on Stage: Nietzsche's Materialism*. Tr. Jamie Owen Daniel. Minneapolis: University of Minnesota Press, 1989

Sloterdijk, Peter. *You Must Change Your Life: On Anthropotechnics*. Tr. Wieland Hoban. Cambridge, UK: Polity, 2013.

Soreanu, Raluca. "The Psychic Life of Fragments: Splitting from Ferenczi to Klein," 421–444 *The American Journal of Psychoanalysis*, Vol. 78, 2018.

Snyder, Timothy. *The Road to Unfreedom: Russia, Europe, America*. New York: Tim Duggan Books, 2018.

Spero, Moshe Halevi. "The Civilization of Discontent: Notes on the Hidden Sources of Unbehagen in Freud's Analysis of Civilization," 221–253 *The Psychoanalytic Study of the Child*, Vol. 63, 2008.

Stäheli, Urs. "Seducing the Crowd: The Leader in Crowd Psychology," Tr. Erich Saroth. *New German Critique*, Vol. 63-77, Iss. 114, Fall 2011.

Steinbach, Oscar. "Aggression, the Death Drive and the Problem of Sado-Masochism: A Re-Interpretation," 857–881 *Psychoanalytic Review*, Vol. 93, Iss. 6, Dec. 2006.

Steiner, John. *Psychic Retreats: Pathological Organization in Psychotic, Neurotic and Borderline Patients*. London: Routledge, 1993.

Strauss, Leo. *What is Political Philosophy?* Chicago: The University of Chicago Press, 1959.

Stroumsa, Guy G. "Myth Into Novel: The Late Freud on Early Religion," *New Perspectives on Freud's Moses and Monotheism*. Eds. Ruth Ginsburg and Ilana Pardes, 2006.

Symington, Neville. *The Blind Man Sees: Freud's Awakening and Other Essays*. London: Karnac, 2004.

Symington, Neville. *Emotion and Spirit: Questioning the Claims of Psychoanalysis of Religion*. London: Karnac, 1998.

Symington, Neville. "Freud's Social Theory: Modernist and postmodernist revisions," 43–72 *History of the Human Sciences*, Vol. 25, Iss. 4, 2012.

Symington, Neville. *Requiem for the Ego: Freud and the Origins of Postmodernism*. Stanford: Stanford University Press, 2013.

Tauber, Alfred I. *Freud, the Reluctant Philosopher*. Princeton: Princeton University Press, 2010.

Taubes, Jacob. *The Political Theology of Paul*. Ed. Aleida Assmann and Jan Assmann, in conjunction with Horst Volkers, Wolf-Daniel Hartwich, and Christoph Schulte. Stanford: Stanford University Press, 2004.

Taylor, Charles. *A Secular Age*. Cambridge, Massachusetts: Harvard University Press, 2007.

Terry, Paul. "Working with Psychosis: Part 2 – encounters with an omnipotent superego," 45–59 *Psychodynamic Practice*, Vol. 10, Iss. 1, 2004.

Thompson, M. Guy. "Happiness and Chance: A Reappraisal of the Psychoanalytic Concept of Suffering," 134–153 *Psychoanalytic Psychology*, Vol. 21, Iss. 1, 2004.

Turner, Stephen. "Freud in Many Contexts," 269–275 *Society*, Vol. 57, Iss. 3, Jun. 2020.

Van Egmond, J.J. "Beyond Secondary Gain," 167–177 *The American Journal of Psychoanalysis*, Vol. 65, Iss. 2, June 2005.

Van Ginneken, Jaap. "The Killing of the Father: The Background of Freud's Group Psychology," 391–414 *Political Psychology*, Vol. 5, Iss. 3, Sep., 1984.

Villa, François. "The Psychoanalytical Method and Disaster of Totalitarianism," 267–287 *Critical Inquiry*, Vol. 40, Iss. 2, Winter 2014.

Viney, Wayne and Parker, Elizabeth. "Necessity as a Nightmare or a Pathway to Freedom: Freud's Dilemma, A Human Dilemma," 299–311 *Psychoanalytic Psychology*, Vol. 33, Iss. 2, 2016, 305.

Virsida, Anthony R. "The Death Drive: psychic construction or destruction," 511–523 *Psychoanalytic Review*, Vol. 88. Iss. 4, Aug. 2001.

Volkan, Vamik D. *Psychoanalysis, International Relations, and Diplomacy: A Sourcebook on Large-Group Psychology*. London: Karnac, 2014.

Voruz, Véronique. "Culpability and the Politics of Love," 205–226 *Law and Critique*, Vol. 22, Iss. 3, Nov. 2011.

Wahl, William H. "Pathologies of Desire and Duty: Freud, Ricoeur and Castoriadis on Transforming Religious Culture," 398–414 *Journal of Religion and Health*, Vol. 47, Iss. 3, Sep 2008.

Webster, Jamieson. "Critique and Cure: A Dream of Uniting Psychoanalysis and Philosophy," 138–157 *American Journal of Psychoanalysis*. Vol. 73, Iss. 2, Jun. 2013.

Weiss, Heinz. "A brief history of the super-ego with an introduction to three papers," 724–734 *International Journal of Psychoanalysis*, Vol. 101, Iss. 4, 2020.

Weiss, Heinz. "Three Papers on Splitting: A Brief Introduction," 119–122 *International Journal of Psychoanalysis*, Vol. 96, 2015.

Werman, David. "Freud's "Civilization and its Discontents" – A Reappraisal" 239–254 *Psychoanalytic Review*, Vol. 7, Iss. 2, Summer 1985.

Winnicott, D.W. "Metapsychological and Clinical Aspects of Regression with the Psychoanalytical Set-Up," 16–26, *International Journal of Psycho-Analysis*, 1955.

Winnicott, D.W. *Playing and Reality*. London: Routledge, 1971.

Wood, Sarah. *Without Mastery: Reading and Other Forces*. Edinburgh: Edinburgh University Press, 2014.

Wurmser, Léon. "Superego Revisited – relevant or irrelevant?" *Psychoanalytic Inquiry*, Vol. 24, 2004.

Young-Bruehl, Elisabeth. *The Clinic and the Context: Historical Essays*. London: Karnac, 2015.

Zaretsky, Eli. *Political Freud: A History*. New York: Columbia University Press, 2015.

Zepf, Siegfried. "Modes of Identification: Freud's Concepts Reorganized," 44–55 in *The Scandinavian Psychoanalytic Review*, Vol. 32, Iss. 1.

Zilbersheid, Uri. "The Historical Character of Human Nature in Freud's Theory," 184–204 *American Journal of Psychoanalysis*, Vol. 93, Iss. 2, Jun 2013.

Žižek, Slavoj. *The Fragile Absolute, or, Why is the Christian Legacy worth Fighting For*. London: Verso, 2000.

Žižek, Slavoj. *The Sublime Object of Ideology*. London: Verso, 1989.

INDEX

Page numbers followed by "n" indicate notes.